Current Management of Invasive Bladder and Upper Tract Urothelial Cancer

Editor

JEFFREY M. HOLZBEIERLEIN

UROLOGIC CLINICS
OF NORTH AMERICA

www.urologic.theclinics.com

Consulting Editor
SAMIR S. TANEJA

May 2018 • Volume 45 • Number 2

ELSEVIER

1600 John F. Kennedy Boulevard • Suite 1800 • Philadelphia, Pennsylvania, 19103-2899

http://www.theclinics.com

UROLOGIC CLINICS OF NORTH AMERICA Volume 45, Number 2
May 2018 ISSN 0094-0143, ISBN-13: 978-0-323-58378-7

Editor: Kerry Holland
Developmental Editor: Sara Watkins

Urologic Clinics of North America (ISSN 0094-0143) is published quarterly by Elsevier Inc., 360 Park Avenue South, New York, NY 10010-1710. Months of issue are February, May, August, and November. Business and Editorial Offices: 1600 John F. Kennedy Blvd., Suite 1800, Philadelphia, PA 19103-2899. Periodicals postage paid at New York, NY and additional mailing offices. Subscription prices are $374.00 per year (US individuals), $721.00 per year (US institutions), $100.00 per year (US students and residents), $431.00 per year (Canadian individuals), $901.00 per year (Canadian institutions), $515.00 per year (foreign individuals), $901.00 per year (foreign institutions), and $240.00 per year (Canadian and foreign students/residents). Foreign air speed delivery is included in all *Clinics* subscription prices. All prices are subject to change without notice. **POSTMASTER:** Send address changes to *Urologic Clinics of North America*, Elsevier Health Sciences Division, Subscription Customer Service, 3251 Riverport Lane, Maryland Heights, MO 63043. **Customer Service: 1-800-654-2452 (US). From outside the United States, call 1-314-447-8871. Fax: 1-314-447-8029. E-mail: JournalsCustomerServiceusa@elsevier.com (for print support) and JournalsOnlineSupport-usa@elsevier.com (for online support).**

Reprints. For copies of 100 or more, of articles in this publication, please contact the Commercial Reprints Department, Elsevier Inc., 360 Park Avenue South, New York, New York 10010-1710. Tel.: 212-633-3874; Fax: 212-633-3820; E-mail: reprints@elsevier.com.

Urologic Clinics of North America is covered in MEDLINE/PubMed (*Index Medicus*), *Excerpta Medica*, *Current Contents/Clinical Medicine*, *Science Citation Index,* and *ISI/BIOMED*.

PROGRAM OBJECTIVE

The goal of *Urologic Clinics of North America* is to keep practicing urologists and urology residents up to date with current clinical practice in urology by providing timely articles reviewing the state of the art in patient care.

TARGET AUDIENCE

Practicing urologists, urology residents and other healthcare professionals practicing in the discipline of urology.

LEARNING OBJECTIVES

Upon completion of this activity, participants will be able to:
- Review preoperative, intraoperative, and follow up management of the cystectomy patient
- Discuss current approaches to staging, surgical management, and adjuvant therapy for muscle invasive bladder cancer and upper tract urothelial cell carcinoma
- Recognize the role and indications of radical cystectomy including patient selection, counselling, and quality of life

ACCREDITATION

The Elsevier Office of Continuing Medical Education (EOCME) is accredited by the Accreditation Council for Continuing Medical Education (ACCME) to provide continuing medical education for physicians.

The EOCME designates this enduring material for a maximum of 15 *AMA PRA Category 1 Credit*(s)™. Physicians should claim only the credit commensurate with the extent of their participation in the activity.

All other healthcare professionals requesting continuing education credit for this enduring material will be issued a certificate of participation.

DISCLOSURE OF CONFLICTS OF INTEREST

The EOCME assesses conflict of interest with its instructors, faculty, planners, and other individuals who are in a position to control the content of CME activities. All relevant conflicts of interest that are identified are thoroughly vetted by EOCME for fair balance, scientific objectivity, and patient care recommendations. EOCME is committed to providing its learners with CME activities that promote improvements or quality in healthcare and not a specific proprietary business or a commercial interest.

The planning committee, staff, authors and editors listed below have identified no financial relationships or relationships to products or devices they or their spouse/life partner have with commercial interest related to the content of this CME activity:

Tala Achkar, MD; Svetlana Avulova, MD; Daniel A. Barocas, MD, MPH; Jack Griffin Campbell, MD; Steven L. Chang, MD, MS; Sam S. Chang, MD, MBA; Siamak Daneshmand, MD; Scott E. Delacroix Jr, MD; Jianjun Gao, MD, PhD; Jessie Gills, MD; Kerry Holland; Jeffrey M. Holzbeierlein, MD, FACS; Karim Kader, MD, PhD; Ashish M. Kamat, MD; Alison Kemp; Adam S. Kibel, MD; Simon Kimm, MD; Roger Li, MD; Danica May, MD; Matthew Mossanen, MD; Rahul A. Parikh, MD, PhD; Firas G. Petros, MD; Madhumitha Reddy, DO; Michael C. Risk, MD, PhD; Niranjan J. Sathianathen, MBBS; Douglas S. Scherr, MD; Ankeet Shah, MD; Woodson Wade Smelser, MD; Guru P. Sonpavde, MD; William Tabayoyong, MD, PhD; Samir S. Taneja, MD; Benjamin L. Taylor, MD; Min Yuen Teo, MD; Mark D. Tyson II, MD; Vignesh Viswanathan; Daniel Zainfeld, MD.

The planning committee, staff, authors and editors listed below have identified financial relationships or relationships to products or devices they or their spouse/life partner have with commercial interest related to the content of this CME activity:

Badrinath R. Konety, MD, FACS, MBA: has received research grant support from Photocure, Inc., F. Hoffmann-La Roche Ltd, Genomic Health, Inc., MDxHealth, and Bristol-Myers Squibb
Eugene K. Lee, MD, FACS: is a consultant for Pacira Pharmaceuticals, Inc.
Surena F. Matin, MD: serves as consultant for TARIS Biomedical, LLC, UroGen Corp, C-SATS, Inc., and Peloton Therapeutics; receives research grant support from the AT&T Foundation and Specialized Programs in Oncology Research (SPORE).
Jonathan E. Rosenberg, MD: serves as a consultant for Merck & Co., Inc., F. Hoffmann-La Roche Ltd, Bristol-Myers Squibb, Seattle Genetics, Inc., AstraZeneca, and EMD Serono, Inc. He has received research grant support from F. Hoffmann-La Roche Ltd, Seattle Genetics, Inc., and Astellas Pharma US, Inc.

UNAPPROVED/OFF-LABEL USE DISCLOSURE

The EOCME requires CME faculty to disclose to the participants:
1. When products or procedures being discussed are off-label, unlabelled, experimental, and/or investigational (not US Food and Drug Administration [FDA] approved); and
2. Any limitations on the information presented, such as data that are preliminary or that represent ongoing research, interim analyses, and/or unsupported opinions. Faculty may discuss information about pharmaceutical agents that is outside of FDA-approved labelling. This information is intended solely for CME and is not intended to promote off-label use of these medications. If you have any questions, contact the medical affairs department of the manufacturer for the most recent prescribing information.

TO ENROLL

To enroll in the *Urologic Clinics of North America* Continuing Medical Education program, call customer service at 1-800-654-2452 or sign up online at http://www.theclinics.com/home/cme. The CME program is available to subscribers for an additional annual fee of USD $280.80.

METHOD OF PARTICIPATION

In order to claim credit, participants must complete the following:

1. Complete enrolment as indicated above.
2. Read the activity.
3. Complete the CME Test and Evaluation. Participants must achieve a score of 70% on the test. All CME Tests and Evaluations must be completed online.

CME INQUIRIES/SPECIAL NEEDS

For all CME inquiries or special needs, please contact elsevierCME@elsevier.com.

Contributors

CONSULTING EDITOR

SAMIR S. TANEJA, MD
The James M. Neissa and Janet Riha Neissa,
Professor of Urologic Oncology, Professor of
Urology and Radiology, Director, Division of
Urologic Oncology, Co-Director, Department
of Urology, Smilow Comprehensive Prostate
Cancer Center, NYU Langone Medical Center,
New York, New York

EDITOR

JEFFREY M. HOLZBEIERLEIN, MD, FACS
John W Weigel Endowed Professor and Chair,
Director of Urologic Oncology, Department of
Urology, University of Kansas Medical Center,
Kansas City, Kansas

AUTHORS

TALA ACHKAR, MD
University of Pittsburgh Medical Center,
Pittsburgh, Pennsylvania

SVETLANA AVULOVA, MD
Department of Urologic Surgery, Vanderbilt
University Medical Center, Nashville, Tennessee

DANIEL A. BAROCAS, MD, MPH
Department of Urologic Surgery, Vanderbilt
University Medical Center, Nashville, Tennessee

JACK GRIFFIN CAMPBELL, MD
Resident Physician, Department of Urology,
University of Kansas Medical Center,
Kansas City, Kansas

SAM S. CHANG, MD, MBA
Department of Urologic Surgery, Vanderbilt
University Medical Center, Nashville, Tennessee

STEVEN L. CHANG, MD, MS
Assistant Professor, Department of Surgery,
Division of Urology, Brigham and Women's
Hospital, Instructor, Harvard Medical School,
Boston, Massachusetts

SIAMAK DANESHMAND, MD
Director of Urologic Oncology, Department of
Urology, Keck School of Medicine of USC,
USC Norris Comprehensive Cancer Center,
Los Angeles, California

SCOTT E. DELACROIX JR, MD
Assistant Professor of Urology, Co-Director
Urologic Oncology, Louisiana State
University Healthcare Network, New Orleans,
Louisiana

JIANJUN GAO, MD, PhD
Assistant Professor, Genitourinary Medical
Oncology, The University of Texas MD
Anderson Cancer Center, Houston, Texas

JESSIE GILLS, MD
Assistant Professor Urology, Co-Director
Urologic Oncology, Louisiana State University
Healthcare Network, New Orleans, Louisiana

KARIM KADER, MD, PhD
Professor of Urology, Moores Cancer Center,
UC San Diego, La Jolla, California

ASHISH KAMAT, MD
Professor, Urology, The University of Texas
MD Anderson Cancer Center, Houston, Texas

ADAM S. KIBEL, MD
Professor and Chief of Urology, Division of
Urology, Department of Surgery, Brigham and
Women's Hospital, Dana-Farber Cancer
Institute, Harvard Medical School, Boston,
Massachusetts

SIMON KIMM, MD
Urologic Ocologist, Palo Alto Medical
Foundation, Palo Alto, California

BADRINATH R. KONETY, MD, FACS, MBA
Department of Urology, University of
Minnesota, Minneapolis, Minnesota

EUGENE K. LEE, MD, FACS
Assistant Professor, Department of Urology,
University of Kansas Medical Center,
Kansas City, Kansas

ROGER LI, MD
Urologic Oncology Fellow, Department
of Urology, The University of Texas MD
Anderson Cancer Center, Houston, Texas

SURENA F. MATIN, MD
Professor, Department of Urology, The
University of Texas MD Anderson Cancer
Center, Houston, Texas

DANICA MAY, MD
Urology Resident, Louisiana State University
Health Sciences Center, New Orleans,
Louisiana

MATTHEW MOSSANEN, MD
Division of Urology, Department of Surgery,
Brigham and Women's Hospital, Instructor,
Harvard Medical School, Boston,
Massachusetts

RAHUL A. PARIKH, MD, PhD
University of Kansas Medical Center,
Westwood, Kansas

FIRAS G. PETROS, MD
Urologic Oncology Fellow, Department of
Urology, The University of Texas MD
Anderson Cancer Center, Houston, Texas

MADHUMITHA REDDY, DO
Urologic Oncology Fellow, Moores Cancer
Center, UC San Diego, La Jolla, California

MICHAEL C. RISK, MD, PhD
Department of Urology, University of
Minnesota, Minneapolis, Minnesota

JONATHAN E. ROSENBERG, MD
Associate Attending Physician, Department of
Medicine, Genitourinary Oncology Service,
Memorial Sloan Kettering Cancer Center,
New York, New York

NIRANJAN J. SATHIANATHEN, MBBS
Department of Urology, University of
Minnesota, Minneapolis, Minnesota

DOUGLAS S. SCHERR, MD
Professor, Department of Urology, Clinical
Director of Urologic Oncology, Weill Cornell
Medicine, NewYork-Presbyterian, New York,
New York

ANKEET SHAH, MD
Resident, Department of Urology, Keck School
of Medicine of USC, USC Norris Comprehensive
Cancer Center, Los Angeles, California

WOODSON WADE SMELSER, MD
Resident Physician, Department of Urology,
University of Kansas Medical Center, Kansas
City, Kansas

GURU P. SONPAVDE, MD
Genitourinary Medical Oncologist, Bladder
Cancer Director, Dana-Farber Cancer Institute,
Boston, Massachusetts

WILLIAM TABAYOYONG, MD, PhD
Fellow, Urology, The University of Texas
MD Anderson Cancer Center, Houston, Texas

BENJAMIN L. TAYLOR, MD
Fellow, Urologic Oncology, Department
of Urology, Weill Cornell Medicine,
NewYork-Presbyterian, New York, New York

MIN YUEN TEO, MD
Assistant Attending Physician, Department of
Medicine, Genitourinary Oncology Service,
Memorial Sloan Kettering Cancer Center,
New York, New York

MARK D. TYSON II, MD
Department of Urology, Mayo Clinic, Mayo
Clinic Hospital, Phoenix, Arizona

DANIEL ZAINFELD, MD
Urologic Oncology Fellow, Department of
Urology, Keck School of Medicine of USC,
Norris Comprehensive Cancer Center, Los
Angeles, California

Contents

outcomes, care pathways, access to high-volume care centers, and efforts to decrease complications may prove as important as the technique itself.

Upper tract urothelial carcinoma is a rare malignancy that has an abundance of surgical treatment options, including open, laparoscopic, robotic, and endoscopic approaches. As advances in technology allow for shorter, less morbid operations, the variation in care of this uncommon disease has raised concerns about compromising oncologic principles. Many institutions have described their experience with promising results; however, there is a paucity of high-quality data that support the use of robotic surgery as a new gold standard. This article describes how to perform the operation using a single-dock method and reviews the contemporary literature on perioperative and oncologic outcomes.

Organ-sparing cystectomy remains an operation for a highly selected patient population that can offer similar oncologic outcomes but improved sexual function in men and women. Occult prostate cancer in men may occur even with screening, but the majority is of clinical insignificance. Paramount to patient selection are oncologic concerns, but preoperative sexual function, age, performance status, and postoperative expectations must also be evaluated during patient selection. Improved diagnostic and surveillance tools may facilitate and improve patient selection in the future.

There are currently no reported randomized trials that characterize the staging or therapeutic benefit of performing a lymph node dissection in either bladder cancer or upper tract urothelial carcinoma. Several unanswered questions remain in this domain focused on the indications and patient selection for pelvic lymph node dissection, extent of dissection, its impact on outcome, and potential risks. However, the results of observational studies suggest that the burden of metastasis is high in both diseases when muscle invasive and performing a lymphadenectomy can provide prognostic information and yield therapeutic benefit.

Radical cystectomy remains the gold standard therapy for the treatment of muscle-invasive urothelial carcinoma, yet it is accompanied by significant rates of perioperative complications and readmission. Enhanced recovery protocols aim to apply evidence-based principles of care to ameliorate the morbidity of this procedure by enabling better tolerance of and recovery from radical cystectomy. Multiple patient series have demonstrated the capacity for enhanced-recovery-after-surgery (ERAS) principles to improve outcomes among patients undergoing radical cystectomy through decreased incidence of gastrointestinal complications and decreased length of hospitalization without increased readmissions or overall morbidity. Opportunities remain for adoption of established ERAS principles.

Bladder cancer is the sixth leading cancer in the United States. Radical cystectomy is a lifesaving procedure for bladder cancer with or without muscle invasion. Radical cystectomy is performed on 39% of these patients, and 35% will have a life-threatening recurrence. Distant metastases are the most common; local, upper tract, and urethral recurrence can also occur. Surveillance after cystectomy is critical to diagnosing recurrence early. Functional complications after urinary diversion include bowel dysfunction, vitamin B_{12} deficiency, acidosis, electrolyte abnormalities, osteopenia, nephrolithiasis, urinary tract infections, renal functional decline, and urinary obstruction, which can be reversed when diagnosed early.

Approximately 1 in 5 new cases of clinically localized bladder cancer is muscle invasive and requires the patient to choose from 1 of 2 prevailing options for treatment: radical cystectomy or radiation to the bladder. However, these treatments are associated with detrimental effects on patient well-being and quality of life, particularly with respect to functional independence, urinary and sexual function, social and emotional health, body image, and psychosocial stress. Compared with the literature on other malignancies, such as breast or prostate cancer, high-quality studies evaluating the effects of bladder cancer treatment on quality of life are lacking.

This article summarizes the role of adjuvant chemotherapy in muscle-invasive and transitional cell carcinoma of the bladder and upper urinary tract.

 Video content accompanies this article at http://www.urologic.theclinics.com.

A select group of patients with upper tract urothelial carcinoma (UTUC) may meet indications for endoscopic management. Strategies for disease management are provided, based on a comprehensive review of the data using PubMed and Medline databases and marrying this with our experience with endoscopic management of UTUC. Endoscopic management of UTUC via retrograde or antegrade approaches is a viable treatment option for appropriately selected patients with low-risk UTUC, including those with low-grade, low-volume, and solitary tumors. However, recurrence risk limits these procedures to compliant patients under a vigilant surveillance program. Efficacious adjuvant therapies are needed to reduce local recurrences.

Min Yuen Teo and Jonathan E. Rosenberg

Neoadjuvant chemotherapy improves survival in patients with muscle-invasive bladder cancer. However, a significant proportion of patients are ineligible for cisplatin owing to renal impairment or other medical comorbidities. The introduction of anti-programmed cell death protein 1/programmed death-ligand 1(PD1/PD-L1) checkpoint inhibitors has redefined the therapeutic landscape for platinum-resistant urothelial cancers; their clinical efficacy and favorable toxicity render these agents attractive therapeutic options either as monotherapy or in combination with other agents in earlier disease states, including muscle-invasive disease. The authors review potential perioperative immunotherapy strategies, ongoing clinical trials, and areas of unmet needs, including upper tract disease and nonurothelial cancers.

UROLOGIC CLINICS OF NORTH AMERICA

THE CLINICS ARE AVAILABLE ONLINE!
Access your subscription at:
www.theclinics.com

Erratum

The authors wish to update content in the November 2017 issue of *Urologic Clinics* on pages 520 and 521, in "Whom to Biopsy: Prediagnostic Risk Stratification with Biomarkers, Nomograms, and Risk Calculators" by Stacy Loeb and Hasan Dani.

The original paragraph on page 521 reads: "Using these measurements in combination with clinical variables such as PSA, age, race, and family history, this assay predicts risk of high-grade PCA in men undergoing their first biopsy. In a validation study of 519 men undergoing initial or repeat biopsy, the urine exosome gene expression assay outperformed the base model of clinical variables (AUC 0.73 vs 0.63, *P*<.001)."

It has been corrected to: "This assay predicts risk of high-grade PCA in men undergoing their first biopsy and can also be used in a multivariable approach with clinical variables such as PSA, age, race and family history. In a validation study of 519 men age ≥50 with PSA 2-10 ng/ml undergoing initial biopsy, the urine exosome gene expression assay outperformed the base model of clinical variables alone (AUC 0.71 exosome alone; AUC 0.73 exosome + clinical variablesvs 0.63 clinical variables alone, *P*<.001).66."

The authors also wish to clarify the following statement on page 520, "Future studies are needed to evaluate the comparative performance of the multiple new urine-based markers," by noting that AUC's are not comparable across marker studies in different populations, and future studies are needed to directly evaluate the comparative performance of the multiple new urine-based markers.

In addition, on page 521, "Examples of such tests include the 4Kscore, MiPS, SelectMDx, and ExoDx Prostate (IntelliScore). By contrast, other tests like phi and PCA3 do not include clinical variables into their formula, but the results of these tests can be incorporated into external nomogram," has been corrected to, "Examples of such tests include the 4Kscore, MiPS, and SelectMDx. By contrast, other tests like phi, PCA3, and ExoDx Prostate (IntelliScore "EPI") do not include clinical variables into their formula, but the results of these tests can be incorporated into external nomograms."

Urol Clin N Am 45 (2018) xiii
https://doi.org/10.1016/j.ucl.2018.03.002
0094-0143/18

Preface

Current Management of Invasive Bladder and Upper Tract Urothelial Cancer

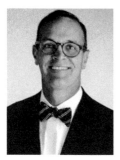

Jeffrey M. Holzbeierlein, MD, FACS
Editor

As the landscape for the management of urothelial cell carcinoma (UCC) is rapidly changing, it is particularly timely that this issue of *Urologic Clinics* focuses on "The Current Management of Invasive Bladder and Upper Tract Urothelial Cancer." Experts in the fields of bladder cancer and upper tract urothelial cell cancer present the latest management strategies and research in these areas. This will be extremely relevant to the practicing urologist who manages these challenging, and all too often, lethal diseases.

As our population ages, the incidence of bladder cancer is likely to increase in the next several decades. Therefore, it will be critical to understand the management of these complex patients. An area of evolution in the evaluation of the patient with newly diagnosed UCC is the initial staging, as this directs therapy. The role of standard imaging and novel imaging techniques is discussed and will help to guide the practitioner in the initial evaluation of the patient with UCC. The topic of neoadjuvant chemotherapy in these disease processes is also covered. Despite Level 1 evidence to support the use of neoadjuvant chemotherapy, the adoption of this practice in the United States has been quite slow. Therefore, the indications and contraindications to its use are presented in this issue. Furthermore, data regarding when neoadjuvant chemotherapy might not be necessary or not helpful are covered.

Radical cystectomy remains the cornerstone for the treatment of muscle-invasive bladder cancer.

Unfortunately, morbidity remains high with this procedure, and the increasing age and frailty of many of these patients make them an especially vulnerable group of patients. A great deal of work is ongoing to reduce the morbidity associated with cystectomy. This encompasses various aspects of the procedure, including patient optimization through nutrition, robotic cystectomy, organ-sparing cystectomy, and enhanced recovery after surgery pathways. This issue covers the latest topics focusing on improving outcomes associated with radical cystectomy. The reader is sure to find valuable information to guide their practice in the latest patient optimization techniques.

Another critical aspect in the comprehensive care of the patient with UCC is survivorship. This includes the follow-up care of these patients involving imaging, management of issues related to their urinary diversion, and issues that affect quality of life. Authors in this issue cover these important topics.

As upper tract UCC carries its own management challenges, a special article is devoted to understanding the latest treatment strategies. This includes endoscopic management as well as discussions throughout this issue of the indications for chemotherapy, follow-up, and surgical approaches.

Finally, one of the hottest topics in UCC is the role of adjuvant chemotherapy and immunotherapy in advanced UCC. Experts in these areas

Urol Clin N Am 45 (2018) xv–xvi
https://doi.org/10.1016/j.ucl.2018.01.002
0094-0143/18/© 2018 Published by Elsevier Inc.

review the latest data for the use of these forms of therapy and explore possible future indications. This area in the management of UCC is one of the most exciting and rapidly evolving parts of UCC treatment and will be extremely informative to the reader.

As the editor of this review, I believe we have assembled some of the world's experts on the management of UCC. In addition, this issue covers a wide array of topics for the treatment of patients with UCC, and I believe that anyone involved in the treatment of these patients will find useful information to help guide their practice.

Jeffrey M. Holzbeierlein, MD, FACS
Department of Urology
University of Kansas Medical Center
3901 Rainbow Boulevard, MS 3016
Kansas City, KS 66160, USA

E-mail address:
jholzbeierlein@kumc.edu

Current Staging Strategies for Muscle-Invasive Bladder Cancer and Upper Tract Urothelial Cell Carcinoma

Matthew Mossanen, MD[a],*, Steven L. Chang, MD, MS[a],
Simon Kimm, MD[b], Guru P. Sonpavde, MD[c],
Adam S. Kibel, MD[a]

KEYWORDS

- Muscle-invasive bladder cancer • Staging • Imaging in bladder cancer
- Upper tract urothelial cell cancer

KEY POINTS

- Staging in bladder cancer is critical because it informs prognosis and management options.
- Current staging methods can help identify patients with localized or metastatic disease but are subject to inherent limitations.
- Upper tract urothelial cell carcinoma staging in large part parallels that of bladder cancer.

STAGING SYSTEMS INFORM PATIENT PROGNOSIS

Staging is important because it informs prognosis and allows providers to determine survival. This information is often communicated to patients while discussing their diagnosis and management. The 5-year disease-specific survival of patients undergoing radical cystectomy without neoadjuvant chemotherapy can be determined by T and N stages with pT0/1 being 92%, pT2 being 73%, pT3 being 66%, pT4 being 46%, and pTx N+ being 22%.[1] A study by Madersbacher and colleagues[2] examined a 15-year experience of 575 cystectomy patients with TxN0M0 staging and examined patterns in survival based on stage.

Given that nodal involvement portends such a poor prognosis, determining the incidence of nodal involvement is important. Based on pathologic stage, 12% of patients with pT2a disease, 32% with pT2b disease, and 49% with pT3 disease will have nodal involvement.[3] Moreover, occult lymph node involvement may occur in 25% of patients that receive cystectomy without chemotherapy, which again confers a dismal 26% 5-year OS.[2] Last, proper staging is important because it may detect patients with metastatic disease that can drastically alter management.

STAGING SYSTEMS CLASSIFY LOCAL, REGIONAL, AND DISTANT TUMOR BURDEN
Muscle-Invasive Bladder Cancer Staging

The American Joint Committee on Cancer (AJCC) provides a staging system for bladder,

Disclosure Statement: The authors have nothing to disclose.
[a] Division of Urology, Department of Surgery, Brigham and Women's Hospital, Harvard Medical School, 45 Francis Street, Boston, MA 02111, USA; [b] Department of Surgery, Palo Alto Medical Foundation, 300 Pasteur Drive, Palo Alto, CA 94304, USA; [c] Department of Genitourinary Oncology, Dana Farber Cancer Institute (DFCI), 450 Brookline Avenue, Boston, MA 0221, USA
* Corresponding author. Division of Urology, Department of Surgery, Brigham and Women's Hospital, Harvard Medical School, 45 Francis Street, Boston, MA 02115.
E-mail address: mmossanen@partners.org

Urol Clin N Am 45 (2018) 143–154
https://doi.org/10.1016/j.ucl.2017.12.001

and the 8th edition was updated in 2017.[4] The National Comprehensive Cancer Network (NCCN) relies on the AJCC staging system,[5] which is based on the primary tumor (T), nodes (N), and metastatic (M) involvement. Anatomic staging in bladder cancer is based upon the AJCC staging system, and the TNM status informs assignment to a category. Stage 0 disease constitutes either 0a (Ta) or 0is (Tis). A stage I classification includes T1 tumors, whereas a stage II tumor includes T2 tumors. Patients with stage III disease can either have T3 disease or T4a disease (prostatic stroma, uterus, vagina). Stage IV disease includes patients with T4b with any N, N1-3 disease, or M1 involvement. **Table 1** displays the TNM staging system for bladder cancer. **Fig. 1** illustrates the anatomic layers of the bladder wall and corresponds to the T stage based on the depth of tumor involvement.

Renal Pelvis and Ureteral Cancer Staging

Staging of the renal pelvis and ureter, in large part, parallels staging of the bladder for T-stage and M-stage components. Similar to bladder cancer, stage I disease corresponds to a T1 tumor, stage II corresponds to a T2 tumor, stage III corresponds to a T3 tumor, and stage IV disease equates to a T4, or any N, or metastatic disease. **Table 2** displays the TNM staging system for renal pelvis and ureteral cancer.

COMPONENTS OF INITIAL CLINICAL STAGING

Thorough clinical staging is essential in order to properly evaluate the extent of disease. In the clinic setting, all patients should have a detailed history and physical examination. Discussing duration of urinary or constitutional symptoms, any smoking history, and other risk potential factors for bladder cancer are important parts of the initial evaluation. The NCCN guidelines state that patients with muscle-invasive bladder cancer (MIBC) should receive a laboratory evaluation with a complete blood count (CBC), basic metabolic panel (BMP), and alkaline phosphatase.[5] Initially, patients with bladder cancer should undergo either a computed tomographic (CT) scan or MRI with contrast to evaluate local extent of disease and assess the upper tracts. Imaging can be completed with a chest radiograph (CXR) or CT of the chest, a bone scan if there is concern based on a clinical picture consistent with bone metastases or elevated alkaline phosphatase, and PET/CT if imaging is equivocal for metastases or there is concern for metastatic disease based on clinical symptoms. Also, for patients who complain of neurologic symptoms, an MRI of the brain may be obtained. After imaging is done, providers may choose to forego office cystoscopy if it is clear a biopsy with resection is necessary.

In the operating room, an examination under anesthesia and transurethral resection of the bladder tumor (TURBT) are performed to determine initial clinical staging. A bimanual examination should be performed because it allows for evaluation of tumor bulk and determination of potential invasion into adjacent organs. However, an important consideration is that an examination under anesthesia may be subject to limitations in accuracy and variability among providers.[6] Based on the TURBT specimen, patients can be assigned cT2 or greater disease, and this presumptive clinical stage of MIBC warrants additional evaluation.

Table 1	
TNM staging for bladder cancer	
Stage	**Primary Tumor (T)**
0	TX: Primary tumor cannot be assessed
	T0: No evidence of tumor
0is	Tis: Carcinoma in situ
I	T1: Tumor invades subepithelial connective tissue
II	T2: Tumor invades muscularis propria T2a: Inner half T2b: Outer half
III	T3: Tumor invades perivesical tissue T3a: Microscopically T3b: Macroscopically
III	T4: Tumor invades adjacent structures T4a: Prostatic stroma, seminal vesicles, uterus, vagina
IV	T4b: Pelvic wall, abdominal wall
Stage	**Regional Nodes (N)**
0	N0: No lymph node metastasis
IV	N1: Single node in the true pelvis (hypogastric, obturator, external iliac, presacral)
IV	N2: Multiple regional nodes in the true pelvis
IV	N3: Lymph node metastasis to the common iliac lymph nodes
Stage	**Distant Metastasis (M)**
0	M0: No distant metastasis
IV	M1: Distant metastasis

Data from Amin MB, Edge SB, Greene FL, et al, editors. AJCC cancer staging manual. 8th edition. New York: Springer; 2017.

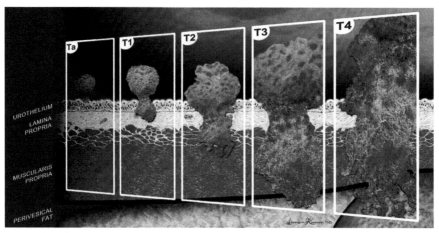

Fig. 1. An illustration of tumor stages in bladder cancer. (*Courtesy of* Simon Kimm, MD, Palo Alto, CA.)

Table 2			
American Joint Committee on Cancer TNM staging for renal pelvis and ureteral cancer			
Stage	**Primary Tumor (T)**		
	TX: Primary tumor cannot be assessed		
0	T0: No evidence of tumor		
0is	Tis: Carcinoma in situ		
I	T1: Tumor invades subepithelial connective tissue		
II	T2: Tumor invades muscularis		
III	T3: Renal pelvis, invades beyond muscularis into peripelvic fat or renal parenchyma Ureteral, invades beyond muscularis into perivesical fat		
IV	T4: Tumor invades adjacent organs or through the kidney into perinephric fat		
Stage	**Regional Nodes (N)**		
0	NX: Lymph nodes cannot be assessed		
IV	N0: No regional lymph node metastasis		
IV	N1: single node 2 cm or smaller in largest dimension		
IV	N2: single node between 2 and 5 cm or multiple nodes with none larger than 5 cm		
IV	N3: node larger than 5 cm		
Stage	**Metastasis (M)**		
0	M0: No distant metastasis		
IV	M1: Distant metastasis		

Data from Amin MB, Edge SB, Greene FL, et al, editors. AJCC cancer staging manual. 8th edition. New York: Springer; 2017.

THE ROLE OF REPEAT TRANSURETHRAL RESECTION OF THE BLADDER TUMORIN THE CLINICAL STAGING OF BLADDER CANCER

An important consideration in the staging of patients with presumptive superficial disease is to rule out occult invasive disease. In order to determine the clinical stage of patients with bladder cancer, a sample of the bladder wall involved with tumor is excised. However, not all tumors may be visible on cystoscopic examination or completely resected during the initial procedure.[7,8] Therefore, a repeat resection to restage these patients is an important component in the initial management of patients suspected but not proven to have MIBC.

Several clinical scenarios warrant an additional biopsy in the staging of patients with bladder cancer. For tumors that appear to be invasive or sessile on cystoscopy, the NCCN guidelines state that TURBT can be repeated for (1) any T1 lesion, (2) an inadequate specimen that precludes pathologic staging, (3) any specimen that lacks the presence of muscularis propria, and (4) tumors that were incompletely resected if bladder preservation therapy is being implemented.[5] Ensuring that muscularis propria is present in a TURBT specimen allows the pathologist to determine if there is cT2 disease. In fact, as many of 50% of TURBT specimens may be missing muscularis propria.[9] Also, if muscle was not present in the original specimen (for example, Tis, Ta, or T1), then upstaging to muscle-invasive disease may occur in up to 10% to 29% of cases.[7,10–12] A repeat TURBT may be needed because it detects residual disease anywhere from 26% to 83% of cases and may upstage tumors originally classified as cT1 to cT2 disease in 2% to 28% of cases, thereby changing management.[7,12] Based on the results of a repeat TURBT, treatment options can be significantly impacted. For example, intravesical therapy may no longer be appropriate, and consideration of neoadjuvant chemotherapy followed by radical cystectomy may be a more appropriate option.

Last, repeating a TURBT may help identify patients at higher risk for progression, which may direct the provider to pursue more aggressive upfront therapy such as early cystectomy. In one study by Herr and colleagues[13] of 352 patients with cT1 bladder cancer on initial TURBT, 66% recurred and 35% progressed in stage within 5 years. When they separated the cohort into patients with residual cT1 disease on repeat resection and patients with no disease or lower stage disease on the repeat resection, they found that the progression rate at 5 years was 82% and 19%, respectively. This data from Herr et al provides a strong rationale for earlier aggressive intervention on patients with residual high grade T1 disease (**Box 1**).

RENAL PELVIS AND URETERAL CANCER STAGING CHALLENGES AND CONSIDERATIONS

A challenge in the staging of patients with upper tract urothelial cell carcinoma (UTUC) occurs with ureteroscopy. During the initial clinical staging, UTUC often occurs with imaging and then is confirmed with ureteroscopic visualization and biopsy, which is recommended in order to accurately assess grade and extent of tumor involvement. Information regarding grade and especially stage is frequently limited because access to the renal pelvis and ureter is associated with the technical challenges of poorly accessible tumors, limited visualization, and difficulties obtaining a deep enough biopsy to accurately stage patients.[14] Clinical judgment of muscle invasion may be reasonable in the presence of high-grade disease with or without radiographic visualization

---

Box 1
Clinical bottom line: the role of repeat transurethral resection of the bladder tumor in the clinical staging of bladder cancer

In bladder cancer, clinical stage is informed by examination under anesthesia, imaging, and TURBT. Patients with high-grade T1 tumors should undergo repeat resection because of the high rate of understaging and the risk of recurrence and progression in patients with residual disease. Ureteroscopic inspection with biopsy is used in the assessment of the upper tracts in patients suspected of having UTUC.

---

of a mass.[15] A correlation with visual appearance of an upper tract tumor along with histologic grade to clinical stage is reportedly accurate up to 70% of the time.[16]

Imaging in the Staging of Patients with Bladder Cancer

Use of computed tomography imaging in the initial evaluation

CT urography (CTU) is recommended as the initial imaging test for patients with hematuria, and this imaging sequence includes a CT scan of the abdomen and pelvis (with and without contrast) and also excretory phase imaging.[17] As a result, before formal staging with a TURBT, most patients with bladder cancer have undergone a CTU during their initial evaluation for hematuria.[18] CT may provide useful staging information during the initial evaluation. For example, CT may be able to detect hydronephrosis that can signal pT2 disease or greater.[17] Also, CT is clinically useful because it may be able to detect perivesical fat involvement, which can be consistent with the presence of pT3 disease.[19,20] As the initial imaging study, CTU has a reported sensitivity of 85% to 96% and specificity of 83% to 94% for bladder cancer.[18,21,22]

Although CT is used to initially evaluate most patients found to have bladder cancer, it also has several limitations. Determining bladder cancer staging depends on determining which layers of the bladder contain disease, and CT is unable to reliably delineate these layers individually.[6,17,23,24] As a result, CT is thought to have an accuracy of 40% to 60% for local staging of bladder cancer.[25,26] If the CT is obtained following TURBT, there may be local inflammation that can cause local perivesical fat stranding, which can be confusing and may lead one to think there is more advanced disease. Last, another consideration in the use of CT for local staging of bladder cancer is that interobserver variability may result in discrepancies in staging.[24] Thus, CT may not be able to accurately capture the extent of invasion of the primary tumor because of a limited capacity to identify the layers of the bladder wall.[6,23]

MRI in the local staging of muscle-invasive bladder cancer

Given the limitations of CT, MRI of the pelvis with and without intravenous contrast may be considered to assist with staging, in addition to CTU, for patients with bladder cancer.[5] In particular, MRI has been hypothesized to be valuable in the local staging of bladder cancer because it provides more detailed differentiation of the layers of the bladder.[27] In comparison to CT, MRI has been shown to have better demonstration of intramural tumor invasion, extravesical extension, and characterization of muscle invasive versus non-muscle-invasive disease.[23,27] Part of the advantage of MRI is that it can provide superior soft tissue resolution and can assist with local staging by providing a T2-weighted image, which allows enhancement of tumor in relation to adjacent tissue[6,23] as well as evidence of extravesical spread.[23,28] Optimally, MRI should be performed before resection to provide a clearer assessment of depth of invasion because, as stated previously, TURBT may result in perivesical inflammation, making the findings confusing on whether extravesical disease exists.

For determining local staging, MRI is dependent on the type of imaging sequences obtained. The appropriate MRI sequences can add significant information in the evaluation of local extent of disease.[26,27,29–32] MRI with dynamic contrast enhancement evaluates tissues before, during, and after contrast administration. Tissue perfusion and vessel permeability are determined, and this information can be used to categorize tissue as benign or malignant. MRI with diffusion weighted imaging (DWI) uses differences in water diffusion between various tissues and can therefore be conducted without contrast. Cancerous tissue may have denser cellular structures that can result in lower water diffusion. Although DWI uses motion of water molecules, within this sequence, apparent diffusion coefficient (ADC) is quantitatively determined and has been shown to be a quantitative imaging biomarker with value in differentiating benign lesions versus cancerous tumors.[33,34] DWI may provide enhanced capacity to visualize bladder cancer in relation to adjacent tissues.[35,36] Specificity for cT2 disease using MRI with DWI may be as high as 93%.[37] Another study reported that DWI MRI is more accurate than T2-weighted images for staging ≤cT2 disease, and comparable for higher-stage tumors.[38]

Combinations of imaging sequences may be more useful than any single sequence alone, and this is now an area of active investigation. One study examined the added benefit of combining 3 different MRI imaging sequences examining patients with cT2 disease.[39] In this study, the investigators reported improved accuracy as more imaging sequences were combined: 67% for T2 alone, 88% for T2 with DWI, and 92% for T2, DWI, and contrast-enhanced images. Also, the investigators found that ADC may help predict histologic grade with mean ADC being significantly lower for high-grade tumors as compared with lower-grade tumors (P<.01).

The use of MRI in bladder cancer is an evolving area of study, and the optimal MRI sequence for bladder cancer staging has yet to be established. A recent meta-analysis examined the diagnostic accuracy of MRI for distinguishing clinical T1 or lower tumors from T2 or greater tumors.[40] This study included a total of 17 studies that represented 1449 patients with bladder cancer and reported a pooled sensitivity of 90% (95% confidence interval [CI] 83%–94%) and specificity of 88% (95% CI 77%–94%). They also reported that DWI and using a 3-T device resulted in improved sensitivity (92% with 95% CI 86%–96%) and specificity (96% with 95% CI 93%–98%). Last, although MRI is a superior imaging study for determination of local disease, it is also subject to limitations, including (1) suboptimal bladder distention may not allow adequate visualization, (2) artifacts from prior TURBT resections can obscure true disease extent, and (3) biological heterogeneity in tumor size or dimensions may pose challenges to accurately imaging tumor burden[36] (**Box 2**).

Computed tomography or MRI can be used to determine nodal involvement in muscle-invasive bladder cancer

Another goal in accurate clinical staging is detecting lymph node involvement preoperatively. When evaluating the abdomen and pelvis for potential lymph node involvement, it is especially important to examine the obturator nodes, which are the most common site of nodal metastases for patients with MIBC.[27] Importantly, up to 40% of patients with a unilateral bladder tumor may have involvement of lymph nodes on the contralateral side, which means that either side of the pelvis may be involved.[41]

Both CT and MRI rely primarily on size criteria to detect lymph node involvement, and overall are thought to be roughly equivalent in the ability to detect lymph node metastases from bladder cancer.[6] Both imaging modalities are limited in their ability to detect metastatic involvement in nodes that are smaller than 1 cm.[27] However, multiple

---

Box 2
Clinical bottom line: computed tomography and MRI for local staging

Most patients receive a CTU during their initial hematuria evaluation. MRI of the pelvis can serve as a useful adjunctive modality to potentially provide additional staging information especially about the local extent of disease. In those cases when MRI is ordered, more detailed information about bladder wall anatomy can be obtained and used to improve accuracy of staging for patients with MIBC. The optimal MRI sequence has yet to be established, and useful sequences to obtain include contrast-enhanced, T2, and DWI.

studies have proposed different size criteria to indicate if nodes are malignant. Barentsz and colleagues[42] reported that pelvic nodes that are longer than 8 mm and abdominal nodes that are larger than 1 cm in the shortest axis may be considered malignant. Another study by Wollin and colleagues[43] reported that nodal features in patients with bladder cancer undergoing cystectomy on DWI measured short axis as greater than 5 mm (sensitivity 88%, specificity 75%) and long axis as greater than 6 mm (sensitivity 88% and specificity 71%). Although the optimal size criterion to define lymph node involvement is not well defined, in clinical practice, lymph nodes measuring greater than 1 cm in diameter in the short axis on imaging are often classified as malignant.[44]

There are also other characteristics of lymph nodes that can be used to determine if they are malignant. Identifying lymph nodes with irregular contours that suggest extracapsular extension may also be useful in identifying malignant involvement.[44] Additional nodal characteristics that may suggest malignancy include internal nodal heterogeneity, more rounded contour (as opposed to ovoid, which is more likely benign), and nonuniform fat density within the node.[44] Furthermore, nodes that demonstrate heterogeneous contrast enhancement are more likely to be malignant.[45] The absence of a fatty hilum on DWI MRI has also been reported (sensitivity 75%, specificity 71%) to be associated with metastatic lymphadenopathy in bladder cancer.[43]

In the evaluation of lymph node involvement for metastatic disease, CT may have an accuracy of 70% to 90%, which is roughly equivalent to MRI, which has an accuracy of 64% to 92%.[20,27,46,47] Ultimately, for detection of nodal involvement, clinicians often use their clinical judgment and should work with the radiologists in their local institution to determine if either CT or MRI, or both studies, are needed to perform preoperative clinical staging (**Box 3**).

Additional studies evaluating extent of metastatic disease in muscle-invasive bladder cancer

In addition to determining the T and N stage of patients with MIBC, it is essential to evaluate patients for additional sites of involvement. Accurately identifying patients with metastatic disease can allow providers to either assign patients to receive neoadjuvant chemotherapy or potentially avoid cystectomy on patients with extensive metastatic disease. After determining the extent of local tumor invasion and spread to lymph nodes, additional evaluations should be directed at determining if there is involvement of the upper urinary tract or other distant organs.

The role of bone scintigraphy A bone scan or bone scintigraphy may be ordered in patients that are suspected of having bone metastases due to laboratory abnormalities or clinical symptoms.[5] An elevated alkaline phosphatase may signify the presence of bone involvement. Among patients with bone metastases, serum alkaline phosphatase was significantly higher ($P = .01$), and on multivariate analysis, alkaline phosphatase (cutoff value 116 U/L) was an independent risk factor for bone metastases. In addition to laboratory studies, patients who complain of focal bone pain should also be evaluated with a bone scan. It is also important to note that after regional lymph nodes, bones are one of the most common sites of metastatic disease, accounting for up to 24% to 35% of metastatic lesions.[48,49] Last, approximately 4% to 27%[50–53] of patients with bladder cancer may develop bone metastases, with the most common sites being the bony pelvis followed by spine.[52]

Obtaining a bone scan if bone involvement is suspected allows clinicians to detect the presence of metastatic disease before treatment selection. The advantages of a bone scan include that it is usually readily available at most centers and is low cost.[54] In patients with bladder cancer, bone scintigraphy may have a sensitivity of 82%, a specificity of 64%, a positive predictive value of 56%, a negative predictive value of 87%, and an accuracy of 71%.[55] However, the overall usefulness of bone scans may be limited. Because of its low specificity and sensitivity and potentially the low prevalence of bone metastases without any other sites of metastatic disease, bone scans may not need to be routinely obtained. In fact, the likelihood of a true positive bone scan may be as low as 2.8% in patients with bladder cancer without symptoms, laboratory test result abnormalities, or other sites of metastases,[56] and bone scans may lead to unnecessary or costly procedures.[55] In patients whereby bone scan findings are concerning for metastatic disease, an MRI may be obtained for further clarification because it can be more sensitive and specific for clarifying suspected lesions.[57,58] Alternatively, a PET/CT

Box 3
Clinical bottom line: nodal staging

CT and MRI have roughly equivalent accuracy for the detection of lymph node involvement in MIBC and rely primarily on size criteria (with a cutoff of >1 cm) and other characteristics (such as irregular contours or extracapsular extension) to detect suspicious nodes.

scan is also more sensitive and specific than a bone scan and may also be obtained to further evaluate for bone metastases.[55] In clinical practice, there is heterogeneity in patterns of preoperative use of bone scans based in part on regional and provider variation.[59] One study using Surveillance, Epidemiology, and End Results (SEER)-Medicare data found that approximately 31% of patients undergoing radical cystectomy receive a bone scan with most studies being ordered by urologists.[59] However, as noted in the MIBC guidelines, in the absence of clinical symptoms, an elevated alkaline phosphatase, or evidence of other metastatic lesions, bone scans should not be ordered routinely (**Box 4**).

Chest imaging In MIBC, chest imaging is essential because bladder cancer may metastasize to several locations, but the chest is among one of the most common sites of spread for patients with pT2 or greater disease. After lymph nodes and bone involvement, the lungs are the next most common site of metastatic disease for patients with pT2-4 bladder cancer.[60]

Initial evaluation of patients with MIBC should include chest imaging, which can be done with a CRX or CT. According to the NCCN guidelines, anterior-posterior and lateral views CXR can be done initially. CT of the chest can be done if an abnormality is seen on the CXR or in higher-risk patients or in patients already undergoing a CT of the abdomen and pelvis.[5] The European Urology Association guidelines are more explicit, recommending a CT scan as the study of choice to detect lung metastases.[61] Moreover, in patients that are active or former smokers (such as those that have smoked for more than 30 pack-years, continue to smoke, or have quit within 15 years), a CT scan of the chest is recommended by the American College of Chest Physicians to detect lung cancer.[62]

Although chest imaging is an important part of the staging in MIBC, in current practice there is debate regarding which imaging study is obtained in the evaluation of patients with bladder cancer.[53] Although a CXR is less costly than a chest CT, it is also less sensitive and specific.[61] Therefore, a CT

may be more likely to detect disease but also may detect incidental nodules that may not necessarily represent metastatic disease. There is considerable variation in preoperative chest imaging in patients with MIBC, and up to 16% of patients may have no chest imaging before cystectomy.[53] However, over time, rates of chest imaging have increased significantly. According to one study examining trends between 1994 and 2008, the percent of patients receiving CXRs increased from 55% to 63% and the number of patients undergoing chest CT increased from 10% to 21%.[53] Despite the variation in practice patterns, obtaining at least some type of chest imaging remains an important component of staging in bladder cancer (**Box 5**).

The role of PET/computed tomography Although PET/CT is not mandatory as the initial staging strategy for cT2 or greater disease, evidence has emerged that it can be valuable when MRI or CT is equivocal or if there is suspicion of metastatic disease. PET/CT has been shown to have superior ability in detecting bone metastases in patients with bladder cancer when compared with conventional bone scan. One study compared these 2 modalities and found that 18-fluorodeoxyglucose (^{18}F-FDG) PET/CT had higher sensitivity, specificity, positive predictive value, negative predictive value, and accuracy when compared with bone scan with respective values of 100%, 87%, 81%, 100%, and 92%.[55] Moreover, a recent meta-analysis of 6 studies examined the diagnostic accuracy of PET/CT in patients with bladder cancer and reported a pooled sensitivity of 82%, specificity of 89%, and diagnostic accuracy of 92%.[63] Of note, limitations of the meta-analysis include a small number of studies available, differences in study designs, and heterogeneity in study quality.

Two studies have examined the utility of PET/CT in the evaluation of patients with bladder cancer. Drieskens and colleagues[47] examined 55 patients with nonmetastatic MIBC to evaluate the utility of PET/CT in detecting metastatic disease in the preoperative setting. The investigators examined

---

Box 4
Clinical bottom line: the role of bone scintigraphy

A bone scan can be done routinely when evaluating patients with MIBC; however, the accuracy is suboptimal. Patients with elevated alkaline phosphatase or local symptoms, such as pain, should have a bone scan.

Box 5
Clinical bottom line: chest imaging

Ultimately, at a minimum, patients with cT2 or greater bladder cancer should undergo a CXR. However, clinicians may choose to obtain CT imaging of the chest based on their clinical discretion. Patients with extensive smoking histories may also require a chest CT. If patients require a CT of the abdomen and pelvis, adding a chest sequence is also a reasonable option.

patients for evidence of nodal or metastatic involvement using ^{18}F-FDG PET/CT. Imaging results were compared with histologic examination after lymphadenectomy or guided biopsy. The investigators reported a sensitivity of 60%, specificity of 88%, and accuracy of 78% for detecting patients with nodal or metastatic disease. Finally, median survival for those with N or M involvement detected on PET/CT was 13 months compared with 32 months for those with a negative PET/CT. Obviously, the utility of this should be first determined by stage as well as the presence of any other abnormalities on CT, CXR, or bone scintigraphy.

Another study by Kibel and colleagues[64] studied the value of ^{18}F-FDG PET/CT in 43 patients with cT2-T3N0 disease to detect occult metastatic disease. In this study, all patients had negative CT and bone scans and were scheduled to undergo cystectomy. Imaging results were confirmed with either percutaneous biopsy or surgical resection. The investigators reported a positive predictive value of 78% (7 of 9), a negative predictive value of 91% (30 of 33), a sensitivity of 70% (7 of 10), and a specificity of 94% (30 of 32). For those patients in whom PET/CT scan demonstrated lymph node involvement, there were significant differences in recurrence-free survival, OS, and disease-specific survival (**Fig. 2**).

PET/CT was compared with MRI for the ability to detect lymph node–positive disease in 48 patients with bladder cancer that ultimately underwent cystectomy with pelvic lymph node dissection.[65] The investigators compared imaging results with final pathologic results. Specificities of MRI versus PET/CT for the detection of nodal metastases were 80% and 93%, respectively. Although no statistically significant difference was observed between ^{18}F-FDG PET/CT and MRI, there was a trend favoring ^{18}F-FDG PET/CT. To date, there are no established guidelines for when to obtain a PET/CT, and the MIBC guidelines recommend obtaining PET/CT only to adjudicate equivocal findings on CT that would change management. Future studies are needed to establish the role of this imaging modality and its optimal application.

The role of lymph node dissection in the staging of muscle invasive bladder cancer

An important component of staging in MIBC is determining involvement of regional lymph nodes. According to the NCCN guidelines, patients undergoing radical cystectomy should receive a bilateral pelvic lymphadenectomy and include at a minimum the common, internal, and external iliac nodes as well as the obturator nodes.[5] A thorough lymph node dissection can provide valuable staging information and may provide a therapeutic

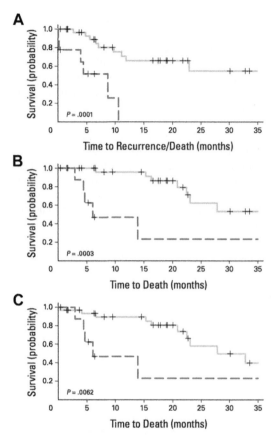

Fig. 2. Kaplan-Meier plots demonstrate differences in recurrence-free survival (*A*), disease-specific survival (*B*), and OS (*C*) for 9 patients with negative PET/CT results (*solid line*) and 33 patients with positive PET/CT results (*dashed line*). (*From* Kibel AS, Dehdashti F, Katz MD, et al. Prospective study of fluorodeoxyglucose positron emission tomography/computed tomography for staging of muscle-invasive bladder carcinoma. J Clin Onc 2009;27(26):4314–20; *Reprinted with permission.* © American Society of Clinical Oncology. All rights reserved.)

benefit via removal of micrometastatic or overt macroscopic disease. Herr and colleagues[66] conducted an analysis of 322 patients with MIBC and reported that at least 9 lymph nodes needed to be studied in order to determine accurate nodal staging. Moreover, the investigators found a statistically significant survival ($P = .004$) benefit in node-positive patients with at least 11 lymph nodes removed.[66] Work by Wright and colleagues[67] using the SEER registry found that for patients who underwent cystectomy and had at least one positive node, the removal of more than 10 lymph nodes was associated with increased OS. Finally, another study reported improved prognosis in both node-positive and -negative patients with MIBC that had 16 or more lymph nodes removed.[3]

The optimal extent of lymph node dissection boundaries in radical cystectomy remains debated. For example, the cephalad-most extent of the dissection is controversial, and multiple limits have been described.[68–73] One particular challenge to studying the impact of lymph node dissection is the variability of templates. A meta-analysis of greater than 25 studies including 41,400 patients with bladder cancer found a large degree of heterogeneity across the studies examined.[74] Although no level I evidence exists and yields may vary because of multiple factors, including surgeon technique, and pathologic processing, 2 prospective randomized trials are underway to assess whether extended pelvic lymph node dissection is associated with improved OS.[75] A more complete discussion of the value of lymphadenectomy is covered by Niranjan J. Sathianathen and colleagues' article, "Lymphadenectomy for Muscle-Invasive Bladder Cancer and Upper Tract Urothelial Cell Carcinoma," in this issue.

Evaluation of the upper tracts in muscle-invasive bladder cancer

It is important to ensure that the upper urinary tract has been imaged properly in patients with bladder cancer because the prevalence of upper urinary tract cancer occurring concomitantly with bladder cancer ranges from 0.75% to 6.4%.[76–78] A CTU is useful because it has the highest diagnostic accuracy for detecting cancer with a sensitivity of 67% to 100% and specificity of 93% to 99%.[17,79] In clinical practice, most patients presenting with hematuria have already been evaluated with CT or MR urogram and have already been evaluated for upper tract involvement. For patients with lesions detected on imaging that are concerning for

malignancy, a ureteroscopy for visual examination with biopsy is needed to obtain a histologic diagnosis.[14,16]

Renal pelvis and ureteral cancer staging additional considerations

The staging of UTUC in large part parallels that of bladder cancer. Patients suspected of having renal pelvis or ureteral tumors should receive imaging of the upper urinary tract, which has typically already been performed because of concern for disease with CT or MR urogram both being reasonable options. Additional components of the initial evaluation may include cytology, cystoscopy, CBC, BMP, CXR, and if clinically indicated, a bone scan. Consideration of renal function in patients scheduled to undergo nephroureterectomy is important because patients with a solitary kidney are at risk for chronic kidney disease, and preoperative glomerular filtration rate can help predict chronic kidney disease after surgery.[80] In patients undergoing staging studies for renal pelvis and ureteral cancer, a nuclear medicine scan may help evaluate renal function and help to determine eligibility for additional therapies, such as chemotherapy. In cases whereby there is concern for a significant decline in renal function after nephroureterectomy, preoperative consultation with a nephrologist may help optimize and address any concomitant contributing comorbidities, such as hypertension and diabetes.[81]

SUMMARY

Staging is a critical element in the evaluation of patients with MIBC and UTUC. **Fig. 3** highlights several key elements in the staging of patients with MIBC and UTUC. The initial clinical evaluation should include a determination of the local extent

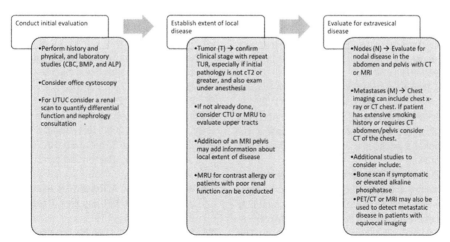

Fig. 3. Summary of staging for MIBC and UTUC: staging algorithm for a patient with concern for MIBC or UTUC. ALP, alkaline phosphatase; MRU, MR urogram; TUR, transurethral resection.

of disease and the presence of distant disease. Although CT and MRI are valuable and widely used, some limitations exist and must be considered. Bone scan, comprehensive metabolic panel, and chest imaging are also part of the routine evaluation. Advanced imaging, such as PET/CT, hold promise, but additional work is needed to continue to refine and develop the capacity to more accurately capture the extent of disease in patients with MIBC and UTUC seeking oncologic care. Future research into novel imaging techniques and indications for more specific imaging is sorely needed.

REFERENCES

1. Hautmann RE, de Petriconi RC, Pfeiffer C, et al. Radical cystectomy for urothelial carcinoma of the bladder without neoadjuvant or adjuvant therapy: long-term results in 1100 patients. Eur Urol 2012; 61(5):1039–47.
2. Madersbacher S, Hochreiter W, Burkhard F, et al. Radical cystectomy for bladder cancer today–a homogeneous series without neoadjuvant therapy. J Clin Oncol 2003;21(4):690–6.
3. Leissner J, Hohenfellner R, Thuroff JW, et al. Lymphadenectomy in patients with transitional cell carcinoma of the urinary bladder; significance for staging and prognosis. BJU Int 2000;85(7): 817–23.
4. Amin MB, Greene FL, Edge SB, et al. The eighth edition AJCC cancer staging manual: continuing to build a bridge from a population-based to a more "personalized" approach to cancer staging. CA Cancer J Clin 2017;67(2):93–9.
5. Spiess PE, Agarwal N, Bangs R, et al. Bladder cancer, version 5.2017, NCCN clinical practice guidelines in oncology. J Natl Compr Canc Netw 2017; 15(10):1240–67.
6. MacVicar AD. Bladder cancer staging. BJU Int 2000;86(Suppl 1):111–22.
7. Herr HW. The value of a second transurethral resection in evaluating patients with bladder tumors. J Urol 1999;162(1):74–6.
8. Herr HW. Role of re-resection in non-muscle-invasive bladder cancer. ScientificWorldJournal 2011;11:283–8.
9. Maruniak NA, Takezawa K, Murphy WM. Accurate pathological staging of urothelial neoplasms requires better cystoscopic sampling. J Urol 2002; 167(6):2404–7.
10. Gill TS, Das RK, Basu S, et al. Predictive factors for residual tumor and tumor upstaging on relook transurethral resection of bladder tumor in non-muscle invasive bladder cancer. Urol Ann 2014;6(4):305–8.
11. Schwaibold HE, Sivalingam S, May F, et al. The value of a second transurethral resection for T1 bladder cancer. BJU Int 2006;97(6):1199–201.

12. Miladi M, Peyromaure M, Zerbib M, et al. The value of a second transurethral resection in evaluating patients with bladder tumours. Eur Urol 2003;43(3):241–5.
13. Herr HW, Donat SM, Dalbagni G. Can restaging transurethral resection of T1 bladder cancer select patients for immediate cystectomy? J Urol 2007; 177(1):75–9 [discussion: 79].
14. Vashistha V, Shabsigh A, Zynger DL. Utility and diagnostic accuracy of ureteroscopic biopsy in upper tract urothelial carcinoma. Arch Pathol Lab Med 2013;137(3):400–7.
15. Baard J, de Bruin DM, Zondervan PJ, et al. Diagnostic dilemmas in patients with upper tract urothelial carcinoma. Nat Rev Urol 2017;14(3):181–91.
16. El-Hakim A, Weiss GH, Lee BR, et al. Correlation of ureteroscopic appearance with histologic grade of upper tract transitional cell carcinoma. Urology 2004;63(4):647–50 [discussion: 650].
17. Cowan NC. CT urography for hematuria. Nat Rev Urol 2012;9(4):218–26.
18. Martingano P, Stacul F, Cavallaro M, et al. 64-Slice CT urography: 30 months of clinical experience. Radiol Med 2010;115(6):920–35.
19. Hodson NJ, Husband JE, MacDonald JS. The role of computed tomography in the staging of bladder cancer. Clin Radiol 1979;30(4):389–95.
20. Morgan CL, Calkins RF, Cavalcanti EJ. Computed tomography in the evaluation, staging, and therapy of carcinoma of the bladder and prostate. Radiology 1981;140(3):751–61.
21. Capalbo E, Kluzer A, Peli M, et al. Bladder cancer diagnosis: the role of CT urography. Tumori 2015; 101(4):412–7.
22. Blick CG, Nazir SA, Mallett S, et al. Evaluation of diagnostic strategies for bladder cancer using computed tomography (CT) urography, flexible cystoscopy and voided urine cytology: results for 778 patients from a hospital haematuria clinic. BJU Int 2012;110(1):84–94.
23. Hafeez S, Huddart R. Advances in bladder cancer imaging. BMC Med 2013;11:104.
24. Tritschler S, Mosler C, Tilki D, et al. Interobserver variability limits exact preoperative staging by computed tomography in bladder cancer. Urology 2012;79(6):1317–21.
25. Beyersdorff D, Zhang J, Schoder H, et al. Bladder cancer: can imaging change patient management? Curr Opin Urol 2008;18(1):98–104.
26. Zhang J, Gerst S, Lefkowitz RA, et al. Imaging of bladder cancer. Radiol Clin North Am 2007;45(1): 183–205.
27. Verma S, Rajesh A, Prasad SR, et al. Urinary bladder cancer: role of MR imaging. Radiographics 2012; 32(2):371–87.
28. Saksena MA, Dahl DM, Harisinghani MG. New imaging modalities in bladder cancer. World J Urol 2006; 24(5):473–80.

29. Tekes A, Kamel I, Imam K, et al. Dynamic MRI of bladder cancer: evaluation of staging accuracy. AJR Am J Roentgenol 2005;184(1):121–7.

30. Matsuki M, Inada Y, Tatsugami F, et al. Diffusion-weighted MR imaging for urinary bladder carcinoma: initial results. Eur Radiol 2007;17(1):201–4.

31. Halefoglu AM, Sen EY, Tanriverdi O, et al. Utility of diffusion-weighted MRI in the diagnosis of bladder carcinoma. Clin Imaging 2013;37(6):1077–83.

32. El-Assmy A, Abou-El-Ghar ME, Refaie HF, et al. Diffusion-weighted MR imaging in diagnosis of superficial and invasive urinary bladder carcinoma: a preliminary prospective study. TheScientificWorldJournal 2008;8:364–70.

33. Sun Y, Tong T, Cai S, et al. Apparent diffusion coefficient (ADC) value: a potential imaging biomarker that reflects the biological features of rectal cancer. PLoS One 2014;9(10):e109371.

34. Koh DM, Collins DJ. Diffusion-weighted MRI in the body: applications and challenges in oncology. AJR Am J Roentgenol 2007;188(6):1622–35.

35. Giannarini G, Petralia G, Thoeny HC. Potential and limitations of diffusion-weighted magnetic resonance imaging in kidney, prostate, and bladder cancer including pelvic lymph node staging: a critical analysis of the literature. Eur Urol 2012;61(2):326–40.

36. Lin WC, Chen JH. Pitfalls and limitations of diffusion-weighted magnetic resonance imaging in the diagnosis of urinary bladder cancer. Transl Oncol 2015;8(3):217–30.

37. Watanabe H, Kanematsu M, Kondo H, et al. Preoperative T staging of urinary bladder cancer: does diffusion-weighted MRI have supplementary value? AJR Am J Roentgenol 2009;192(5):1361–6.

38. El-Assmy A, Abou-El-Ghar ME, Mosbah A, et al. Bladder tumour staging: comparison of diffusion- and T2-weighted MR imaging. Eur Radiol 2009;19(7):1575–81.

39. Takeuchi M, Sasaki S, Ito M, et al. Urinary bladder cancer: diffusion-weighted MR imaging–accuracy for diagnosing T stage and estimating histologic grade. Radiology 2009;251(1):112–21.

40. Huang L, Kong Q, Liu Z, et al. The diagnostic value of MR imaging in differentiating T staging of bladder cancer: a meta-analysis. Radiology 2017;286(2):502–11.

41. Mills RD, Turner WH, Fleischmann A, et al. Pelvic lymph node metastases from bladder cancer: outcome in 83 patients after radical cystectomy and pelvic lymphadenectomy. J Urol 2001;166(1):19–23.

42. Barentsz JO, Engelbrecht MR, Witjes JA, et al. MR imaging of the male pelvis. Eur Radiol 1999;9(9):1722–36.

43. Wollin DA, Deng FM, Huang WC, et al. Conventional and diffusion-weighted MRI features in diagnosis of metastatic lymphadenopathy in bladder cancer. Can J Urol 2014;21(5):7454–9.

44. Ganeshalingam S, Koh DM. Nodal staging. Cancer Imaging 2009;9:104–11.

45. Barentsz JO, Jager GJ, van Vierzen PB, et al. Staging urinary bladder cancer after transurethral biopsy: value of fast dynamic contrast-enhanced MR imaging. Radiology 1996;201(1):185–93.

46. Paik ML, Scolieri MJ, Brown SL, et al. Limitations of computerized tomography in staging invasive bladder cancer before radical cystectomy. J Urol 2000;163(6):1693–6.

47. Drieskens O, Oyen R, Van Poppel H, et al. FDG-PET for preoperative staging of bladder cancer. Eur J Nucl Med Mol Imaging 2005;32(12):1412–7.

48. Sengelov L, Kamby C, von der Maase H. Pattern of metastases in relation to characteristics of primary tumor and treatment in patients with disseminated urothelial carcinoma. J Urol 1996;155(1):111–4.

49. Bianchi M, Roghmann F, Becker A, et al. Age-stratified distribution of metastatic sites in bladder cancer: a population-based analysis. Can Urol Assoc J 2014;8(3–4):E148–58.

50. Taher AN, Kotb MH. Bone metastases in muscle-invasive bladder cancer. J Egypt Natl Canc Inst 2006;18(3):203–8.

51. Bienz M, Saad F. Management of bone metastases in prostate cancer: a review. Curr Opin Support Palliat Care 2015;9(3):261–7.

52. Huang P, Lan M, Peng AF, et al. Serum calcium, alkaline phosphotase and hemoglobin as risk factors for bone metastases in bladder cancer. PLoS One 2017;12(9):e0183835.

53. McInnes MD, Siemens DR, Mackillop WJ, et al. Utilisation of preoperative imaging for muscle-invasive bladder cancer: a population-based study. BJU Int 2016;117(3):430–8.

54. Heidenreich A, Albers P, Classen J, et al. Imaging studies in metastatic urogenital cancer patients undergoing systemic therapy: recommendations of a multidisciplinary consensus meeting of the Association of Urological Oncology of the German Cancer Society. Urol Int 2010;85(1):1–10.

55. Chakraborty D, Bhattacharya A, Mete UK, et al. Comparison of 18F fluoride PET/CT and 99mTc-MDP bone scan in the detection of skeletal metastases in urinary bladder carcinoma. Clin Nucl Med 2013;38(8):616–21.

56. Brismar J, Gustafson T. Bone scintigraphy in staging of bladder carcinoma. Acta Radiol 1988;29(2):251–2.

57. Lauenstein TC, Goehde SC, Herborn CU, et al. Whole-body MR imaging: evaluation of patients for metastases. Radiology 2004;233(1):139–48.

58. Guimaraes MD, Schuch A, Hochhegger B, et al. Functional magnetic resonance imaging in oncology: state of the art. Radiol Bras 2014;47(2):101–11.

59. Turner RM 2nd, Yabes JG, Davies BJ, et al. Variations in preoperative use of bone scan among Medicare beneficiaries undergoing radical cystectomy. Urology 2017;103:84–90.

60. Shinagare AB, Ramaiya NH, Jagannathan JP, et al. Metastatic pattern of bladder cancer: correlation with the characteristics of the primary tumor. AJR Am J Roentgenol 2011;196(1):117–22.

61. Girvin F, Ko JP. Pulmonary nodules: detection, assessment, and CAD. AJR Am J Roentgenol 2008;191(4):1057–69.

62. Detterbeck FC, Lewis SZ, Diekemper R, et al. Executive summary: diagnosis and management of lung cancer, 3rd ed: American College of Chest Physicians evidence-based clinical practice guidelines. Chest 2013;143(5 Suppl):7S–37S.

63. Lu YY, Chen JH, Liang JA, et al. Clinical value of FDG PET or PET/CT in urinary bladder cancer: a systemic review and meta-analysis. Eur J Radiol 2012; 81(9):2411–6.

64. Kibel AS, Dehdashti F, Katz MD, et al. Prospective study of [18F]fluorodeoxyglucose positron emission tomography/computed tomography for staging of muscle-invasive bladder carcinoma. J Clin Oncol 2009;27(26):4314–20.

65. Jensen TK, Holt P, Gerke O, et al. Preoperative lymph-node staging of invasive urothelial bladder cancer with 18F-fluorodeoxyglucose positron emission tomography/computed axial tomography and magnetic resonance imaging: correlation with histopathology. Scand J Urol Nephrol 2011;45(2):122–8.

66. Herr HW, Bochner BH, Dalbagni G, et al. Impact of the number of lymph nodes retrieved on outcome in patients with muscle invasive bladder cancer. J Urol 2002;167(3):1295–8.

67. Wright JL, Lin DW, Porter MP. The association between extent of lymphadenectomy and survival among patients with lymph node metastases undergoing radical cystectomy. Cancer 2008;112(11):2401–8.

68. Jensen JB, Ulhoi BP, Jensen KM, et al. Lymph node mapping in patients with bladder cancer undergoing radical cystectomy and lymph node dissection to the level of the inferior mesenteric artery: how high is "high enough"? Radical cystectomy and extended pelvic lymphadenectomy: survival of patients with lymph node metastasis above the bifurcation of the common iliac vessels treated with surgery only. BJU Int 2010;106(2):199–205.

69. Stein JP, Skinner DG. The role of lymphadenectomy in high-grade invasive bladder cancer. Urol Clin North Am 2005;32(2):187–97.

70. Stein JP, Quek ML, Skinner DG. Lymphadenectomy for invasive bladder cancer. II. Technical aspects and prognostic factors. BJU Int 2006;97(2): 232–7.

71. Stein JP, Quek ML, Skinner DG. Lymphadenectomy for invasive bladder cancer: I. Historical perspective and contemporary rationale. BJU Int 2006;97(2): 227–31.

72. Steven K, Poulsen AL. Radical cystectomy and extended pelvic lymphadenectomy: survival of patients with lymph node metastasis above the bifurcation of the common iliac vessels treated with surgery only. J Urol 2007;178(4 Pt 1):1218–23 [discussion 1223–4].

73. Karl A, Carroll PR, Gschwend JE, et al. The impact of lymphadenectomy and lymph node metastasis on the outcomes of radical cystectomy for bladder cancer. Eur Urol 2009;55(4):826–35.

74. Li F, Hong X, Hou L, et al. A greater number of dissected lymph nodes is associated with more favorable outcomes in bladder cancer treated by radical cystectomy: a meta-analysis. Oncotarget 2016;7(38):61284–94.

75. Sundi D, Svatek RS, Nielsen ME, et al. Extent of pelvic lymph node dissection during radical cystectomy: is bigger better? Rev Urol 2014;16(4): 159–66.

76. Picozzi S, Ricci C, Gaeta M, et al. Upper urinary tract recurrence following radical cystectomy for bladder cancer: a meta-analysis on 13,185 patients. J Urol 2012;188(6):2046–54.

77. Sanderson KM, Cai J, Miranda G, et al. Upper tract urothelial recurrence following radical cystectomy for transitional cell carcinoma of the bladder: an analysis of 1,069 patients with 10-year followup. J Urol 2007;177(6):2088–94.

78. Gakis G, Black PC, Bochner BH, et al. Systematic review on the fate of the remnant urothelium after radical cystectomy. Eur Urol 2017;71(4):545–57.

79. Roupret M, Babjuk M, Comperat E, et al. European Association of Urology guidelines on upper urinary tract urothelial carcinoma: 2017 update. Eur Urol 2018;73(1):111–22.

80. Wu FM, Tay MH, Chen Z, et al. Postoperative risk of chronic kidney disease in radical nephrectomy and donor nephrectomy patients: a comparison and analysis of predictive factors. Can J Urol 2014; 21(4):7351–7.

81. Li L, Lau WL, Rhee CM, et al. Risk of chronic kidney disease after cancer nephrectomy. Nat Rev Nephrol 2014;10(3):135–45.

Optimal Timing of Chemotherapy and Surgery in Patients with Muscle-Invasive Bladder Cancer and Upper Urinary Tract Urothelial Carcinoma

William Tabayoyong, MD, PhD[a], Roger Li, MD[a],
Jianjun Gao, MD, PhD[b], Ashish Kamat, MD[a],*

KEYWORDS

- Bladder cancer • Upper tract urothelial cancer • Neoadjuvant chemotherapy
- Adjuvant chemotherapy

KEY POINTS

- Survival post-radical cystectomy/nephroureterectomy is closely associated with final pathologic staging, with survival decreasing with increasing pT stage, which is attributed to associated occult micrometastases indicating the need for systemic chemotherapy.
- A multidisciplinary approach is necessary for patients with surgically resectable disease, including cisplatin-based neoadjuvant chemotherapy followed by radical cystectomy with pelvic lymph node dissection.
- The data show that neoadjuvant chemotherapy is much more beneficial than adjuvant chemotherapy for patients with bladder cancer.
- For patients who have surgically resectable disease and are noncisplatin candidates, expedient surgery is necessary; there is no role for carboplatin-based regimens in this situation.
- Advances in molecular biology, genetic subtyping, and immunotherapy are promising but cannot yet be used to supplant the role of neoadjuvant chemotherapy.

INTRODUCTION

There will be an estimated 79,030 new cases diagnosed and 16,870 deaths attributed to bladder cancer in the United States in 2017.[1] The standard of care for patients with clinically localized muscle-invasive bladder cancer (MIBC) has been radical cystectomy with bilateral pelvic lymph node dissection.[2] Survival after radical cystectomy is closely associated with final pathologic staging: patients who are pT0 have 5-year recurrence-free survival of 92%, with survival decreasing with increasing pT stage to where patients with nonorgan-confined disease have 5-year recurrence-free survival ranges between 53% and 62% for pT3b N0 and even lower (<50%) for

Disclosure: The authors have nothing to disclose.
[a] Urology, University of Texas MD Anderson Cancer Center, 1515 Holcombe Boulevard, Unit 1373, Houston, TX 77030, USA; [b] Genitourinary Medical Oncology, University of Texas MD Anderson Cancer Center, 1515 Holcombe Boulevard, Unit 1374, Houston, TX 77030, USA
* Corresponding author.
E-mail address: akamat@mdanderson.org

Urol Clin N Am 45 (2018) 155–167
https://doi.org/10.1016/j.ucl.2017.12.002
0094-0143/18/© 2018 Elsevier Inc. All rights reserved.

urologic.theclinics.com

pT4 and (<35%) for pN$^+$ (lymph node positive) disease.[3,4] One cause for this stage-dependent reduction in survival is thought to be the presence of occult micrometastases indicating the need for systemic chemotherapy to improve survival.[2,5] Systemic chemotherapy is delivered perioperatively either as neoadjuvant therapy in the preoperative period, or as adjuvant therapy in the postoperative period. Recent expert panels have advocated for a multidisciplinary approach to the treatment of nonmetastatic MIBC that includes coordination of the timing of administration of perioperative cisplatin-based chemotherapy and radical cystectomy with pelvic lymph node dissection.[6] Unfortunately, despite these recommendations, perioperative chemotherapy is still underused in the management of surgically resectable bladder cancer.[7,8]

In this article, we review the major neoadjuvant and adjuvant chemotherapy trials for the treatment of MIBC and upper urinary tract urothelial carcinoma (UTUC) and offer recommendations based on the results of these trials and the recently updated clinical guidelines.

NEOADJUVANT CHEMOTHERAPY

Neoadjuvant chemotherapy is, by definition, the administration of chemotherapy to patients with the intent of consolidation with definitive local therapy (eg, radical cystectomy). This is in contrast with preoperative chemotherapy, which includes patients who receive chemotherapy for metastatic/unresectable disease but then ultimately become surgical candidates. Thus, strictly speaking, patients with clinical T2-T3N0M0 and T4 (prostate or vaginal wall) MIBC are candidates for neoadjuvant chemotherapy. Administration of chemotherapy in the neoadjuvant setting has several advantages.[2,5] Patients typically have better performance status and are better able to tolerate chemotherapy before surgery. Neoadjuvant chemotherapy allows for in vivo drug sensitivity testing (response of bladder tumor) and radiographic response is a significant prognostic indicator. Additionally, neoadjuvant chemotherapy could downstage tumors, which can make surgery easier and less morbid in some situations.

The major disadvantage of neoadjuvant chemotherapy is that one still cannot predict who will not respond to chemotherapy and the potential for delay to cystectomy in these patients could allow growth of tumor and further metastasis because it has been demonstrated that a delay in surgery of greater than 12 weeks from the time of diagnosis is associated with advanced pathologic stage and decreased survival.[9,10] This is especially true for variant histology bladder cancers with plasmacytoid, sarcomatoid, and pure squamous cell carcinoma variants being poorly responsive to chemotherapy, associated with advanced stage, distant metastases, local progression, and worse survival and disease-specific survival when compared with conventional urothelial carcinoma.[11]

Another disadvantage of neoadjuvant chemotherapy is the overtreatment of patients with organ-confined disease and no micrometastatic disease. However, this can be reduced using certain risk-adapted selection criteria (discussed later). Lastly, one theoretic disadvantage of neoadjuvant chemotherapy is the possibility of increased perioperative morbidity; however, a study of integrated neoadjuvant chemotherapy before cystectomy followed by additional administration of adjuvant chemotherapy after cystectomy demonstrated that neoadjuvant chemotherapy did not increase perioperative morbidity.[12]

Randomized Trials of Neoadjuvant Chemotherapy

Several randomized trials have attempted to determine whether neoadjuvant chemotherapy before radical cystectomy improves overall survival compared with radical cystectomy alone. With the exception of two studies mentioned later, many of these trials showed either minimal benefit or no benefit.[13–17] These trials were limited by their suboptimal chemotherapy combinations, small sample size, premature closure, and inadequate follow-up. In response to these shortcomings, a meta-analysis was performed to explain and interpret these data.[18] Combining the data of a total of 3005 patients included in 11 randomized neoadjuvant chemotherapy trials, it was determined that a 5% absolute improvement in overall survival at 5 years was associated with platinum-based combination chemotherapy. Moreover, a 9% absolute improvement in disease-free survival at 5 years was associated with platinum-based combination chemotherapy. These results represent the best available evidence in favor of the use of neoadjuvant platinum-based combination chemotherapy for patients with MIBC.

The two largest trials included in the meta-analysis that did show significant survival benefit for neoadjuvant platinum-based combination chemotherapy when their data were analyzed individually are the MRC BA06/EORTC 30894 and the SWOG 8710 trials. The MRC BA06/EORTC 30894 study was a large trial, randomizing 976 patients with locally advanced MIBC to receive either three cycles of cisplatin, methotrexate, and vinblastine neoadjuvant chemotherapy or no chemotherapy followed by definitive therapy with either radical cystectomy or radiotherapy.[19,20] The first report from this study at a median of only 4 years of follow-up demonstrated a 15% reduction in the risk of death attributed to neoadjuvant chemotherapy but did not reach statistical significance[19]; however, after 8-year follow-up, statistical significance was achieved with patients receiving neoadjuvant cisplatin, methotrexate, and vinblastine chemotherapy showing improvement in absolute survival of 6% and a relative reduction in the risk of death resulting from bladder cancer of 16% at 10 years.[20]

The SWOG 8710 trial randomized 317 patients with MIBC (stage T2 to T4a) to radical cystectomy alone or three cycles of methotrexate, vinblastine, doxorubicin, and cisplatin (MVAC) followed by radical cystectomy.[21] Median survival was 77 months in patients assigned to the MVAC arm versus 46 months in patients receiving cystectomy alone ($P = .06$ by a two-sided stratified log-rank test), and the estimated risk of death from bladder cancer was reduced by 33%. In both groups, improved survival was associated with the absence of residual cancer (pT0) in the cystectomy specimen and 85% of patients who were pT0 at cystectomy were alive at 5 years. Importantly, significantly more patients who received MVAC neoadjuvant chemotherapy were found to be pT0 at the time of cystectomy (38% vs 15%; $P<.001$).

Alternate Chemotherapy Regimens to Methotrexate, Vinblastine, Doxorubicin, and Cisplatin

In the late 1970s and 1980s, single-agent cisplatin was the standard chemotherapy agent for patients with metastatic bladder cancer. Loehrer and colleagues[22] performed a randomized comparison of single-agent cisplatin or in combination with methotrexate, vinblastine, and doxorubicin. From a total of 246 patients with metastatic bladder cancer, 126 were randomized to cisplatin alone and 120 were randomized to MVAC. The overall response rate (39% vs 12%; $P<.0001$) and overall survival (12.5 vs 8.2 months; $P = .0002$) were significantly superior for MVAC, and the MVAC regimen subsequently became the new standard.

The traditional MVAC regimen takes 12 weeks to complete and is associated with significant toxicity often leading to treatment interruption, delays, and early termination, thus compromising benefit. To address the toxicity and time delay limitations, accelerated dose-dense MVAC (ddMVAC) regimens have been proposed. Plimack and colleagues[23] performed a single-arm phase II trial of 44 patients with cT2-T4 and N0-1 MIBC who received three cycles of neoadjuvant accelerated MVAC before cystectomy. At the time of cystectomy, 38% of evaluable patients achieved complete pT0 pathologic response, and another 14% showed partial pathologic response with downstaging to nonmuscle-invasive disease. There were no grade 3 or 4 renal toxicities and no treatment-related deaths and all patients were able to proceed to cystectomy within 8 weeks after last chemotherapy. This study demonstrated that ddMVAC was well tolerated and achieved similar pT0 rates with 6 weeks of treatment compared with the standard 12-week MVAC regimen. Similarly, Choueiri and colleagues[24] performed a single-arm phase II study of 39 patients with T2-T4 N0-1 M0 MIBC who received four cycles of ddMVAC followed by radical cystectomy. After a median follow-up of 2 years, 49% achieved a pathologic response less than or equal to pT1N0M0, with 26% achieving pT0. Additionally, 82% of patients identified with CN1 disease on staging imaging studies were pN0 at cystectomy following ddMVAC. High-grade (grade ≥ 3) toxicities were observed in 10% of patients with no treatment-related deaths. In this study, neoadjuvant ddMVAC was well tolerated and resulted in significant pathologic and radiologic downstaging.

The combination of ddMVAC plus additional agents targeting the vascular endothelial growth factor pathway does not seem to provide any significant benefit. McConkey and colleagues[25] performed a single arm study of patients with advanced urothelial cancer treated with ddMVAC plus bevacizumab in a neoadjuvant setting. Bevacizumab had no appreciable impact on pathologic response or survival outcomes.

In addition to ddMVAC, the gemcitabine-cisplatin (GC) combination has also been successful for the treatment of bladder cancer. The first study comparing GC with MVAC was performed by von der Maase and colleagues.[26] This was a noninferiority randomized phase III trial comparing GC and MVAC for patients with metastatic bladder cancer demonstrating that the survival benefit of GC (13.8 months) was similar to that of MVAC (14.8 months) with a better safety profile and tolerability. Data from this trial were used to support use of GC in the neoadjuvant setting without a randomized trial. Two retrospective studies have since investigated the role of GC in the neoadjuvant setting in comparison with neoadjuvant MVAC. Yeshchina and colleagues[27] performed a retrospective review of 114 patients with T2-T4N0-N2M0 bladder cancer who received either neoadjuvant GC or neoadjuvant MVAC followed by cystectomy. No statistically significant difference was found between the two neoadjuvant regimens with respect to pathologic complete response at cystectomy or cystoscopy. Similarly, Galsky and colleagues[28] reported a retrospective review of 212 patients with T2-T4N0-N2M0 bladder cancer who received either neoadjuvant GC or neoadjuvant MVAC followed by cystectomy. Again, no significant difference in the pathologic complete response between GC or MVAC regimens was identified. Taken together, these studies have provided the rationale for the use of GC as a suitable alternative to MVAC for neoadjuvant chemotherapy; however, there are no prospective, randomized comparisons between GC and MVAC in the neoadjuvant setting.

Alternate Chemotherapy Regimens for Platinum-Ineligible Patients

Although MVAC and GC combinations have become the mainstay of neoadjuvant therapy, it is important to consider what options are available to those patients who are ineligible for cisplatin. Patients who meet at least one of the following criteria are considered unfit for cisplatin-based chemotherapy: (1) World Health Organization or Eastern Cooperative Oncology Group performance status of 2, or Karnofsky performance status of 60% to 70%; (2) creatinine clearance (calculated or measured) less than 60 mL/min, equivalent to an estimated glomerular filtration rate less than 60 mL/min; (3) Common Terminology Criteria for Adverse Events version 4 grade 2 or higher audiometric hearing loss; (4) Common Terminology Criteria for Adverse Events version 4 grade 2 or higher peripheral neuropathy; or (5) New York Heart Association class III heart failure.[29] Although carboplatin has been substituted for cisplatin in several chemotherapy regimens for other solid tumors, there are insufficient data to recommend carboplatin-based regimens for neoadjuvant chemotherapy. Several randomized trials in the metastatic setting have clearly demonstrated that carboplatin-based therapy is inferior for MIBC with respect to complete response and overall response.

Bellmunt and colleagues[30] performed a randomized trial of 47 patients with surgically incurable advanced bladder cancer, with 23 patients receiving carboplatin-based chemotherapy and 24 patients receiving cisplatin-based chemotherapy. The overall response rate with carboplatin was lower at 39% compared with 52% for cisplatin, with zero complete responses in the carboplatin group and three complete responses in the cisplatin group. There was also a statistically significant difference in disease-specific survival in favor of the cisplatin-based regimen (16 months)

compared with carboplatin (9 months). Petrioli and colleagues[31] reported a phase II randomized trial comparing the efficacy and toxicity of a cisplatin-based regimen with a carboplatinum-based regimen for patients with recurrent or metastatic bladder cancer. A total of 57 patients were randomized, with 29 receiving the cisplatin regimen and 28 receiving the carboplatin regimen. A statistically significant difference in clinical response rate was observed in favor of the cisplatin regimen, 71% overall (25% complete responses) compared with 41% (11% complete responses) with carboplatin.

In addition, Dogliotti and colleagues[32] assessed the efficacy and toxicity of GC compared with gemcitabine-carboplatin in a randomized phase 2 trial. A total of 110 patients with locally advanced or metastatic bladder cancer were randomized with 55 patients in each group. The overall response rate was higher at 49% in the GC group compared with 40% in the gemcitabine-carboplatin group. Median time to progression and median survival were also higher for the GC group compared with the gemcitabine-carboplatin group at 8.3 months and 12.8 months versus 7.7 months and 9.8 months, respectively. Taken together, the data from the three previously mentioned trials clearly demonstrate that carboplatin is inferior to cisplatin for the treatment of MIBC; therefore, carboplatin combination therapy is not recommended for cisplatin-ineligible patients in the neoadjuvant setting.

Other regimens have been studied including a phase 2 clinical trial at MD Anderson in cisplatin-ineligible patients with locally advanced urothelial cancer investigating sequential neoadjuvant chemotherapy with ifosfamide, doxorubicin, and gemcitabine followed by reduced-dose cisplatin (50 mg/m^2 compared with conventional dosing of 70 mg/m^2), gemcitabine, and ifosfamide before radical cystecomy.[33] In this setting, sequential ifosfamide, doxorubicin, and gemcitabine followed by reduced-dose cisplatin, gemcitabine, and ifosfamide resulted in pathologic downstaging to pT1 disease or lower in 50% of patients, similar to the results from the SWOG 8710 trial discussed previously.

Immune checkpoint inhibitor therapy may also be a promising alternative to cisplatin-based regimens. In a recent phase 2 trial, Balar and colleagues[34] demonstrated that for cisplatin-ineligible patients with locally advanced or metastatic urothelial carcinoma, treatment with atezolizumab, a monoclonal antibody targeting programmed dealth-ligand-1, resulted in a 23% objective response rate per Response Evaluation Criteria in Solid Tumors version 1.1, and a 9% complete response rate. However, the role of atezolizumab has yet to be tested in the neoadjuvant setting.

Recommendations for the Use of Neoadjuvant Chemotherapy

In March 2017, the American Urological Association, American Society of Clinical Oncology, American Society for Radiation Oncology, and the Society of Urologic Oncology released a joint clinical guideline for the treatment of nonmetastatic MIBC.[35] These guidelines highlight that before initiating neoadjuvant chemotherapy, patients should undergo complete evaluation including examination under anesthesia at the time of transurethral resection of bladder tumor (TURBT), imaging of the chest, and cross-sectional imaging of the abdomen and pelvis with intravenous contrast. A multidisciplinary approach should be adopted with standard four-cycle cisplatin-based neoadjuvant chemotherapy offered to eligible patients before radical cystectomy (**Fig. 1**). Importantly, repeat imaging studies are recommended after the third chemotherapy cycle to assess for response to therapy. If

it is determined at that time that the patient has had disease progression or no response, the fourth cycle may be held and the patient could proceed directly to cystectomy (or in certain cases, the regimen can be altered). Cystectomy should be performed within an appropriate time frame from the completion of neoadjuvant chemotherapy.

Patients who are ineligible for cisplatin-based combination neoadjuvant chemotherapy because of renal insufficiency should not be offered carboplatin-based neoadjuvant chemotherapy because no benefit has been demonstrated with this treatment.[35] Patients who are ineligible for cisplatin should proceed directly to cystectomy. Alternatively, enrollment into an immunotherapy clinical trial could be considered. Refer Min Yuen Teo and Jonathan E. Rosenberg's article, "Perioperative Immunotherapy in Muscle-Invasive Bladder Cancer and Upper Tract Urothelial Carcinoma," in this issue for further details.

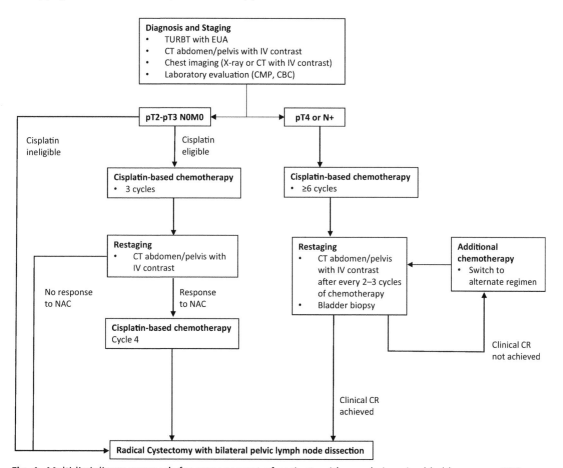

Fig. 1. Multidisciplinary approach for management of patients with muscle-invasive bladder cancer. CBC, complete blood count; CMP, comprehensive metabolic panel; CR, complete response; CT, computed tomography; EUA, exam under anesthesia; IV, intravenous; TURBT, transurethral resection of bladder tumor; NAC, neoadjuvant chemotherapy.

Upfront presurgical cisplatin-based chemotherapy should also be offered to patients with pT4 or N+ disease, because treatment with chemotherapy could result in clinical downstaging, which would allow the option for surgical intervention. In this scenario six cycles of cisplatin-based combination therapy, or more if necessary, are given with the intent to proceed to surgery once the patient demonstrates a radiographic response and repeat biopsy shows pathologic response. Patients are restaged with computed tomography scans after every two to three cycles of chemotherapy, and if no significant response is noted, an alternative chemotherapy regimen is initiated.[36] In support of this strategy, Zargar-Shoshtari and colleagues[37] demonstrated in a multi-institutional study assessing pathologic and survival outcomes in 304 patients with bladder cancer with cT1-4a N1-N3 disease treated with induction chemotherapy followed by radical cystectomy that a pN0 rate of 48% could be achieved. The combination of induction chemotherapy followed by consolidative surgery achieved a 14.5% complete pathologic response rate and a 27% partial pathologic response rate.

In addition, Ho and colleagues[38] reported a series of 55 patients with bladder cancer with concurrent node-positive disease who underwent preoperative chemotherapy followed by consolidative surgery. For the entire cohort, cancer-specific survival (CSS) was 26%, and 55% of patients achieved pathologic N0 disease at the time of surgical extirpation. For patients who achieved pathologic N0 disease, 5-year CSS rate was 66%; therefore, a multimodality treatment approach with upfront chemotherapy followed by consolidative surgery can result in a 66% 5-year CSS for patients rendered pN0 at the time of cystectomy despite initially presenting with node-positive disease. Similarly, in a larger study of 149 patients with node-positive bladder cancer who received induction chemotherapy followed by surgery, Meijer and colleagues[39] demonstrated that median CSS was 20 months and 5-year CSS was 29.2%. In this study, a complete pathologic response was achieved in 26.8% of patients, and for these patients a significant CSS benefit up to 127 months and 5-year CSS of 63.5% was observed.

Further evidence was provided by Galsky and colleagues[40] who performed a review of the National Cancer Database and identified 1104 patients with bladder cancer with lymph node involvement that had been treated with chemotherapy alone, cystectomy alone, or preoperative chemotherapy followed by cystectomy. For lymph node–positive patients, preoperative chemotherapy followed by cystectomy was associated with a significant improvement in 5-year overall survival compared with either chemotherapy or cystectomy alone (14% chemotherapy alone, 19% cystectomy alone, and 31% preoperative chemotherapy followed by cystectomy).

After completion of neoadjuvant chemotherapy, restaging studies may demonstrate that some patients have achieved clinical T0 responses; however, it is imperative that all patients proceed to radical cystectomy with bilateral pelvic lymphadenopathy in a timely fashion, even those who are cT0. In support of this recommendation, the SWOG S0219 phase II study reported that in 34 patients who achieved cT0 after neoadjuvant chemotherapy, 10 patients proceeded to immediate cystectomy.[41] In 6 of these 10 patients (60%) deemed cT0, final pathology of the cystectomy specimen demonstrated pT2-4 disease. Furthermore, Herr[42] reported on the outcome of 63 patients who refused cystectomy after achieving cT0 response after neoadjuvant chemotherapy. In this study, 23 patients (36%) who refused cystectomy died of bladder cancer and 19 (30%) relapsed with invasive cancer in the bladder. The risk of death was high (75%) in patients who experienced recurrent invasive disease. There are ongoing studies to potentially allow clinicians to identify which patients might be spared radical surgery after neoadjuvant chemotherapy but until such time as this is validated, these data demonstrate that even after cT0 response to chemotherapy, the risk of residual undetected muscle invasive disease and the high risk of death preclude further observation as a safe option in these cases and prompt cystectomy should be completed.

ADJUVANT CHEMOTHERAPY

In contrast to neoadjuvant chemotherapy, the major advantage of adjuvant chemotherapy is the avoidance of a delay to cystectomy.[2,5] This also avoids overtreatment of patients with tumor confined to the bladder with no micrometastases, and patients at highest risk of recurrence are identified for adjuvant chemotherapy based on the final pathologic evaluation of the cystectomy specimen. The major disadvantage of adjuvant chemotherapy is the delay in starting systemic therapy in patients who might harbor occult metastases. Furthermore, patients may no longer be eligible for chemotherapy following surgery because of postoperative complications or prolonged recovery. It is also well documented that many patients develop decreased renal function following radical cystectomy.[43,44] A recent study demonstrated that

25% of patients who were initially eligible for cisplatin-based neoadjuvant chemotherapy before radical cystectomy were no longer eligible for cisplatin-based adjuvant chemotherapy after radical cystectomy because of renal insufficiency.[45] Furthermore, a retrospective review of 1142 consecutive radical cystectomies at a high-volume tertiary cancer center demonstrated that 30% of patients undergoing radical cystectomy would not have been able to receive adjuvant chemotherapy because of postoperative complications.[46]

Adjuvant Chemotherapy Trials for Muscle-Invasive Bladder Cancer

The data supporting the use of adjuvant chemotherapy are not as strong as that for neoadjuvant chemotherapy. The role of adjuvant chemotherapy in MIBC has been evaluated in several small series that showed marginal to no benefit[47–51]; furthermore these studies were criticized for their considerable methodologic flaws including low accrual with insufficient sample sizes, inappropriate early stopping of patient entry, inappropriate statistical analyses, and overreaching conclusions that were poorly supported by data.[52] These trials were then included in a meta-analysis published in 2005 where the authors concluded that the included trials were small and underpowered and the meta-analysis was limited with insufficient evidence to guide treatment decisions, despite a reduction in the risk of death of 25% attributed to adjuvant chemotherapy after cystectomy compared with cystectomy alone.[53]

In a recent Italian multicenter phase III trial, patients with cT2G3, pT3-4, pN0-2 bladder cancer received cystectomy and were then randomized to receive either four courses of GC adjuvant chemotherapy or observation.[54] The study was designed to enroll 610 patients but closed early because of poor accrual after randomizing 194 patients over 83 months. In the adjuvant treatment arm, only 62% of patients completed four courses of chemotherapy, and at a median follow-up of 35 months there was no significant difference in overall survival between the two arms. The Spanish Oncology Group then presented preliminary results of a randomized phase III trial comparing adjuvant paclitaxel, gemcitabine, and cisplatin therapy to observation following cystectomy in patients with high-risk MIBC at the American Society of Clinical Oncology annual meeting in 2010.[55] This trial also closed early because of poor accrual; however, preliminary data were promising, showing a significant increase in overall survival because of adjuvant chemotherapy (5-year

survival 60% vs 30%; hazard ratio [HR], 0.44). Final data from this trial have yet to be published.

In 2009, an update to the 2005 adjuvant chemotherapy meta-analysis was published, including the previously mentioned trials.[56] The update included nine trials with a total of 945 patients and demonstrated that cisplatin-based combination adjuvant chemotherapy provided a 23% reduction in risk of death ($P = .049$) and 34% reduction in risk of progression ($P = .014$) compared with cystectomy alone, with the same caveats.

To date, the largest adjuvant chemotherapy trial for bladder cancer is the EORTC 30994 phase III trial of immediate versus deferred cisplatin-based combination chemotherapy following radical cystectomy and extended lymph node dissection in patients with pT3-pT4 or pN+ M0 bladder cancer.[57] Patients were randomized to receive either four cycles of cisplatin-based combination chemotherapy immediately after cystectomy or six cycles of cisplatin-based combination chemotherapy at the time of disease progression. Similar to prior adjuvant trials, the EORTC trial was stopped early because of slow accrual after randomization of 284 patients. No significant difference in overall survival was identified between groups; however, immediate adjuvant chemotherapy did show a statistically significant improvement in progression-free survival compared with delayed therapy (47.6% vs 31.8%; $P<.0001$).

There are currently no randomized trials comparing neoadjuvant chemotherapy with adjuvant chemotherapy. The closest study to evaluate this scenario was a phase 3 randomized trial from MD Anderson that compared patients who received two cycles of MVAC before cystectomy followed by three cycles of MVAC postoperatively versus patients who underwent initial cystectomy followed by five cycles of adjuvant MVAC.[12] There were no significant differences in overall survival observed between the two groups; however, this trial was not a direct comparison of neoadjuvant with adjuvant chemotherapy.

Recommendations for the Use of Adjuvant Chemotherapy

Because the evidence for the benefit of adjuvant chemotherapy is not as strong as that for neoadjuvant chemotherapy, adjuvant chemotherapy should not supplant neoadjuvant chemotherapy as the standard of care. Adjuvant chemotherapy does, however, provide some benefit, and in the case where a patient has had a radical cystectomy but did not receive cisplatin-based neoadjuvant chemotherapy, then adjuvant cisplatin-based chemotherapy should be offered if they are eligible.[35]

Immune checkpoint inhibitor therapy may also be a promising alternative; however, immune checkpoint inhibitors have yet to be tested in the adjuvant setting.

UPPER TRACT UROTHELIAL CARCINOMA

UTUC is a distinct disease entity from urothelial carcinoma of the bladder based on phenotypic and genotypic differences with greater than 60% of UTUC presenting with invasion at diagnosis compared with 15% to 25% for bladder cancer.[58] Invasive UTUC has a poor prognosis with 5-year survival rates of 73% for T2 disease and 40% for T3 disease, and a median 6-month survival for T4 disease.[59] Radical nephroureterectomy is the standard of care for high-grade UTUC; however, systemic recurrences are common suggesting a role for perioperative chemotherapy. Unfortunately, there are currently no level 1 data from prospective randomized trials regarding neoadjuvant or adjuvant chemotherapy for invasive UTUC and most of the following recommendations are made based on smaller single-center studies or retrospective larger cohort database type analyses.

Neoadjuvant Chemotherapy for Upper Urinary Tract Urothelial Carcinoma

Similar to bladder cancer, neoadjuvant treatment of invasive UTUC has the potential to downstage tumors and treat occult micrometastatic disease. Importantly, in the neoadjuvant setting, patients are more likely to tolerate chemotherapy with two functioning kidneys before radical nephroureterectomy. A particular challenge with UTUC is obtaining sufficient tissue during ureteroscopic biopsy for pathologic analysis and risk stratification. For most specimens, only tumor grade is accurately assessed because sufficient tissue to identify muscle invasion is not available due to the technical challenges of ureteroscopic biopsy. To address this issue, Brown and colleagues[60] investigated whether tumor grade at the time of biopsy could predict pathologic stage with a retrospective review of 184 patients undergoing nephroureterectomy for UTUC. The authors determined that patients with grade 3 UTUC on preoperative diagnostic biopsy had a 66% positive predictive value of having invasive UTUC on final pathology of the nephroureterectomy specimen. Conversely, patients with grade 1 or 2 UTUC on biopsy had a negative predictive value of 72% for invasive disease; therefore, tumor

grade at biopsy could serve as a surrogate for pathologic invasion and inform which patients would benefit the most from neoadjuvant therapy.

There is no level 1 data comparing neoadjuvant chemotherapy plus radical nephroureterectomy with nephroureterectomy alone. A phase 2 clinical trial at MD Anderson in patients with locally advanced urothelial cancer investigating sequential neoadjuvant chemotherapy with ifosfamide, doxorubicin, and gemcitabine followed by cisplatin, gemcitabine, and ifosfamide before surgery did include five patients with high-grade upper tract cancer of the ureter or renal pelvis.[33] After neoadjuvant therapy and radical nephroureterectomy three of five patients (60%) showed pathologic downstaging to less than or equal to pT1 disease, proving the efficacy of neoadjuvant chemotherapy for UTUC.

Three recent retrospective reviews have also demonstrated a benefit for neoadjuvant chemotherapy before radical nephroureterectomy. Igawa and colleagues[61] reported that in a series of 15 patients with locally advanced UTUC who were treated with either MVAC or MVEC before radical nephroureterectomy, 13% achieved a complete pathologic response and an associated survival advantage was observed for these patients. Porten and colleagues[62] performed a retrospective review on a series of 31 patients with high-risk UTUC who received neoadjuvant cisplatin-based combination chemotherapy followed by radical nephroureterectomy compared with a historical matched cohort control of 81 patients. Patients who received neoadjuvant chemotherapy had significantly improved 5-year overall and disease-specific survival at 80.2% and 90.1%, respectively, compared with 57.6% 5-year overall survival and 57.6% 5-year disease-specific survival for patients receiving upfront nephroureterectomy. Kobayashi and colleagues[63] reported that in a series of 55 patients, the 24 patients who received neoadjuvant chemotherapy before radical nephroureterectomy had significantly longer 5-year overall survival versus surgery alone (44% vs 29%; $P = .047$). Although the number of patients in these three studies is small, the data support the idea that neoadjuvant chemotherapy can downstage tumors and provide a survival advantage.

Adjuvant Chemotherapy for Upper Urinary Tract Urothelial Carcinoma

Similar to bladder cancer, adjuvant chemotherapy for UTUC has the benefit of possible avoidance of overtreatment; however, its major disadvantage is the inability to deliver cisplatin-based combination adjuvant chemotherapy because of surgically induced poor renal function.

There are no randomized trials investigating the role of adjuvant chemotherapy for UTUC. A recent systematic review and meta-analysis combined one prospective study and nine retrospective studies for analysis.[64] The prospective study included 36 patients receiving adjuvant carboplatin-paclitaxel and the nine retrospective studies included 482 patients who received cisplatin-based or noncisplatin-based adjuvant chemotherapy after nephroureterectomy and 1300 patients who received nephroureterectomy alone. The analysis demonstrated that for the cisplatin-based regimens adjuvant chemotherapy conferred an overall survival benefit with a pooled HR of 0.43 (95% confidence interval, 0.21–0.89; $P = .023$) and a disease-free survival benefit with a pooled HR of 0.49 (95% confidence interval, 0.24–0.99; $P = .048$). No benefit was seen for noncisplatin-based regimens.

FUTURE DIRECTIONS

Neoadjuvant and adjuvant chemotherapy benefit patients with MIBC; however, there is a significant portion of patients who do not respond to these treatments and are subject to unnecessary toxicity and delay to surgery. Future research is needed to further refine the selection process to identify those patients with high-risk disease who would benefit the most from neoadjuvant chemotherapy. To that end, at MD Anderson we have adopted a risk-adapted algorithm to select individuals with high-risk features to receive neoadjuvant chemotherapy, sparing those patients without high-risk features from treatment toxicity and delay. High-risk features in our algorithm (**Fig. 2**) include hydroureteronephrosis, cT3b-T4a disease, lymphovascular

invasion, and neuroendocrine or micropapillary variant histologies, and patients with high-risk features exhibit decreased 5-year overall survival (47.0% vs 64.8%), disease-specific survival (64.3% vs 83.5%), and progression-free survival (62.0% vs 84.1%) compared with patients without high-risk features (P<.001).[65] Importantly, patients without high-risk features who do not receive neoadjuvant chemotherapy according to our algorithm achieve a 5-year disease-specific survival of 80% after cystectomy, comparable with patients with organ-confined pT2 disease.[65]

Recent advances in genomic sequencing technology may allow us to tailor our neoadjuvant chemotherapy regimens to the genetic code of a patient's tumor. The recently developed CO eXpression ExtrapolatioN (COXEN) computer algorithm is a novel tool for drug discovery that combines genetic profiling of a patient's tumor and compares it with the genetic profile of known cancer cell lines with well-defined chemosensitivities. The COXEN algorithm shows promise in being able to predict what chemotherapy agent is most efficacious for a patient's tumor. A SWOG-sponsored neoadjuvant clinical trial evaluating the role of this assay in the setting of GC and MVAC is currently underway.[66] Results of this trial are eagerly anticipated especially because it will provide well annotated tissue to analyze for genomic profiling. As outlined in Matthew Mossanen and colleagues' article, "Current Staging Strategies for Muscle Invasive Bladder Cancer and Upper Tract Urothelial Cell Carcinoma," in this issue, genomic sequencing has demonstrated that patients with the basal molecular subtype of MIBC may receive the most survival benefit with cisplatin-based neoadjuvant chemotherapy.[25,67] These findings warrant validation in larger prospective studies.

Immune checkpoint inhibitor therapy has also shown great promise as second-line treatment of

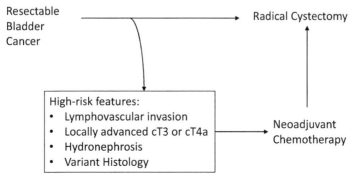

Fig. 2. MD Anderson risk-adapted algorithm to select individuals with high-risk features to receive neoadjuvant chemotherapy. (*Adapted from* Karam JA, Kamat AM. Optimal timing of chemotherapy and cystectomy. F1000 Med Rep 2010;2:[pii:48], under a Creative Commons Attribution 4.0 License.)

Box 1
Summary points

- Survival after radical cystectomy is closely associated with final pathologic staging, with survival decreasing with increasing pT stage.
- Stage-dependent reduction in survival is caused by the presence of occult micrometastases indicating the need for systemic chemotherapy.
- In a meta-analysis, neoadjuvant cisplatin-based chemotherapy regimens provide a 5% absolute improvement in survival at 5 years.
- Neoadjuvant MVAC significantly improves the number of patients who achieve pT0 status at the time of cystectomy.
- MVAC and GC are the standard neoadjuvant chemotherapy regimens.
- Carboplatin-based regimens are inferior to cisplatin and are not recommended for neoadjuvant therapy.
- A multidisciplinary approach should be offered to patients with pT2-pT3 N0M0 disease including cisplatin-based neoadjuvant chemotherapy followed by radical cystectomy with pelvic lymph node dissection.
- Patients who are ineligible for cisplatin should proceed directly to radical cystectomy
- Patients with pT4 or N$^+$ disease should be offered presurgical cisplatin-based chemotherapy with the intent of consolidation surgery should the patient respond to chemotherapy.
- The evidence for adjuvant chemotherapy is weaker than that for neoadjuvant chemotherapy; therefore adjuvant chemotherapy should not supplant neoadjuvant chemotherapy as the standard of care.
- In the circumstance that a patient has had a radical cystectomy without neoadjuvant chemotherapy, then adjuvant chemotherapy should be offered if they are cisplatin-eligible.
- For UTUC, cisplatin-based neoadjuvant chemotherapy can downstage tumors and provide a survival advantage.
- For UTUC, the evidence for adjuvant chemotherapy is weaker; however, a meta-analysis of pooled data showed that adjuvant cisplatin-based chemotherapy may confer an overall survival benefit, whereas noncisplatin regimens do not.
- Continued research is needed to refine selection criteria for patients who would benefit the most from neoadjuvant chemotherapy to prevent overtreatment and delays to radical cystectomy for nonresponders.

---

patients with metastatic bladder cancer and first-line treatment of patients ineligible for cisplatin-containing chemotherapy regimen. At the time of writing, there are five approved immune-oncologic agents for bladder cancer, which is the most of any tumor type. Although immune checkpoint inhibitors do not have a solidly defined role in the neoadjuvant or adjuvant setting, clinical trials using immune checkpoint inhibitors in the neoadjuvant and adjuvant space are forthcoming (**Box 1**).

REFERENCES

1. Siegel RL, Miller KD, Jemal A. Cancer statistics, 2017. CA Cancer J Clin 2017;67(1):7–30.
2. Calabro F, Sternberg CN. Neoadjuvant and adjuvant chemotherapy in muscle-invasive bladder cancer. Eur Urol 2009;55(2):348–58.
3. Stein JP, Lieskovsky G, Cote R, et al. Radical cystectomy in the treatment of invasive bladder cancer: long-term results in 1,054 patients. J Clin Oncol 2001;19(3):666–75.
4. Hautmann RE, Gschwend JE, de Petriconi RC, et al. Cystectomy for transitional cell carcinoma of the bladder: results of a surgery only series in the neobladder era. J Urol 2006;176(2):486–92 [discussion: 491–2].
5. Trenta P, Calabro F, Cerbone L, et al. Chemotherapy for muscle-invasive bladder cancer. Curr Treat Options Oncol 2016;17(1):6.
6. Apolo AB, Grossman HB, Bajorin D, et al. Practical use of perioperative chemotherapy for muscle-invasive bladder cancer: summary of session at the Society of Urologic Oncology annual meeting. Urol Oncol 2012;30(6):772–80.
7. David KA, Milowsky MI, Ritchey J, et al. Low incidence of perioperative chemotherapy for stage III bladder cancer 1998 to 2003: a report from the National Cancer Data Base. J Urol 2007;178(2):451–4.
8. Zaid HB, Patel SG, Stimson CJ, et al. Trends in the utilization of neoadjuvant chemotherapy in muscle-

invasive bladder cancer: results from the National Cancer Database. Urology 2014;83(1):75–80.

9. Sanchez-Ortiz RF, Huang WC, Mick R, et al. An interval longer than 12 weeks between the diagnosis of muscle invasion and cystectomy is associated with worse outcome in bladder carcinoma. J Urol 2003; 169(1):110–5 [discussion: 115].

10. Chang SS, Hassan JM, Cookson MS, et al. Delaying radical cystectomy for muscle invasive bladder cancer results in worse pathological stage. J Urol 2003; 170(4 Pt 1):1085–7.

11. Willis D, Kamat AM. Nonurothelial bladder cancer and rare variant histologies. Hematol Oncol Clin North Am 2015;29(2):237–52, viii.

12. Millikan R, Dinney C, Swanson D, et al. Integrated therapy for locally advanced bladder cancer: final report of a randomized trial of cystectomy plus adjuvant M-VAC versus cystectomy with both preoperative and postoperative M-VAC. J Clin Oncol 2001; 19(20):4005–13.

13. Wallace DM, Raghavan D, Kelly KA, et al. Neoadjuvant (pre-emptive) cisplatin therapy in invasive transitional cell carcinoma of the bladder. Br J Urol 1991;67(6):608–15.

14. Martinez-Pineiro JA, Gonzalez Martin M, Arocena F, et al. Neoadjuvant cisplatin chemotherapy before radical cystectomy in invasive transitional cell carcinoma of the bladder: a prospective randomized phase III study. J Urol 1995;153(3 Pt 2):964–73.

15. Malmstrom PU, Rintala E, Wahlqvist R, et al. Five-year followup of a prospective trial of radical cystectomy and neoadjuvant chemotherapy: Nordic Cystectomy Trial I. The Nordic Cooperative Bladder Cancer Study Group. J Urol 1996;155(6):1903–6.

16. Sherif A, Holmberg L, Rintala E, et al. Neoadjuvant cisplatinum based combination chemotherapy in patients with invasive bladder cancer: a combined analysis of two Nordic studies. Eur Urol 2004; 45(3):297–303.

17. Sherif A, Rintala E, Mestad O, et al. Neoadjuvant cisplatin-methotrexate chemotherapy for invasive bladder cancer: Nordic Cystectomy Trial 2. Scand J Urol Nephrol 2002;36(6):419–25.

18. Advanced Bladder Cancer (ABC) Meta-analysis Collaboration. Neoadjuvant chemotherapy in invasive bladder cancer: update of a systematic review and meta-analysis of individual patient data advanced bladder cancer (ABC) meta-analysis collaboration. Eur Urol 2005;48(2):202–5 [discussion: 205–6].

19. Neoadjuvant cisplatin, methotrexate, and vinblastine chemotherapy for muscle-invasive bladder cancer: a randomised controlled trial. International collaboration of trialists. Lancet 1999;354(9178): 533–40.

20. International Collaboration of Trialists, Medical Research Council Advanced Bladder Cancer Working Party (now the National Cancer Research Institute Bladder Cancer Clinical Studies Group), European Organisation for Research and Treatment of Cancer Genito-Urinary Tract Cancer Group, Australian Bladder Cancer Study Group, National Cancer Institute of Canada Clinical Trials Group, Finnbladder, Norwegian Bladder Cancer Study Group, Club Urologico Espanol de Tratamiento Oncologico Group, Griffiths G, Hall R, Sylvester R, et al. International phase III trial assessing neoadjuvant cisplatin, methotrexate, and vinblastine chemotherapy for muscle-invasive bladder cancer: long-term results of the BA06 30894 trial. J Clin Oncol 2011;29(16):2171–7.

21. Grossman HB, Natale RB, Tangen CM, et al. Neoadjuvant chemotherapy plus cystectomy compared with cystectomy alone for locally advanced bladder cancer. N Engl J Med 2003;349(9):859–66.

22. Loehrer PJ Sr, Einhorn LH, Elson PJ, et al. A randomized comparison of cisplatin alone or in combination with methotrexate, vinblastine, and doxorubicin in patients with metastatic urothelial carcinoma: a cooperative group study. J Clin Oncol 1992;10(7):1066–73.

23. Plimack ER, Hoffman-Censits JH, Viterbo R, et al. Accelerated methotrexate, vinblastine, doxorubicin, and cisplatin is safe, effective, and efficient neoadjuvant treatment for muscle-invasive bladder cancer: results of a multicenter phase II study with molecular correlates of response and toxicity. J Clin Oncol 2014;32(18):1895–901.

24. Choueiri TK, Jacobus S, Bellmunt J, et al. Neoadjuvant dose-dense methotrexate, vinblastine, doxorubicin, and cisplatin with pegfilgrastim support in muscle-invasive urothelial cancer: pathologic, radiologic, and biomarker correlates. J Clin Oncol 2014; 32(18):1889–94.

25. McConkey DJ, Choi W, Shen Y, et al. A prognostic gene expression signature in the molecular classification of chemotherapy-naive urothelial cancer is predictive of clinical outcomes from neoadjuvant chemotherapy: a phase 2 trial of dose-dense methotrexate, vinblastine, doxorubicin, and cisplatin with bevacizumab in urothelial cancer. Eur Urol 2016; 69(5):855–62.

26. von der Maase H, Hansen SW, Roberts JT, et al. Gemcitabine and cisplatin versus methotrexate, vinblastine, doxorubicin, and cisplatin in advanced or metastatic bladder cancer: results of a large, randomized, multinational, multicenter, phase III study. J Clin Oncol 2000;18(17):3068–77.

27. Yeshchina O, Badalato GM, Wosnitzer MS, et al. Relative efficacy of perioperative gemcitabine and cisplatin versus methotrexate, vinblastine, adriamycin, and cisplatin in the management of locally advanced urothelial carcinoma of the bladder. Urology 2012;79(2):384–90.

28. Galsky MD, Pal SK, Chowdhury S, et al. Comparative effectiveness of gemcitabine plus cisplatin versus methotrexate, vinblastine, doxorubicin, plus cisplatin as neoadjuvant therapy for muscle-invasive bladder cancer. Cancer 2015;121(15):2586–93.

29. Galsky MD, Hahn NM, Rosenberg J, et al. A consensus definition of patients with metastatic urothelial carcinoma who are unfit for cisplatin-based chemotherapy. Lancet Oncol 2011;12(3):211–4.

30. Bellmunt J, Ribas A, Eres N, et al. Carboplatin-based versus cisplatin-based chemotherapy in the treatment of surgically incurable advanced bladder carcinoma. Cancer 1997;80(10):1966–72.

31. Petrioli R, Frediani B, Manganelli A, et al. Comparison between a cisplatin-containing regimen and a carboplatin-containing regimen for recurrent or metastatic bladder cancer patients. A randomized phase II study. Cancer 1996;77(2):344–51.

32. Dogliotti L, Carteni G, Siena S, et al. Gemcitabine plus cisplatin versus gemcitabine plus carboplatin as first-line chemotherapy in advanced transitional cell carcinoma of the urothelium: results of a randomized phase 2 trial. Eur Urol 2007;52(1):134–41.

33. Siefker-Radtke AO, Dinney CP, Shen Y, et al. A phase 2 clinical trial of sequential neoadjuvant chemotherapy with ifosfamide, doxorubicin, and gemcitabine followed by cisplatin, gemcitabine, and ifosfamide in locally advanced urothelial cancer: final results. Cancer 2013;119(3):540–7.

34. Balar AV, Galsky MD, Rosenberg JE, et al. Atezolizumab as first-line treatment in cisplatin-ineligible patients with locally advanced and metastatic urothelial carcinoma: a single-arm, multicentre, phase 2 trial. Lancet 2017;389(10064):67–76.

35. Chang SS, Bochner BH, Chou R, et al. Treatment of non-metastatic muscle-invasive bladder cancer: AUA/ASCO/ASTRO/SUO guideline. J Urol 2017;198(3):552–9.

36. Siefker-Radtke AO. Surgical consolidation of initially unresectable urothelial carcinoma: an incremental opportunity to cure. Expert Rev Anticancer Ther 2009;9(12):1701–3.

37. Zargar-Shoshtari K, Zargar H, Lotan Y, et al. A multi-institutional analysis of outcomes of patients with clinically node positive urothelial bladder cancer treated with induction chemotherapy and radical cystectomy. J Urol 2016;195(1):53–9.

38. Ho PL, Willis DL, Patil J, et al. Outcome of patients with clinically node-positive bladder cancer undergoing consolidative surgery after preoperative chemotherapy: the M.D. Anderson cancer center experience. Urol Oncol 2016;34(2):59.e1-8.

39. Meijer RP, Mertens LS, van Rhijn BW, et al. Induction chemotherapy followed by surgery in node positive bladder cancer. Urology 2014;83(1):134–9.

40. Galsky MD, Stensland K, Sfakianos JP, et al. Comparative effectiveness of treatment strategies for bladder cancer with clinical evidence of regional lymph node involvement. J Clin Oncol 2016;34(22):2627–35.

41. White RWD, Lara PN, Goldman B, et al. A sequential treatment approach to myoinvasive urothelial cancer: a phase II southwest oncology group trial (S0219). J Urol 2009;181(6):2476–80.

42. Herr HW. Outcome of patients who refuse cystectomy after receiving neoadjuvant chemotherapy for muscle-invasive bladder cancer. Eur Urol 2008;54(1):126–32.

43. Eisenberg MS, Thompson RH, Frank I, et al. Long-term renal function outcomes after radical cystectomy. J Urol 2014;191(3):619–25.

44. Dash A, Galsky MD, Vickers AJ, et al. Impact of renal impairment on eligibility for adjuvant cisplatin-based chemotherapy in patients with urothelial carcinoma of the bladder. Cancer 2006;107(3):506–13.

45. Thompson RH, Boorjian SA, Kim SP, et al. Eligibility for neoadjuvant/adjuvant cisplatin-based chemotherapy among radical cystectomy patients. BJU Int 2014;113(5b):E17–21.

46. Donat SM, Shabsigh A, Savage C, et al. Potential impact of postoperative early complications on the timing of adjuvant chemotherapy in patients undergoing radical cystectomy: a high-volume tertiary cancer center experience. Eur Urol 2009;55(1):177–85.

47. Skinner DG, Daniels JR, Russell CA, et al. The role of adjuvant chemotherapy following cystectomy for invasive bladder cancer: a prospective comparative trial. J Urol 1991;145(3):459–64 [discussion: 464–7].

48. Stockle M, Meyenburg W, Wellek S, et al. Advanced bladder cancer (stages pT3b, pT4a, pN1 and pN2): improved survival after radical cystectomy and 3 adjuvant cycles of chemotherapy. Results of a controlled prospective study. J Urol 1992;148(2 Pt 1):302–6 [discussion: 306–7].

49. Stockle M, Meyenburg W, Wellek S, et al. Adjuvant polychemotherapy of nonorgan-confined bladder cancer after radical cystectomy revisited: long-term results of a controlled prospective study and further clinical experience. J Urol 1995;153(1):47–52.

50. Studer UE, Bacchi M, Biedermann C, et al. Adjuvant cisplatin chemotherapy following cystectomy for bladder cancer: results of a prospective randomized trial. J Urol 1994;152(1):81–4.

51. Freiha F, Reese J, Torti FM. A randomized trial of radical cystectomy versus radical cystectomy plus cisplatin, vinblastine and methotrexate chemotherapy for muscle invasive bladder cancer. J Urol 1996;155(2):495–9 [discussion: 499–500].

52. Sylvester R, Sternberg C. The role of adjuvant combination chemotherapy after cystectomy in locally

advanced bladder cancer: what we do not know and why. Ann Oncol 2000;11(7):851–6.

53. Advanced Bladder Cancer (ABC) Meta-analysis Collaboration. Adjuvant chemotherapy in invasive bladder cancer: a systematic review and meta-analysis of individual patient data Advanced Bladder Cancer (ABC) Meta-analysis Collaboration. Eur Urol 2005;48(2):189–99 [discussion: 199–201].

54. Cognetti F, Ruggeri EM, Felici A, et al. Adjuvant chemotherapy with cisplatin and gemcitabine versus chemotherapy at relapse in patients with muscle-invasive bladder cancer submitted to radical cystectomy: an Italian, multicenter, randomized phase III trial. Ann Oncol 2012;23(3):695–700.

55. Paz-Ares LG, Solsona E, Eseban E, et al. Randomized phase III trial comparing adjuvant paclitaxel/gemcitabine/cisplatin (PGC) to observation in patients with resected invasive bladder cancer: results of the Spanish Oncology Genitourinary Group (SOGUG) 99/01 study. J Clin Oncol 2010;28:18s.

56. Leow JJ, Martin-Doyle W, Rajagopal PS, et al. Adjuvant chemotherapy for invasive bladder cancer: a 2013 updated systematic review and meta-analysis of randomized trials. Eur Urol 2014;66(1):42–54.

57. Sternberg CN, Skoneczna I, Kerst JM, et al. Immediate versus deferred chemotherapy after radical cystectomy in patients with pT3-pT4 or N+ M0 urothelial carcinoma of the bladder (EORTC 30994): an intergroup, open-label, randomised phase 3 trial. Lancet Oncol 2015;16(1):76–86.

58. Leow JJ, Chong KT, Chang SL, et al. Upper tract urothelial carcinoma: a different disease entity in terms of management. ESMO Open 2016;1(6):e000126.

59. Audenet F, Yates DR, Cussenot O, et al. The role of chemotherapy in the treatment of urothelial cell carcinoma of the upper urinary tract (UUT-UCC). Urol Oncol 2013;31(4):407–13.

60. Brown GA, Matin SF, Busby JE, et al. Ability of clinical grade to predict final pathologic stage in upper urinary tract transitional cell carcinoma: implications for therapy. Urology 2007;70(2):252–6.

61. Igawa M, Urakami S, Shiina H, et al. Neoadjuvant chemotherapy for locally advanced urothelial cancer of the upper urinary tract. Urol Int 1995;55(2):74–7.

62. Porten S, Siefker-Radtke AO, Xiao L, et al. Neoadjuvant chemotherapy improves survival of patients with upper tract urothelial carcinoma. Cancer 2014;120(12):1794–9.

63. Kobayashi K, Saito T, Kitamura Y, et al. Effect of preoperative chemotherapy on survival of patients with upper urinary tract urothelial carcinoma clinically involving regional lymph nodes. Int J Urol 2016;23(2):153–8.

64. Leow JJ, Martin-Doyle W, Fay AP, et al. A systematic review and meta-analysis of adjuvant and neoadjuvant chemotherapy for upper tract urothelial carcinoma. Eur Urol 2014;66(3):529–41.

65. Culp SH, Dickstein RJ, Grossman HB, et al. Refining patient selection for neoadjuvant chemotherapy before radical cystectomy. J Urol 2014;191(1):40–7.

66. Dinney CP, Hansel D, McConkey D, et al. Novel neoadjuvant therapy paradigms for bladder cancer: results from the National Cancer Center Institute Forum. Urol Oncol 2014;32(8):1108–15.

67. Seiler R, Ashab HAD, Erho N, et al. Impact of molecular subtypes in muscle-invasive bladder cancer on predicting response and survival after neoadjuvant chemotherapy. Eur Urol 2017;72(4):544–54.

Contemporary Preoperative and Intraoperative Management of the Radical Cystectomy Patient

Jack Griffin Campbell, MD, Woodson Wade Smelser, MD, Eugene K. Lee, MD*

KEYWORDS

- Bladder cancer • Radical cystectomy • Preoperative optimization • Intraoperative optimization
- Outcomes

KEY POINTS

- Smoking remains a key risk factor for muscle-invasive bladder cancer and despite often long smoking history, preoperative smoking cessation is necessary because it can contribute to better outcomes.
- Patient education remains crucial for this intensive surgery.
- Immunonutrition is an emerging area in surgery showing promise to reduce both early and late complications.
- Peripherally acting μ-opioid antagonists and avoidance of opioid-based analgesia promotes earlier return of bowel function.
- Restrictive intraoperative fluid administration significantly reduces transfusion requirements.

INTRODUCTION

Bladder cancer continues to be a prevalent, morbid, and lethal disease accounting for approximately 80,00 new cases per year and 16,000 deaths per year in the United states.[1] Of this number, approximately 15% to 20% of patients with bladder present with muscle-invasive bladder cancer,[2] which has significantly lower 5-year survival rates (47%) compared with non–muscle invasive disease (81%).[3] Radical cystectomy (RC) after neoadjuvant chemotherapy remains the standard of care in nonmetastatic muscle-invasive bladder cancer based on "Category I" evidence from randomized, controlled trials, where improved overall and disease-specific survival was observed.[4,5] This finding is true despite the increasing popularity of bladder-preserving regimens in which acceptable oncologic outcomes have been observed.[6]

RC is a morbid procedure often performed on a high-risk population. In 1 large cohort, 75% of patients who underwent RC were classified as high risk, as defined by Association of Anesthesiologist score of 3 or 4.[7] Furthermore, RC has been shown to have 90-day complication rates of 64%[8] and

Disclosure: E.K. Lee is a consultant for Pacira Pharmaceuticals. W.W. Smelser and J.G. Campbell have nothing to disclose.
Department of Urology, University of Kansas Medical Center, 3901 Rainbow Boulevard, Kansas City, KS 66160, USA
* Corresponding author.
E-mail address: elee@kumc.edu

Urol Clin N Am 45 (2018) 169–181
https://doi.org/10.1016/j.ucl.2017.12.003
0094-0143/18/© 2017 Elsevier Inc. All rights reserved.

urologic.theclinics.com

90-day mortality rates between 6% and 9%.[9,10] Furthermore, association has been observed between hospital-acquired adverse events and odds of in-hospital death, duration of stay, and total cost.[11] Given the significant morbidity associated with RC, in addition to the emerging reality of transitioning from a traditional fee-for-service payment model to novel reimbursement structures, there has been an ever-growing focus on optimization of the RC patient. This trend is apparent in the development of numerous enhanced recovery pathways,[12–19] and also has been thoroughly highlighted in the context of perioperative care redesign by Matulewicz and colleagues.[20]

The purpose of this article is to discuss preoperative and intraoperative optimization of the RC patient to delineate features associated with high-quality care delivery as evidenced in the literature.

PREOPERATIVE MANAGEMENT
Patient Education

Patient optimization begins in the clinic setting with patient education, which has been known to improve outcomes across multiple surgical specialties, from reducing falls after total knee arthroplasty,[21] to increasing adherence to lifestyle modifications in bariatric surgery.[22] Not only should patient education expand beyond the traditional components of informed consent, but the patient should be an active participant in their care both for improvement of overall health, but also regarding specific components of RC and associated procedures.

Tobacco

Smoking represents the most important modifiable risk factor for bladder cancer. Rink and colleagues[23] observed that not only do past or current smokers account for approximately 80% of RC patients, but cumulative smoking exposure was associated with advanced tumor stages, lymph node metastasis, disease recurrence, and cancer-specific and overall mortality after RC. Although some evidence exists for nicotine as a mediator of chemoresistance,[24] a small retrospective cohort did not observe an association between smoking characteristics and response to neoadjuvant cisplatin-based chemotherapy, recurrence, or cancer-specific survival.[25] Although some evidence suggests that current smoking status affects competing mortality rather than cancer-specific mortality,[26,27] there remains significant value in smoking cessation for numerous aspects of health. In a Cochrane review of 13 randomized, controlled trials evaluating a smoking cessation

intervention and surgical outcomes (including urologic surgery), brief interventions were neither associated with long-term smoking outcomes nor reduced postoperative complications. However, intensive interventions were observed to reduce postoperative complications (relative risk, 0.42; 95% confidence interval, 0.27–0.65).[25] Notably, this review included 1 trial where preoperative varenicline before elective noncardiac surgery was observed to increase abstinence from smoking at 3, 6, and 12 months postoperatively.[28]

Alcohol

Although hazardous drinking is not known to be a specific risk factor for bladder cancer, preoperative alcohol use has been associated with increased complications after surgery, including postoperative infections, cardiopulmonary complications, and bleeding episodes.[29] A 2012 Cochrane Review included 2 randomized, controlled trials where the authors used intensive alcohol cessation programs, one with disulfiram 800 mg twice weekly for 4 weeks preoperatively, and the other with disulfiram 400 mg twice weekly, plus a weekly motivational interview and a 24/7 support line. The review observed a significant reduction in overall complication rates (odds ratio, 0.22; 95% confidence interval, 0.08–0.61), although there was no reduction of in-hospital or 30-day mortality, nor a difference in duration of stay or postoperative alcohol use.[30] Notably, the STOP smoking and alcohol drinking before operation for bladder cancer trial (STOP-OP study; ClinicalTrials.gov, ID: NCT02188446) is a multiinstitutional, randomized clinical trial to investigate changes in smoking and alcohol-related postoperative complications after intervention programs. Interventions will be biochemically validated by blood, urine, and breath tests.[31] Results from this and other trials will further quantify the benefit of lifestyle modification before RC.

Urinary diversion

Clearly, urinary diversion education is a cornerstone of preoperative planning for either incontinent or continent urinary diversion. Decisions should be based on multiple patient-centered factors and with shared decision making with the clinical team. Once a decision is reached, self-care education is paramount to set realistic expectations and maximize postoperative quality of life, both short term and long term. In patients opting for conduit diversion, the Urostomy Education Scale is a validated educational and an assessment tool for developing a patient's skill level regarding changing a urostomy appliance.[32] Furthermore, it may not require specialized personnel to lead this education; it has been found to be reliable regardless of nursing experience using the Urostomy Education Scale.[33] Additionally, these authors recently reported a significant difference in Urostomy Education Scale scores between patients who completed a standardized preoperative stoma education program and those who did not at 1 year postoperatively.[34]

Although there are no randomized, prospective trials investigating preoperative urostomy site marking and outcomes in the RC population, improved quality of life metrics have been observed with preoperative education and site marking.[35] A questionnaire-based study found increased quality-of-life metrics in patients who had received a colostomy, ileostomy, or urostomy and had been marked by a surgeon or wound care nurse preoperatively with patient input.[36] The Wound, Ostomy, and Continence Nurses Society, American Urological Association, and American Society of Colon and Rectal Surgeons official position statement is that "ostomy education and stoma site selection should be performed preoperatively for all patients when an ostomy is a possibility."[37] If possible, it is valuable to offer separate wound/ostomy clinic appointments before surgery for stoma education, site marking, bag teaching, and time for questions and practice.

For patients undergoing orthotopic neobladder, urinary incontinence and/or urinary obstruction can sometimes further challenge an already morbid operation. Currently, there are no studies to support a claim that preoperative or postoperative pelvic floor strengthening exercises improve continence in patients undergoing orthotopic neobladder creation; however, there is little downside to such exercises given their minimal or no cost nature. Clean intermittent catheterization becomes necessary in patients who do not empty their neobladders to completion and without it can lead to infections, increased mucus retention, and stone formation, among other complications. Although clean intermittent catheterization is necessary in a only minority of patients after neobladder creation, it does add bother to the patient.[38] Although the rates of requiring clean intermittent catheterization are minimal, 4.3% to 9.5%, it is critical that patients understand this outcome to be a possibility and preoperative teaching of catheterization techniques and a patient's willingness to perform clean intermittent catheterization is mandatory.[39,40]

Risk Stratification

Risk stratification in radical cystectomy
Although educating patients regarding the risks, benefits, and alternatives during the informed consent process should include quantitative data on certain risks of the procedure, a more individualized risk stratification process can be used to inform them on their risk, in particular, and their possible disposition after surgery. Recently, Atallah and colleagues[34] collected and graded preoperative morbidities for 49 patients 75 years of age and older according to the American Society of Anesthesiologists score system, the Adult Comorbidity Evaluation scale, and the Charlson Comorbidity Index. They found that neither morbidity nor mortality were associated with these scoring indices, but that preoperative malnutrition, renal insufficiency, a greater need of perioperative blood transfusions, and prolonged ileus were risk factors for early and late complications, including surgical site infection, abscess formation, wound dehiscence, pulmonary embolism, and readmission, and that low weight may be an additional association. Another study found that older age and poor preoperative exercise tolerance predicted discharge to a facility, and that those who were discharged to a facility were more likely to die within 90 days.[41]

Frailty
Frailty is defined as a biologic syndrome of decreased reserve and resistance to stressors, resulting from cumulative declines across multiple physiologic systems and causing vulnerability to adverse outcomes.[42] Patients undergoing RC are often of advanced age and have multiple underlying comorbidities; therefore, assessment of frailty is increasingly valued in preoperative risk assessment. The National Surgical Quality Improvement Program database has been analyzed using an 11-point modified Frailty Index (mFI) by multiple studies. Pearl and colleagues[43] analyzed this database for patients undergoing RC between 2011 and 2014, and observed that, among 4330 patients treated with RC, frail patients (mFI ≥ 0.27) were more likely to be discharged to a facility versus robust patients (mFI = 0; odds ratio, 2.33; 95% confidence interval, 1.34–4.03) independent of experiencing a major complication before discharge. Further, Chappidi and colleagues[44] evaluated this database for patients undergoing RC and counted mFI risk factors (0, 1, 2, and ≥ 3). The authors observed that in 2679 patients, those with an mFI of 2 or greater had significantly higher Clavien grade 4 or 5 complications (14.6% vs 8.3%) and overall mortality rate (3.5% vs 1.8%) out to 30 days postoperatively. As part of the preoperative RC evaluation process, it is not only critical to identify patients with frailty, but further effort to modify risk factors should be the focus of further research.

Prehabilitation

One area of significant interest in surgeons who perform RC is the concept of prehabilitation. This is the idea that preoperative optimization of nutrition and exercise tolerance can improve intraoperative and postoperative outcomes. Jensen and colleagues[45] performed a prospective randomized controlled trial whereby RC patients were randomized to either a regular fast tract design, or an intervention group that included preoperative and postoperative strength and endurance exercises with focused postoperative mobilization, starting 2 weeks before RC. In the 50 patients in the intervention arm, adherence to the program was 59% and there was a significant improvement in both walking distance and ability to perform activities of daily living (a 1-day difference), although duration of stay and complications were no different between groups (control arm, n = 57). Further studies in preoperative exercise are necessary but can be limited by the urgency between diagnosis and RC in these patients. Perhaps further studies of increasing exercise during chemotherapy may be a window of opportunity for future studies.

Nutrition

General

It is well-known that preoperative nutritional deficiency contributes to complications and mortality after RC. Gregg and colleagues[7] analyzed a cohort of 538 patients undergoing RC and found that 19% were malnourished, as defined by a preoperative albumin of less than 3.5 g/dL, a body mass index of less than 18.5 kg/m^2, or preoperative weight loss of more than 5% of body weight. In this cohort, there was a 7.3% overall 90-day mortality, but 16.5% in the malnourished population compared with 5.1% otherwise. Additionally, 3-year survival was found to be 44.5% and 67.6% for malnourished and nutritionally adequate patients, respectively. In the American College of Surgeons National Surgical Quality Improvement Program RC cohort, Johnson and colleagues[46] found that only preoperative albumin of less than 3.5 g/dL was predictive of postoperative complications, among body mass index and greater than 10% body weight loss in the last 6 months, similar to a prior study.[47] Another analysis of the National Surgical Quality Improvement Program database focused on preoperative albumin level and duration of stay.[48] Specifically, the authors found that in patients with preoperative albumin below a threshold of 4 g/dL, increase above this threshold was associated with decreased length of stay (hazard ratio, 1.05; 95% confidence interval, 1.01–1.09; P<.004).

Carbohydrate loading

Carbohydrate loading is a component of newer RC pathways that directly contradicts long-standing tradition of overnight fasting, which theoretically reduces the volume of stomach contents, reducing the risk of regurgitation and aspiration. A Cochrane review found no difference in volume or pH of gastric contents between an abbreviated fast (clear liquids up to 2 hours preoperatively) and a standard fast. Counterintuitively, patients given a drink of water preoperatively were found to have a lower volume of gastric contents.[49] Furthermore, this review observed improved patient anxiety, hunger, and thirst in patients permitted an abbreviated fast. Carbohydrate loading programs show mixed results regarding the impact on duration of stay and complication rates; however, they have been shown to reduce postoperative insulin resistance, which theoretically enhances insulin uptake into muscle, reducing infectious and cardiovascular complications.[50,51] Carbohydrate loading is now a part of numerous RC pathways for these reasons.[52]

Immunonutrition

Another component of preoperative nutrition which is emerging in the optimization of RC patients is immunonutrition. Although there is no standardized formulation, generally immunonutrition provides supplemental L-arginine, fish oil, vitamin A, and dietary nucleotides derived from yeast RNA. Cachexia is a physiologic process often associated with inflammation and the increased metabolic demands of cancer, and often acts as a harbinger of cancer-related death. Cuenca and colleagues[53] have demonstrated that myeloid-derived suppressor cell expansion is, in part, responsible for changes in protein and energy metabolism that decrease resistance to infection and contribute to the inflammation-induced organ injury of cachexia, and even death. Before this mechanism had been postulated, arginine and n-fatty acid supplementation had been observed to decrease postoperative infection rates and protection of the intestinal mucosa from damage in surgical patients via improved immune response in colorectal surgical patients.[54,55] Clinically, a Cochrane review relating to preoperative nutrition in patients undergoing gastrointestinal surgery found a relative risk of postoperative complications of 0.67 for studies comparing immunonutrition with traditional preoperative nutrition.[56] Immunonutrition has been investigated in the RC population by Bertrand and colleagues,[57] who performed a prospective, multicenter, pilot, case-control study using 7 days of immunonutrition compared with historical controls. The immunonutrition group had fewer postoperative complications (40% vs 76.7%; P = .008), less ileus at postoperative day 7 (6.6% vs 33%; P = .02), fewer infections (23% vs 60%; P = .008), and less pyelonephritis (16.7% vs 46.7%; P = .03). This study also observed lesser duration of stay by 3 days and lower Clavien grade for complications. In a randomized, controlled trial in RC patients, Hamilton-Reeves and colleagues[58] have demonstrated that immunonutrition reduced postoperative complications by 33%, infections by 39%, and suppressed myeloid-derived suppressor cell expansion. Studies assessing immunonutrition in surgical patients are summarized in **Table 1**. This work has lead to the launch of a multiinstitutional Southwest Oncology Group trial examining the effects of a immunonutrition in an RC population set to open in the spring of 2018.

Gastrointestinal Optimization

Bowel preparation

As thoroughly outlined by Matulewicz and colleagues,[20] there is ample evidence in the

Table 1
Outcome improvement with immunonutrition in the surgical patient

Study	Variable	Arms	Outcomes
Bertrand et al,[57] 2014	SIM vs standard preoperative diet in RC patients	SIM, n = 60 HC, n = 60	37% reduction in postoperative complications with SIM (P = .008) 37% reduction in infection rate with SIM (P = .008)
Hamilton-Reeves et al,[58] 2016	Preoperative SIM vs Standard ONS in RC patients	SIM, n = 14 ONS, n = 15	MDSC count significantly lower in SIM POD2 (P<.001) MDSC count expansion weakly associated with increased infection rate at 90 d (P = .061) SIM 33% reduction postoperative complication rate (P = .060) SIM 29% decrease in infections (P = .027)
Braga et al,[54] 2002	Preoperative SIM vs preoperative and postoperative SIM vs ONS vs SEN for GI cancer surgery	SIM preoperative, n = 50 SIM preoperative and postoperative, n = 50 ONS, n = 50 SEN, n = 50	Significantly lower infection rates with SIM; 12% in preoperative SIM, 10% in preoperative and postoperative SIM, 32% in ONS, 30% in conventional diet (P<.04)
Klek et al,[60] 2008	Enteral vs parenteral; standard vs SIM in patients undergoing bowel resection for GI cancer	SIM, n = 51 SEN, n = 53 SPN, n = 49 IPN, n = 51	No difference infectious complications between SIM and SEN, nor SPN and IPN No difference in overall morbidity, mortality, and LOS
Aida et al,[111] 2014	SIM with 50% reduction in volume vs SEN in pancreatoduodenectomy patients	SIM, n = 25 SEN, n = 25	Significantly lower infection rates with SIM; 28% with SIM, 60% with conventional diet (P = .23)
Drover et al,[59] 2011	Metaanalysis including 12 studies	N/A	Perioperative SIM reduced infections (OR, 0.59; 95% CI, 0.5 to 0.7; P<.0001) SIM also decreased mean LOS (OR, −2.38; 95% CI, −3.39 to −1.36; P<.0001)

Abbreviations: CI, confidence interval; HC, historical control; IPN, immunomodulating parenteral nutrition; LOS, length of stay; MDSC, myeloid-derived suppressor cells; ONS, oral nutrition supplement; OR, odds ratio; POD, postoperative day; RC, radical cystectomy; SEN, standard enteral nutrition; SIM, specialized immunonutrition; SPN, standard parenteral nutrition.

colorectal literature[61–63] and the RC literature[64–71] that mechanical bowel preparation and/or antibiotic bowel preparation do not decrease the risk of infectious, or any complications, and may contribute to patient dissatisfaction and intraoperative dehydration. Therefore, the routine use of bowel preparation should not be used.

Peripherally acting μ-opioid antagonists

There is an increasing body of data in both the colorectal and RC literature supporting the use of preoperative and postoperative alvimopan, a peripherally acting μ-opioid antagonist to benefit bowel recovery and decrease the duration of hospitalization.[72–74] Alvimopan is administered 30 to 90 minutes before surgery, and a phase III multicenter trial of alvimopan in bowel resection surgery demonstrated a decrease in postoperative ileus and decreased duration of stay (5.2 days vs 6.2 days) favoring the alvimopan group. Additionally, Lee and colleagues[73] performed a randomized, double-blind, placebo-controlled trial in patients undergoing RC and receiving postoperative intravenous patient-controlled opioid analgesia, and the alvimopan cohort had a superior time to first bowel movement (5.5 vs 6.8 days) shorter mean duration of stay (7.4 vs 10.1 days), and less postoperative ileus related morbidity (8.4% vs 29.1%). An analysis of this trial estimated a cost-savings benefit in the alvimopan group of $2340 to $2640 per patient owing to the decreased duration of stay and ileus-related morbidity.[74] At our own institution, we demonstrated that alvimopan shortened time to bowel function and hospital stay by approximately 1 day, even within an already established enhanced recovery pathway,[75] and is now a fixture of our RC clinical care pathway.

INTRAOPERATIVE MANAGEMENT
Patient Positioning

Patient positioning for RC has not been studied in a systematic manner. Nevertheless, we typically position men in the supine position with approximately 15% flexion at the level of the anterior-superior iliac spine. We decreased the amount of flexion in patients with a history of spinal fusion or prior lumbar injury. For female patients, we position in the low lithotomy position using stirrups or spreader bars, allowing access to the vagina intraoperatively. We do not use table flexion in female patients. The operative field should be prepared from the upper thighs and genitals to the xiphoid process. We use povidone-iodine preparation solution, because clorhexidine gluonate can be irritating to the genital skin.

Antimicrobial Prophylaxis

The American Urological Association Best Practice Statement on Urologic Surgery Antimicrobial Prophylaxis provides guidance on antimicrobial prophylaxis.[76] These recommendations recommend antimicrobial coverage of the genitourinary tract, skin, and intestine with options including a second- or third-generation cephalosporin, an aminoglycoside plus metronidazole, or clindamycin. We use cefoxitin, except in patients with a history of hypersensitivity, in which case alternative antimicrobials as described are substituted. Antibiotics should be provided within 1 hour of the incision and redosed as indicated if the procedure is prolonged for 24 hours of antimicrobial coverage.

Maintenance of Normothermia

Another important element of intraoperative management during RC is maintenance of a normal core body temperature. Multiple trials and systematic reviews support the maintenance of normothermia as a technique for reducing perioperative morbidity.[77–80] Frank and colleagues[78] observed that, during thoracic, vascular, and abdominal operations, maintaining normothermia using the room thermostat, warmed intravenous fluids and blood, heat-exchanging respiratory circuits, and postoperative blankets, resulted in a decreased relative risk of cardiac events, whereas hypothermia increased the risk of cardiac events by a factor of 2.2. Hypothermia has also been associated with increases in blood loss and transfusion in patients undergoing total hip arthroplasty.[81] Kurz and colleagues[77] examined the effect of maintaining normothermia on surgical wound infections and duration of hospital stay, and found that a 1.9°C difference in body temperature during colorectal surgery resulted in a rate of 19% surgical wound infections in the hypothermia group versus only 6% in the normothermic group. Furthermore, the duration of stay was 2.6 days longer in hypothermic group.

A recent Cochrane Review examined the use of active body surface warming systems for preventing complications caused by perioperative hypothermia, reviewing a total of 67 trials with more than 5400 participants, and concluded that active body surface warming systems had no effect on mortality, but did reduce blood loss and total volume of fluids administered.[80] The investigators did not observe a significant difference in transfusion rates. There was no difference found across different types of active body surface warming system or modes of administration of a particular type of active body surface warming systems. Additionally, another Cochrane Review analyzed

14 trials evaluating the effects of intraoperative use of intravenous nutrients to theoretically increase metabolism and, thus, heat production to help maintain normothermia. The authors observed significant heterogeneity between study protocols and only minimal changes in core body temperature with the use of intravenous nutrients during surgery.[82] Campbell and colleagues[83] also reviewed 24 studies using warmed intravenous and irrigation fluids and noted a 0.5°C difference in core temperature in patients receiving warmed fluids versus room temperature fluids at 30, 60, 90, and 120 minutes and at the end of surgery, but found insufficient evidence to comment on their effect on cardiovascular complications, infections, bleeding, duration of stay, or mortality.

Transfusion of Blood Products and Restrictive Fluid Strategies

Receipt of blood transfusion during RC has been independently associated with increased overall morbidity and mortality.[84–86] Additionally, one study in 2008 noted that transfusion of blood products in rat models may also have a cancer-promoting role and may increase progression.[87] Blood loss during RC most often occurs during dissection and handling of the bladder vasculature and pedicles, dissection of the paravaginal tissues in female patients, and division of the dorsal venous complex in male patients.

Multiple techniques have been described to try to prevent blood loss and minimize transfusion. First, many investigators believe that robotic-assisted cystectomy will prove to significantly decrease intraoperative blood loss and the need for transfusion in a similar to robotic radical prostatectomy. Multiple studies have consistently shown decreased significant blood loss (>500 mL)[88] and transfusion rates (odds ratio, 0.13).[89] Other techniques include preoperative correction of anemia with intravenous iron and erythropoietin,[90] use of a "cell saver" or cell salvage,[91,92] ultrasound-guided intraoperative fluid management,[93] and central venous pressure measurement and stroke volume guided intraoperative fluid administration.[94] Although the use of a cell salvage machine or intraoperative cell saver has been found to significantly reduce allogenic blood transfusion requirements,[91,92] the use of a cell saver in oncologic surgery is limited due to the fear of infusing cancer cells. Small trials have demonstrated that the use of either ultrasound-guided or central venous pressure/stroke volume–guided fluid administration is also effective at reducing perioperative transfusions.[93,94] One trial in the RC population examined the use of a restrictive

intraoperative fluid management strategy with norepinephrine infusion to reduce blood transfusions.[95] Restrictive fluid management was associated with a decreased total median blood loss (800 mL in the restrictive group vs 1200 mL in the control group), rate of transfusion (27/83 [33%] vs 50/83 [60%]), and average number of units of packed red blood cells received (1.8 units vs 2.9 units) during hospitalization. Absolute reduction in transfusions was 28%. Another strategy for reducing perioperative blood transfusion may be the administration of the antifibrinolytic agent tranexamic acid. The Mayo Clinic observed that, in 103 patients who received tranexamic acid during open RC and compared with historic controls, there was a 26% difference in perioperative blood transfusion and no significant increase in perioperative venous thromboembolism.[96]

Interestingly, Burkhard and colleagues[97] examined 1-year postoperative functional outcomes in patients undergoing RC and orthotopic neobladder who were randomized to either a restrictive or standard intraoperative fluid management strategy. They observed improved daytime and nighttime continence rates, as well as improved erectile function in the fluid-restricted group. Long-term oncologic outcomes in patients undergoing a fluid-restricted strategy during RC have not been studied, and may represent an opportunity for future investigation. Regardless of strategies, it is critical to partner with anesthesia colleagues when performing RC. Restrictive fluid management and either ultrasound-guided or central venous pressure/stroke volume–guided fluid management demonstrate evidence for decreasing blood transfusion and should be integral to the RC pathway.

Venous Thromboembolism Prophylaxis

Venous thromboembolism is a highly prevalent perioperative complication after RC, and can account for up to 22% of deaths.[98] The American Urological Association Best Practice Statement for the prevention of deep vein thrombosis in patients undergoing urologic surgery supports that perioperative chemoprophylaxis for venous thromboembolism is the standard of care and is a universally accepted practice.[99] There is limited evidence regarding the timing of administration of chemoprophylaxis. Given the prolonged immobilization during and after cystectomy, as well as increased risk of venous thromboembolism owing to malignancy, patients at our institution receive 5000 units of heparin in the preoperative bay before the case, and we continue chemoprophylaxis daily for 30 days postoperatively with enoxaparin. There are few data on early identification of venous thromboembolism; however, authors from our institution evaluated the use of screening lower extremity ultrasound examination in patients undergoing RC where patients underwent screening ultrasound examination at 2 to 3 days after RC to determine the rate of asymptomatic deep vein thrombosis.[100] Asymptomatic deep vein thrombosis was identified in 9.5% of 221 total patients; however, of the 9 patients (4.5%) who ultimately developed a symptomatic pulmonary embolus, none had a positive postoperative screening ultrasound examination.

Pain Management

Because gastrointestinal complications in the form of postoperative ileus is one of the most common complications after RC, avoidance of opioid medications is a mainstay of current Enhanced Recovery After Surgery pathways. *The Guidelines for Perioperative Care after Radical Cystectomy for Bladder Cancer: ERAS Society Recommendations* report strong evidence for the superiority of thoracic epidural analgesia over systemic opioids in relieving pain.[101] Furthermore, multiple trials

support the use of intraoperative neuraxial or regional anesthesia techniques to help minimize postoperative opioid use and speed recovery.[102–105] The question of superiority of epidural patient-controlled anesthesia versus regional blocks such as transversus abominis plane block remains unanswered. Multiple trials have been completed examining use of either technique for analgesia in abdominal surgery or as a part of Enhanced Recovery After Surgery or fast track protocols.[13,17,19,106–108] No high-quality head-to-head trial has been completed comparing the 2 techniques as part of an enhanced recovery pathway in RC.

Pruthi and colleagues[18] reported on the use of ketorolac as a nonnarcotic analgesic as part of an enhanced recovery protocol, and have noted its efficacy and safety in a series of 362 patients undergoing RC. Some have historically avoided perioperative use of ketorolac owing to theoretic concerns for increased risk of bleeding. However, a recent metaanalysis found no association between ketorolac and perioperative bleeding.[109] Postmarketing surveillance analysis of ketorolac also did not demonstrate an increased risk of peri-operative bleeding.[110] At our institution, we

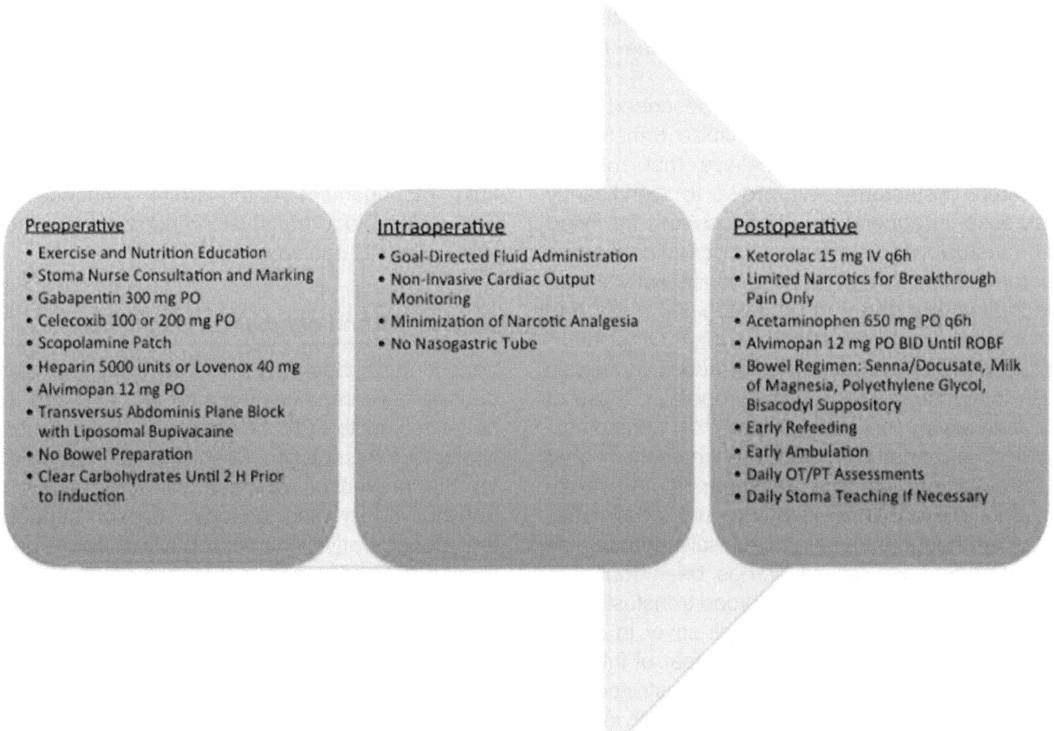

Preoperative
- Exercise and Nutrition Education
- Stoma Nurse Consultation and Marking
- Gabapentin 300 mg PO
- Celecoxib 100 or 200 mg PO
- Scopolamine Patch
- Heparin 5000 units or Lovenox 40 mg
- Alvimopan 12 mg PO
- Transversus Abdominis Plane Block with Liposomal Bupivacaine
- No Bowel Preparation
- Clear Carbohydrates Until 2 H Prior to Induction

Intraoperative
- Goal-Directed Fluid Administration
- Non-Invasive Cardiac Output Monitoring
- Minimization of Narcotic Analgesia
- No Nasogastric Tube

Postoperative
- Ketorolac 15 mg IV q6h
- Limited Narcotics for Breakthrough Pain Only
- Acetaminophen 650 mg PO q6h
- Alvimopan 12 mg PO BID Until ROBF
- Bowel Regimen: Senna/Docusate, Milk of Magnesia, Polyethylene Glycol, Bisacodyl Suppository
- Early Refeeding
- Early Ambulation
- Daily OT/PT Assessments
- Daily Stoma Teaching If Necessary

Fig. 1. Enhanced Recovery After Surgery (ERAS) pathway at the author's institution. BID, 2 times per day; CLD, clear liquid diet; IV, intravenous; OT, occupational therapy; PO, per os; POD, postoperative day; PT, physical therapy; ROBF, return of bowel function.

administer celecoxib 100 to 200 mg, gabapentin 300 mg, and a transverse abdominis plane block, as well as postoperative ketorolac for nonopioid pain management in addition to opioid analgesia on an as-needed basis. We have observed decreased opioid dose requirements, earlier return of bowel function, and decreased duration of stay with standardized implementation of this pain management regimen (Holzbeierlein J, unpublished data, 2016). The Enhanced Recovery After Surgery pathway used at our institution is displayed in **Fig. 1**.

SUMMARY

RC is a morbid procedure performed on an aged population; however, advances in preoperative and perioperative management of these patients can facilitate improved outcomes. Although standardization of this process may never be fully achieved owing to the heterogeneity of population and health care delivery systems, and the need for continued individualized care for every patient, knowledge of the current landscape of surgical optimization of the RC patient is essential.

REFERENCES

1. Siegel RL, Miller KD, Jemal A. Cancer statistics, 2016. CA Cancer J Clin 2016;66(1):7–30.
2. Konety BR, Joyce GF, Wise M. Bladder and upper tract urothelial cancer. J Urol 2007;177(5): 1636–45.
3. Miller KD, Siegel RL, Lin CC, et al. Cancer treatment and survivorship statistics, 2016. CA Cancer J Clin 2016;66(4):271–89.
4. Grossman HB, Natale RB, Tangen CM, et al. Chemotherapy plus cystectomy compared with cystectomy alone for locally advanced bladder cancer. N Engl J Med 2003;349(9):859–66.
5. International Collaboration of Trialists, Medical Research Council Advanced Bladder Cancer Working Party (now the National Cancer Research Institute Bladder Cancer Clinical Studies Group), European Organisation for Research and Treatment of Cancer Genito-Urinary Tract Cancer Group, Australian Bladder Cancer Study Group, National Cancer Institute of Canada Clinical Trials Group, Finnbladder, Norwegian Bladder Cancer Study Group, Club Urologico Espanol de Tratamiento Oncologico Group, Griffiths G, Hall R, Sylvester R, et al. International phase III trial assessing neoadjuvant cisplatin, methotrexate, and vinblastine chemotherapy for muscle-invasive bladder cancer: long-term results of the BA06 30894 trial. J Clin Oncol 2011;29(16):2171–7.
6. Jani AB, Efstathiou JA, Shipley WU. Bladder preservation strategies. Hematol Oncol Clin North Am 2015;29(2):289–300.
7. Gregg JR, Cookson MS, Phillips S, et al. Effect of preoperative nutritional deficiency on mortality after radical cystectomy for bladder cancer. J Urol 2011; 185(1):90–6.
8. Shabsigh A, Korets R, Vora KC, et al. Defining early morbidity of radical cystectomy for patients with bladder cancer using a standardized reporting methodology. Eur Urol 2009;55(1):164–76.
9. Stimson CJ, Chang SS, Barocas DA, et al. Early and late perioperative outcomes following radical cystectomy: 90-day readmissions, morbidity and mortality in a contemporary series. J Urol 2010;184(4):1296–300.
10. Aziz A, May M, Burger M, et al. Prediction of 90-day mortality after radical cystectomy for bladder cancer in a prospective European multicenter cohort. Eur Urol 2014;66(1):156–63.
11. Kim SP, Shah ND, Karnes RJ, et al. The implications of hospital acquired adverse events on mortality, length of stay and costs for patients undergoing radical cystectomy for bladder cancer. J Urol 2012;187(6):2011–7.
12. Djaladat H, Katebian B, Bazargani ST, et al. 90-Day complication rate in patients undergoing radical cystectomy with enhanced recovery protocol: a prospective cohort study. Cochrane Database Syst Rev 2003;(4):CD004423.
13. Dutton TJ, Daugherty MO, Mason RG, et al. Implementation of the Exeter Enhanced Recovery Programme for patients undergoing radical cystectomy. BJU Int 2014;113(5):719–25.
14. Smith J, Meng ZW, Lockyer R, et al. Evolution of the Southampton Enhanced Recovery Programme for radical cystectomy and the aggregation of marginal gains. BJU Int 2014;114(3):375–83.
15. Daneshmand S, Ahmadi H, Schuckman AK, et al. Enhanced recovery protocol after radical cystectomy for bladder cancer. J Urol 2014;192(1):50–6.
16. Karl A, Buchner A, Becker A, et al. A new concept for early recovery after surgery for patients undergoing radical cystectomy for bladder cancer: results of a prospective randomized study. J Urol 2014;191(2):335–40.
17. Maffezzini M, Campodonico F, Capponi G, et al. Fast-track surgery and technical nuances to reduce complications after radical cystectomy and intestinal urinary diversion with the modified Indiana pouch. Surg Oncol 2012;21(3):191–5.
18. Pruthi RS, Nielsen M, Smith A, et al. Fast track program in patients undergoing radical cystectomy: results in 362 consecutive patients. J Am Coll Surg 2010;210(1):93–9.
19. Arumainayagam N, McGrath J, Jefferson KP, et al. Introduction of an enhanced recovery protocol for radical cystectomy. BJU Int 2008;101(6):698–701.

20. Matulewicz RS, Brennan J, Pruthi RS, et al. Radical cystectomy perioperative care redesign. Urology 2015;86(6):1076–86.

21. Clarke HD, Timm VL, Goldberg BR, et al. Preoperative patient education reduces in-hospital falls after total knee arthroplasty. Clin Orthop Relat Res 2012;470(1):244–9.

22. Groller KD. Systematic review of patient education practices in weight loss surgery. Surg Obes Relat Dis 2017;13(6):1072–85.

23. Rink M, Zabor EC, Furberg H, et al. Impact of smoking and smoking cessation on outcomes in bladder cancer patients treated with radical cystectomy. Eur Urol 2013;64(3):456–64.

24. Chen RJ, Ho YS, Guo HR, et al. Long-term nicotine exposure–induced chemoresistance is mediated by activation of Stat3 and downregulation of ERK1/2 via nAChR and beta-adrenoceptors in human bladder cancer cells. Toxicol Sci 2010; 115(1):118–30.

25. Kim PH, Kent M, Zhao P, et al. The impact of smoking on pathologic response to neoadjuvant cisplatin-based chemotherapy in patients with muscle-invasive bladder cancer. World J Urol 2014;32(2):453–9.

26. Froehner M, Koch R, Hübler M, et al. Selection effects may explain smoking-related outcome differences after radical cystectomy. Eur Urol Focus 2017;71(5):710–3.

27. Thomsen T, Villebro N, Møller AM. Interventions for preoperative smoking cessation. Cochrane Database Syst Rev 2010;(7):CD002294.

28. Wong J, Abrishami A, Yang Y, et al. A perioperative smoking cessation intervention with varenicline: a double-blind, randomized, placebo-controlled trial. Anesthesiology 2012;117(4):755–64.

29. Tønnesen H. Alcohol abuse and postoperative morbidity. Dan Med Bull 2003;50(2):139–60.

30. Oppedal K, Møller AM, Pedersen B, et al. Preoperative alcohol cessation prior to elective surgery. Cochrane Database Syst Rev 2012;(7):CD008343.

31. Lauridsen SV, Thomsen T, Thind P, et al. STOP smoking and alcohol drinking before OPeration for bladder cancer (the STOP-OP study), perioperative smoking and alcohol cessation intervention in relation to radical cystectomy: study protocol for a randomised controlled trial. Trials 2017;18(1):329.

32. Kristensen SA, Laustsen S, Kiesbye B, et al. The urostomy education scale: a reliable and valid tool to evaluate urostomy self-care skills among cystectomy patients. J Wound Ostomy Continence Nurs 2013;40(6):611–7.

33. Kristensen SA, Jensen BT. Testing inter-rater reliability of the urostomy education scale. Eur J Oncol Nurs 2016;20:17–23.

34. Atallah F, Letocart P, Malavaud B, et al. Can We Predict Morbidity and Mortality of Patients Aged 75 Years and Older Undergoing Cystectomy? J Frailty Aging 2017;6(2):72–5.

35. Colwell JC, Gray M. Does preoperative teaching and stoma site marking affect surgical outcomes in patients undergoing ostomy surgery? J Wound Ostomy Continence Nurs 2007;34(5): 492–6.

36. Maydick D. A Descriptive study assessing quality of life for adults with a permanent ostomy and the influence of preoperative stoma site marking. Ostomy Wound Manage 2016;62(5):14–24.

37. Salvadalena G, Hendren S, McKenna L, et al. WOCN society and AUA position statement on preoperative stoma site marking for patients undergoing urostomy surgery. J Wound Ostomy Continence Nurs 2015;42(3):253–6.

38. Ahmadi H, Skinner EC, Simma-Chiang V, et al. Urinary functional outcome following radical cystoprostatectomy and ileal neobladder reconstruction in male patients. J Urol 2013;189(5):1782–8.

39. Ji H, Pan J, Shen W, et al. Identification and management of emptying failure in male patients with orthotopic neobladders after radical cystectomy for bladder cancer. Urology 2010;76(3):644–8.

40. Atallah F, Letocart P, Malavaud B, et al. Can we predict morbidity and mortality of patients aged 75 years and older undergoing cystectomy? J Frailty Aging 2017;6(2):72.

41. Aghazadeh MA, Barocas DA, Salem S, et al. Determining factors for hospital discharge status after radical cystectomy in a large contemporary cohort. J Urol 2011;185(1):85–9.

42. Fried LP, Tangen CM, Walston J, et al. Frailty in older adults: evidence for a phenotype. J Gerontol A Biol Sci Med Sci 2001;56(3):M146–57.

43. Pearl JA, Patil D, Filson CP, et al. Patient frailty and discharge disposition following radical cystectomy. Clin Genitourin Cancer 2017;15(4):e615–21.

44. Chappidi MR, Kates M, Patel HD, et al. Frailty as a marker of adverse outcomes in patients with bladder cancer undergoing radical cystectomy. Urol Oncol 2016;34(6):256.e1-6.

45. Jensen BT, Petersen AK, Jensen JB, et al. Efficacy of a multiprofessional rehabilitation programme in radical cystectomy pathways: a prospective randomized controlled trial. Scand J Urol 2015;49(2):133–41.

46. Johnson DC, Riggs SB, Nielsen ME, et al. Nutritional predictors of complications following radical cystectomy. World J Urol 2015;33(8):1129–37.

47. Garg T, Chen LY, Kim PH, et al. Preoperative serum albumin is associated with mortality and complications after radical cystectomy. BJU Int 2014;113(6): 918–23.

48. Bhalla RG, Wang L, Chang SS, et al. Association between preoperative albumin levels and length of stay after radical cystectomy. J Urol 2017; 198(5):1039–45.

49. Brady MC, Kinn S, Stuart P, et al. Preoperative fasting for adults to prevent perioperative complications. Cochrane Database Syst Rev 2003;(4): CD004423.

50. Smith MD, McCall J, Plank L, et al. Preoperative carbohydrate treatment for enhancing recovery after elective surgery. Cochrane Database Syst Rev 2014;(8):CD009161.

51. Awad S, Varadhan KK, Ljungqvist O, et al. A meta-analysis of randomised controlled trials on preoperative oral carbohydrate treatment in elective surgery. Clin Nutr 2013;32(1):34–44.

52. Pang KH, Groves R, Venugopal S, et al. Prospective implementation of enhanced recovery after surgery protocols to radical cystectomy. Eur Urol 2017. [Epub ahead of print].

53. Cuenca AG, Cuenca AL, Winfield RD, et al. Novel role for tumor-induced expansion of myeloid-derived cells in cancer cachexia. J Immunol 2014;192(12):6111–9.

54. Braga M, Gianotti L, Vignali A, et al. Preoperative oral arginine and n-3 fatty acid supplementation improves the immunometabolic host response and outcome after colorectal resection for cancer. Surgery 2002;132(5):805–14.

55. Guo G, Bai X, Cai C, et al. The protective effect of different enteral nutrition combined with growth hormone on intestinal mucosal damage of scalded rats. Burns 2010;36(8):1283–8.

56. Burden S, Todd C, Hill J, et al. Preoperative nutrition in patients undergoing gastrointestinal surgery. Cochrane Database Syst Rev 2014;(8):CD009161.

57. Bertrand J, Siegler N, Murez T, et al. Impact of preoperative immunonutrition on morbidity following cystectomy for bladder cancer: a case–control pilot study. World J Urol 2014;32(1):233–7.

58. Hamilton-Reeves JM, Bechtel MD, Hand LK, et al. Effects of immunonutrition for cystectomy on immune response and infection rates: a pilot randomized controlled clinical trial. Eur Urol 2016;69(3):389–92.

59. Drover JW, Dhaliwal R, Weitzel L, et al. Perioperative use of arginine-supplemented diets: a systematic review of the evidence. J Am Coll Surg 2011; 212(3):385–99.

60. Klek S, Kulig J, Sierzega M, et al. The impact of immunostimulating nutrition on infectious complications after upper gastrointestinal surgery: a prospective, randomized, clinical trial. Ann Surg 2008;248(2):212–20.

61. Contant CM, Hop WC, Van't Sant HP, et al. Mechanical bowel preparation for elective colorectal surgery: a multicentre randomised trial. Lancet 2007;370(9605):2112–7.

62. Cao F, Li J, Li F. Mechanical bowel preparation for elective colorectal surgery: updated systematic review and meta-analysis. Int J Colorectal Dis 2012; 27(6):803–10.

63. Guenaga KK, Matos D, Wille-Jorgensen P. Mechanical bowel preparation for elective colorectal surgery. Cochrane Database Syst Rev 2009;(1):CD001544.

64. Shafii M, Murphy DM, Donovan MG, et al. Is mechanical bowel preparation necessary in patients undergoing cystectomy and urinary diversion? BJU Int 2002;89(9):879–81.

65. Tabibi A, Simforoosh N, Basiri A, et al. Bowel preparation versus no preparation before ileal urinary diversion. Urology 2007;70(4):654–8.

66. Xu R, Zhao X, Zhong Z, et al. No advantage is gained by preoperative bowel preparation in radical cystectomy and ileal conduit: a randomized controlled trial of 86 patients. Int Urol Nephrol 2010; 42(4):947–50.

67. Large MC, Kiriluk KJ, DeCastro GJ, et al. The impact of mechanical bowel preparation on postoperative complications for patients undergoing cystectomy and urinary diversion. J Urol 2012; 188(5):1801–5.

68. Hashad MM, Atta M, Elabbady A, et al. Safety of no bowel preparation before ileal urinary diversion. BJU Int 2012;110(11 Pt C):E1109–13.

69. Raynor MC, Lavien G, Nielsen M, et al. Elimination of preoperative mechanical bowel preparation in patients undergoing cystectomy and urinary diversion. Urol Oncol 2013;31(1):32–5.

70. Yang L, Chen HS, Welk B, et al. Does using comprehensive preoperative bowel preparation offer any advantage for urinary diversion using ileum? A meta-analysis. Int Urol Nephrol 2013;45(1):25–31.

71. Deng S, Dong Q, Wang J, et al. The role of mechanical bowel preparation before ileal urinary diversion: a systematic review and meta-analysis. Urol Int 2014;92(3):339–48.

72. Ludwig K, Enker WE, Delaney CP, et al. Gastrointestinal tract recovery in patients undergoing bowel resection: results of a randomized trial of alvimopan and placebo with a standardized accelerated postoperative care pathway. Arch Surg 2008;143: 1098–105.

73. Lee CT, Chang SS, Kamat AM, et al. Alvimopan accelerates gastrointestinal recovery after radical cystectomy: a multicenter randomized placebo-controlled trial. Eur Urol 2014;66(2):265–72.

74. Kauf TL, Svatek RS, Amiel G, et al. Alvimopan, a peripherally acting μ-opioid receptor antagonist, is associated with reduced costs after radical cystectomy: economic analysis of a phase 4 randomized, controlled trial. J Urol 2014;191(6):1721–7.

75. Hamilton Z, Parker W, Griffin J, et al. Alvimopan in an enhanced recovery program following radical cystectomy. Bladder Cancer 2015;1(2):137–42.

76. Wolf JS, Bennett CJ, Dmochowski RR, et al. Best practice policy statement on urologic surgery antimicrobial prophylaxis. J Urol 2008;179(4): 1379–90.

77. Kurz A, Sessler DI, Lenhardt R. Perioperative normothermia to reduce the incidence of surgical-wound infection and shorten hospitalization. N Engl J Med 1996;334(19):1209–16.

78. Frank SM, Fleisher LA, Breslow MJ, et al. Perioperative maintenance of normothermia reduces the incidence of morbid cardiac events: a randomized clinical trial. JAMA 1997;277(14):1127–34.

79. Harper CM, McNicholas T, Gowrie-Mohan S. Maintaining perioperative normothermia: a simple, safe, and effective way of reducing complications of surgery. BMJ 2003;326(7392):721.

80. Madrid E, Urrútia G, Roqué i Figuls M, et al. Active body surface warming systems for preventing complications caused by inadvertent perioperative hypothermia in adults. Cochrane Database Syst Rev 2016;(4):CD009016.

81. Schmied H, Reiter A, Kurz A, et al. Mild hypothermia increases blood loss and transfusion requirements during total hip arthroplasty. Lancet 1996; 347(8997):289–92.

82. Warttig S, Alderson P, Lewis SR, et al. Intravenous nutrients for preventing inadvertent perioperative hypothermia in adults. Cochrane Database Syst Rev 2016;(11):CD009906.

83. Campbell G, Alderson P, Smith AF, et al. Warming of intravenous and irrigation fluids for preventing inadvertent perioperative hypothermia. Cochrane Database Syst Rev 2015;(4):CD009891.

84. Chang SS, Smith JA, Wells N, et al. Estimated blood loss and transfusion requirements of radical cystectomy. J Urol 2001;166(6):2151–4.

85. Lawrentschuk N, Colombo R, Hakenberg OW, et al. Prevention and management of complications following radical cystectomy for bladder cancer. Eur Urol 2010;57(6):983–1001.

86. Morgan TM, Barocas DA, Chang SS, et al. The relationship between perioperative blood transfusion and overall mortality in patients undergoing radical cystectomy for bladder cancer. Urol Oncol 2013; 31(6):871–7.

87. Atzil S, Arad M, Glasner A, et al. Blood transfusion promotes cancer progression: a critical role for aged erythrocytes. Anesthesiology 2008;109(6): 989–97.

88. Gandaglia G, Karl A, Novara G, et al. Perioperative and oncologic outcomes of robot-assisted vs. open radical cystectomy in bladder cancer patients: a comparison of two high-volume referral centers. Eur J Surg Oncol 2016;42(11):1736–43.

89. Tang K, Xia D, Li H, et al. Robotic vs. open radical cystectomy in bladder cancer: a systematic review and meta-analysis. Eur J Surg Oncol 2014;40(11): 1399–411.

90. Albers P, Heicappell R, Schwaibold H, et al. Erythropoietin in urologic oncology. Eur Urol 2001; 39(1):1–8.

91. Bouras I, Mingo O. Should cell salvage be used in oncological surgery? Br J Hosp Med (Lond) 2010; 71(1):57.

92. Aning J, Dunn J, Daugherty M, et al. Towards bloodless cystectomy: a 10-year experience of intra-operative cell salvage during radical cystectomy. BJU Int 2012;110(11 Pt B):E608–13.

93. Pillai P, McEleavy I, Gaughan M, et al. A double-blind randomized controlled clinical trial to assess the effect of Doppler optimized intraoperative fluid management on outcome following radical cystectomy. J Urol 2011;186(6):2201–6.

94. Kong YG, Kim JY, Yu J, et al. Efficacy and safety of stroke volume variation-guided fluid therapy for reducing blood loss and transfusion requirements during radical cystectomy: a randomized clinical trial. Medicine (Baltimore) 2016;95(19):e3685.

95. Wuethrich PY, Studer UE, Thalmann GN, et al. Intraoperative continuous norepinephrine infusion combined with restrictive deferred hydration significantly reduces the need for blood transfusion in patients undergoing open radical cystectomy: results of a prospective randomised trial. Eur Urol 2014;66(2):352–60.

96. Zaid HB, Yang DY, Tollefson MK, et al. Efficacy and safety of intraoperative tranexamic acid infusion for reducing blood transfusion during open radical cystectomy. Urology 2016;92:57–62.

97. Burkhard FC, Studer UE, Wuethrich PY. Superior functional outcome after radical cystectomy and orthotopic bladder substitution with restrictive intraoperative fluid management: a follow up study of a randomized clinical trial. J Urol 2015;193(1):173–8.

98. Quek ML, Stein JP, Daneshmand S, et al. A critical analysis of perioperative mortality from radical cystectomy. J Urol 2006;175(3):886–90.

99. Forrest JB, Clemens JQ, Finamore P, et al. AUA Best Practice Statement for the prevention of deep vein thrombosis in patients undergoing urologic surgery. J Urol 2009;181(3):1170–7.

100. Murray KM, Parker W, Stephany H, et al. Venous thromboembolism after radical cystectomy: experience with screening ultrasonography. Arab J Urol 2016;14(1):37–43.

101. Cerantola Y, Valerio M, Persson B, et al. Guidelines for perioperative care after radical cystectomy for bladder cancer: enhanced recovery after surgery (ERAS®) society recommendations. Clin Nutr 2013;32(6):879–87.

102. Jorgensen H, Wetterslev J, Moiniche S, et al. Epidural local anaesthetics versus opioid-based analgesic regimens for postoperative gastrointestinal paralysis, PONV and pain after abdominal surgery. Cochrane Database Syst Rev 2000;(4): CD001893.

103. Carli F, Trudel JL, Belliveau P. The effect of intraoperative thoracic epidural anesthesia and

postoperative analgesia on bowel function after colorectal surgery. Dis Colon Rectum 2001;44(8): 1083–9.

104. Winer AG, Sfakianos JP, Puttanniah VG, et al. Comparison of perioperative outcomes for epidural versus intravenous patient-controlled analgesia after radical cystectomy. Reg Anesth Pain Med 2015; 40(3):239.

105. Guay J, Nishimori M, Kopp S. Epidural local anaesthetics versus opioid-based analgesic regimens for postoperative gastrointestinal paralysis, vomiting and pain after abdominal surgery. Cochrane Database Syst Rev 2016;(7): CD001893.

106. McDonnell JG, O'donnell B, Curley G, et al. The analgesic efficacy of transversus abdominis plane block after abdominal surgery: a prospective randomized controlled trial. Anesth Analg 2007; 104(1):193–7.

107. Kadam RV, Field JB. Ultrasound-guided continuous transverse abdominis plane block for abdominal surgery. J Anaesthesiol Clin Pharmacol 2011;27(3):333.

108. Kadam VR, Van Wijk RM, Moran JL, et al. Epidural versus continuous transversus abdominis plane catheter technique for postoperative analgesia after abdominal surgery. Anaesth Intensive Care 2013;41(4):476.

109. Gobble RM, Hoang HL, Kachniarz B, et al. Ketorolac does not increase perioperative bleeding: a meta-analysis of randomized controlled trials. Plast Reconstr Surg 2014;133(3):741–55.

110. Strom BL, Berlin JA, Kinman JL, et al. Parenteral ketorolac and risk of gastrointestinal and operative site bleeding: a postmarketing surveillance study. JAMA 1996;275(5):376–82.

111. Aida T, Furukawa K, Suzuki D, et al. Preoperative immunonutrition decreases postoperative complications by modulating prostaglandin E 2 production and T-cell differentiation in patients undergoing pancreatoduodenectomy. Surgery 2014;155(1): 124–33.

Robotic Cystectomy

Danica May, MD[a], Jessie Gills, MD[b],*, Scott E. Delacroix Jr, MD[b]

KEYWORDS

- Laparoscopic • Robotic • Radical cystectomy • Intracorporeal urinary diversion

KEY POINTS

- Robotic-assisted radical cystectomy (RARC) is a technique and should complement, not substitute, oncologic principles.
- To date, randomized controlled trials have compared 117 RARCs with 122 open radical cystectomies, all of which underwent extracorporeal urinary diversions. These trials have shown lower estimated blood loss, lower blood transfusion rates, increased cost per operation and longer operative times with similar oncologic outcomes, length of hospital stay, and perioperative complications.
- The principal potential benefit of robotic cystectomy is avoidance of gastrointestinal complications by using intracorporeal urinary diversion. Observational studies are promising; however, prospective randomized trials have not studied this aspect.

INTRODUCTION

Robotic-assisted laparoscopic radical cystectomy (RARC) was first described in 2003,[1] predated by case reports of laparoscopic radical cystectomies in 1995[2] and intracorporeal ileal conduit urinary diversion (UD) 5 years later in 2000.[3] Robotic-assisted laparoscopic radical cystectomy (RARC) has been evolving over the last 15 years under close scrutiny, with the first prospective randomized controlled trial of robotic versus open radical cystectomy (ORC) performed in 2009[4] (**Fig. 1**). Since then, 4 additional randomized controlled trials have been completed and, to date, 3 have reported final results. More than 100 articles in the last 2 years and more than 300 articles in the last 5 years have been published on RARC. Given the abundance of literature, the utility of RARC should be well known and accepted or rejected based on scientific merit. Unfortunately, aside from technical feasibility, short-term oncologic outcomes, and intraoperative or perioperative characteristics, much is left unknown. This is partially because the quality and level of evidence for these published articles is extremely variable.

In addition, the rapidly changing, nonstandardized periprocedural care pathways for patients undergoing radical cystectomy likely have as much influence, if not more, on periprocedural outcomes than the technique used.

Unlike open surgery, in which the technical components of the operation remain largely unchanged over time, multiple technologic advances in robotic platforms, instrumentation, and endoscopic training in residency are quickly evolving. This, along with the increasing understanding of disease biology, care pathways, and drivers of patient outcomes are likely to make the utility of a technique, in an ever-changing, multifaceted, disease-management decision tree, only a minor component. This article discusses the known benefits, limitations, and potential future refinements of the surgical technique, RARC.

ROBOTIC-ASSISTED LAPAROSCOPIC RADICAL CYSTECTOMY
Feasibility

Nix and colleagues[4] performed the first randomized controlled trial of RARC versus ORC. Twenty

Disclosure: The authors have nothing to disclose.
[a] Department of Urology, Louisiana State University Health Sciences Center, 1542 Tulane Avenue, Room 547, New Orleans, LA 70112, USA; [b] Department of PI Urology, Louisiana State University Healthcare Network, 1542 Tulane Avenue, Room 547, New Orleans, LA 70112, USA
* Corresponding author.
E-mail address: jgills@lsuhsc.edu

Urol Clin N Am 45 (2018) 183–188
https://doi.org/10.1016/j.ucl.2017.12.012

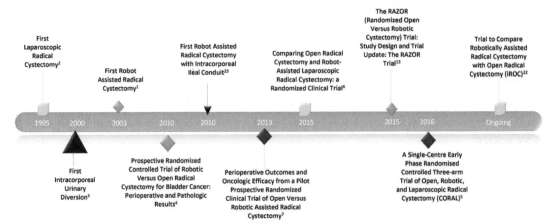

Fig. 1. Evolution of laparoscopic and robotic cystectomy. iROC, International Robotic Cystectomy Consortium.

subjects underwent ORC and 21 underwent RARC, with both groups receiving extracorporeal UDs (ECUDs). Subjects were well-matched in regard to clinicopathologic characteristics. The median operative time was 4.2 hours for RARC and 3.5 hours for ORC. Median estimated blood loss was 258 mL for RARC and 575 mL for ORC. Median time to flatus, bowel movement, and length of stay was 1 day shorter in the RARC arm. Oncologic outcomes were similar in both groups in regard to surgical margins, lymph node count, and pathologic stage.[4] This was the first study to support the safety, feasibility, and transference of oncologic principles with the RARC technique.

Three additional prospective randomized controlled trials on RARC have been completed.[5–7] A recent meta-analysis of these studies included 117 subjects undergoing RARC and 122 subjects undergoing ORC.[8] The meta-analysis revealed that RARC was associated with a longer operative time (17.25–122.12 minutes; P = .009) and 300 mL lower estimated blood loss per case (CI −414.66 to −184.99; P = .00001).[8] All other variables tested were not statistically different between the 2 groups, including length of hospital stay, time to flatus, time to oral diet, lymph node yield, and perioperative complications. Mortality rates and positive surgical margins were also similar between the 2 groups.[8] Despite the heterogeneity among the studies, the results of this meta-analysis support what has been shown in a plethora of retrospective reviews. One interesting factor identified is that, even at high volume centers, surgical technique is variable between surgeons and institutions.[8,9] As mentioned previously, a consistent factor throughout all these studies was the extracorporeal creation of the urinary conduit.

With the demonstration of the feasibility of RARC, its utilization has been steadily increasing. Leow and colleagues,[10] examined a private charge capture research database of more than 600 US hospitals and found that 0.6% of radical cystectomies were being performed using robotic assistance in 2004, increasing to 12.8% in 2010. In an analysis of the National Cancer Database, 26.3% of radical cystectomy subjects underwent minimally invasive radical cystectomy in 2010, which increased to rates of 39.4% in 2013.[11] Despite the lack of evidence for superiority, the prevalence of RARC is certainly increasing.

Oncologic Principles

The goals of minimally invasive and robotic-assisted cystectomy have been to reduce periprocedural morbidity and allow earlier return of normal activity while maintaining oncologic equivalence.[9,12] The Randomized Open Versus Robotic Cystectomy (RAZOR) trial, a multiinstitutional randomized study to compare ORC with RARC for oncologic outcomes, complications, health-related quality of life (HRQOL), pelvic lymph node count, cost, and morbidity, had accrued 306 of the proposed 320 subjects at last update in 2015,[13] with final data expected soon. To date, oncologic outcomes from a variety of studies have not been significantly different between RARC and ORC.[4–7,13]

The presence of positive soft tissue margins (PSMs) is a strong marker of poor prognosis, with 5-year disease-specific survival in the PSM cystectomy group of 32% compared with 72% for negative margins.[14] An analysis of 4410 ORC subjects found the overall incidence of PSM was 6.3% at 12 academic centers.[14] There was some heterogeneity of rates of PSM in RARC subjects among the original randomized controlled trials with rates ranging from 0% to 15%.[4–7] PSM rates of 7% were found in an analysis of 496 subjects undergoing RARC but were extrapolated to drop to a 5% overall PSM rate after completion of the 30th robotic cystectomy.[15] Given the overall poor prognosis of PSM, obtaining negative soft tissue margins should be paramount regardless of technique.

Periprocedural blood transfusion has been shown to decrease overall and cancer-specific mortality.[15,16] It is also associated with a higher incidence of postoperative complications and ileus.[17] One of the touted benefits of robotic compared with open surgery is lower blood loss as evidenced by a weighted mean difference of 300 mL less blood loss per case with RARC (−159 mL to −499 mL).[4–7] This has ranged between studies from no difference in rate of transfusion[6] to 77% reduced odds for blood transfusion between ORC and RARC.[32] A cumulative analysis that looked at 105 papers found transfusion rates of 12% for RARC with extracorporeal conduit versus 14.7% with intracorporeal conduit.[31] Given the decrease in overall and patient-specific survival associated with blood transfusion, attention to hemostasis should be undertaken regardless of approach.

Intracorporeal Diversion

The creation of a UD, regardless of indication, results in most of the significant morbidity that occurs with cystectomy and has been estimated at 11% to 29%.[18–21] All randomized RARC versus ORC trials to date, as well as the anticipated RAZOR trial, included subjects who underwent ECUD. This had caused many proponents of RARC to postulate that extracorporeal diversion negates many of the potential benefits of RARC.[8,9] Proponents of intracorporeal UD (ICUD) cite the potential benefits of a smaller incision, reduction in pain and need for narcotic pain management, improved cosmesis, and decreased bowel exposure, which reduces the risk of fluid imbalances.[3,9,22] Almost all series show an increased operative time with ICUD. The largest consecutive series looked at 100 consecutive RARCs with ICUD and showed that UD in the first quartile took a median of 140 additional minutes to complete, which decreased to a median of 103 additional minutes in the fourth quartile of subjects.[23] The largest analysis of RARC with ICUD versus ECUD included 18 international institutions with 167 subjects undergoing ICUD (106 ileal conduit; 61 neobladder) and 768 ECUD (570 ileal conduit; 198 neobladder).[22] In this large nonrandomized,

retrospective, multicenter, comparative analysis, no significant difference in operative times between the 2 groups was seen, although there was a statistically significant lower transfusion rate (7% vs 16%; $P = .022$) in the ICUD versus the ECUD groups, and lower attributable gastrointestinal complications (10% vs 23%) for the ICUD versus the ECUD groups.[22] Although this is certainly promising, the first multicenter randomized controlled trial (International Robotic Cystectomy Consortium (iROC)) on RARC with ICUD compared with ORC is currently recruiting subjects. It is hoped this trial will answer the question of utility of ICUD.

Surgeon Volume

Just as surgeon and center volume affect intraoperative variables and patient outcomes in ORC,[24,25] the same is true with RARC. The learning curve for RARC has been studied by looking at intraoperative variables of 21 surgeons at 14 institutions during the infancy of RARC, which showed proficiency improving up to 30 cases.[26] Interestingly in this same review, dividing case volume into tertiles of less than 30, 30 to 50, and greater than 50 showed continued improvement in mean operative time (454, 393, 339 minutes, respectively; $P \leq .0001$) and increased lymph node yield.[26] In robotic-assisted prostatectomy, perioperative complications continue to decrease with case volume and plateau after 150 cases with HRQOL metrics improving until after 600 cases.[27,28]

Cost

One randomized trial addressed the cost associated per procedure based on Medicare reimbursement.[6] The study found that subjects who underwent RARC with extracorporeal neobladder generated an average additional cost of $3920 ($P<.0001$), whereas subjects undergoing RARC with ileal conduit generated an additional cost of $1740 ($P<.05$) compared with ORC subjects. When considering the cost of radical cystectomy and perioperative care cited by various institutions, which ranges from $23,451 to greater than $30,000, with cost exponentially increasing with each postoperative complication,[29] these differences are significant but only a fraction of the overall cost of treating muscle invasive bladder cancer.

Technique

The surgical technique for RARC with ICUD or ECUD has been well-described in the literature. Initial descriptions are of cases that used 3 8-mm robotic ports and 1 12-mm camera port.

Additionally, 2 12-mm and 1 5-mm assistant ports are placed. The patient is then placed in the steep Trendelenburg position and the robot is docked. The ureters are then identified and dissected as far as the level of the bladder, proximally and distally. They are then transected distally and clipped on the bladder side. The posterior dissection between the bladder and rectum is performed, followed by lateral dissection to isolate the bladder pedicles. The pedicles are then most commonly taken with an endovascular stapler or thermal sealing device. Next, the bladder is dropped from the anterior abdominal wall. The dorsal venous complex is ligated and the urethra transected. A pelvic lymphadenectomy is then performed.[30]

The ureters are tagged, as well as the terminal ileum. If an orthotopic neobladder is planned, preplaced sutures are placed on the posterior urethra. The robot is then undocked for performance of the ECUD. Ports are removed and a 6-mm to 8-cm incision is made below the umbilicus down to the pubis. The left ureter is passed posterior to the sigmoid for an ileal conduit while the right ureter is passed in the same fashion toward the left for an orthotopic neobladder with left-sided afferent limb. The terminal ileum is identified and harvested. The conduit or neobladder is created and ureteroenteric anastomoses performed. The neobladder to urethra anastomosis is then completed using the preplaced posterior urethral sutures or the stoma is matured for the ileal conduit.

Robotic-assisted intracorporeal conduits may be preferred by some surgeons. A key difference is placement of a 12-mm suprapubic port for bowel reanastomosis after standard RARC and lymph node dissection have been performed. An ileal segment is then harvested using an endovascular stapler via an assistant port. The bowel is tagged to ensure proper anatomic approximation for bowel continuity. Two enterotomies are created in the proximal end of the harvested ileum. The ureter is then prepared for the anastomosis via partial transection and is spatulated. The anastomosis is then begun. A ureteral stent is then placed across the anastomosis before it is completed. The distal ureteral tissue is transected and sent for pathologic evaluation and the anastomosis is finished. This is repeated with the other ureter. Bowel continuity is then achieved via the suprapubic port. The stapler is placed into the enterotomies made in the ileum and fired after opposition of the antimesenteric sides of the bowel. A second stapler is fired across the section of the anastomosis that contains the enterotomies. Finally, the stoma site is opened.

A Forceps is passed into the peritoneum and the distal end of the conduit is externalized and the stoma is matured.[24]

SUMMARY

RARC is a technique gaining wide acceptance as a minimally invasive technique, which seems noninferior to ORC and utilization seems to be increasing yearly. Management of patients with bladder cancer requires a multidisciplinary approach. Cystectomy, whether performed open or robotically, is widely underutilized. The technique applied seems to be only a minor contributor at this time but certainly RARC has the potential to increase cystectomy utilization and to decrease blood loss and, possibly, gastrointestinal complications. Recognition and optimization of comorbid conditions, appropriate staging, timely patient-specific or disease-specific neoadjuvant treatment when indicated, and understanding and instituting care pathways for prevention and early intervention of known complications are all necessary for optimal patient outcomes. Individually and collaboratively, these factors will likely play a larger role in perioperative outcomes when adhering to sound oncologic principles, regardless of technique. RARC does have the potential to continue to evolve, with ICUD possibly reducing gastrointestinal complications, which remains the driver of a sizable proportion of perioperative complications and HRQOL events in this postoperative patient population.

REFERENCES

1. Menon M, Hemal AK, Tewari A, et al. Nerve-sparing robotic-assisted radical cystoprostatectomy and urinary diversion. BJU Int 2003;92(3):232–6.
2. Sánchez de Badajoz E, Gallego Perales JL, Reche Rosado A, et al. Laparoscopic cystectomy and ileal conduit: case report. J Endourol 1995;9(1):59–62.
3. Gill IS, Fergany A, Klein EA, et al. Laparoscopic radical cystoprostatectomy with ileal conduit performed completely intracorporeally: the initial 2 cases. Urology 2000;56(1):26–9 [discussion: 29–30].
4. Nix J, Smith A, Kurpad R, et al. Prospective randomized controlled trial of robotic versus open radical cystectomy for bladder cancer: perioperative and pathologic results. Eur Urol 2010;57(2):196–201.
5. Khan MS, Gan C, Ahmed K, et al. A single-centre early phase randomised controlled three-arm trial of open, robotic, and laparoscopic radical cystectomy (CORAL). Eur Urol 2016;69(4):613–21.

6. Bochner BH, Dalbagni G, Sjoberg DD, et al. Comparing open radical cystectomy and robot-assisted laparoscopic radical cystectomy: a randomized clinical trial. Eur Urol 2015;67(6):1042–50.

7. Parekh DJ, Messer J, Fitzgerald J, et al. Perioperative outcomes and oncologic efficacy from a pilot prospective randomized clinical trial of open versus robotic assisted radical cystectomy. J Urol 2013; 189(2):474–9.

8. Tang J-Q, Zhao Z, Liang Y, et al. Robotic-assisted versus open radical cystectomy in bladder cancer: a meta-analysis of four randomized controlled trails. Int J Med Robot 2017. https://doi.org/10.1002/rcs.1867.

9. Tan WS, Khetrapal P, Tan WP, et al. Robotic assisted radical cystectomy with extracorporeal urinary diversion does not show a benefit over open radical cystectomy: a systematic review and meta-analysis of randomised controlled trials. PLoS One 2016; 11(11):e0166221.

10. Leow JJ, Reese SW, Jiang W, et al. Propensity-matched comparison of morbidity and costs of open and robotic-assisted radical cystectomies: a contemporary population-based analysis in the United States. Eur Urol 2014;66(3):569–76.

11. Bachman AG, Parker AA, Shaw MD, et al. Minimally invasive versus open approach for cystectomy: trends in the utilization and demographic or clinical predictors using the national cancer database. Urology 2017;103:99–105.

12. Tan WS, Lamb BW, Kelly JD. Evolution of the neobladder: a critical review of open and intracorporeal neobladder reconstruction techniques. Scand J Urol 2016;50(2):95–103.

13. Smith ND, Castle EP, Gonzalgo ML, et al. The RAZOR (randomized open vs robotic cystectomy) trial: study design and trial update: the RAZOR trial. BJU Int 2015;115(2):198–205.

14. Novara G, Svatek RS, Karakiewicz PI, et al. Soft tissue surgical margin status is a powerful predictor of outcomes after radical cystectomy: a multicenter study of more than 4,400 patients. J Urol 2010; 183(6):2165–70.

15. Cata JP, Lasala J, Pratt G, et al. Association between perioperative blood transfusions and clinical outcomes in patients undergoing bladder cancer surgery: a systematic review and meta-analysis study. J Blood Transfus 2016;2016. https://doi.org/10.1155/2016/9876394.

16. Chalfin HJ, Liu J-J, Gandhi N, et al. Blood transfusion is associated with increased perioperative morbidity and adverse oncologic outcomes in bladder cancer patients receiving neoadjuvant chemotherapy and radical cystectomy. Ann Surg Oncol 2016;23(8):2715–22.

17. Chang SS, Cookson MS, Baumgartner RG, et al. Analysis of early complications after radical cystectomy: results of a collaborative care pathway. J Urol 2002;167(5):2012–6.

18. Osborn DJ, Dmochowski RR, Kaufman MR, et al. Cystectomy with urinary diversion for benign disease: indications and outcomes. Urology 2014;83(6): 1433–7.

19. Brown KGM, Solomon MJ, Latif ER, et al. Urological complications after cystectomy as part of pelvic exenteration are higher than that after cystectomy for primary bladder malignancy. J Surg Oncol 2017;115(3):307–11.

20. van Hemelrijck M, Thorstenson A, Smith P, et al. Risk of in-hospital complications after radical cystectomy for urinary bladder carcinoma: population-based follow-up study of 7608 patients. BJU Int 2013; 112(8):1113–20.

21. Shabsigh A, Korets R, Vora KC, et al. Defining early morbidity of radical cystectomy for patients with bladder cancer using a standardized reporting methodology. Eur Urol 2009;55(1):164–74.

22. Ahmed K, Khan SA, Hayn MH, et al. Analysis of intracorporeal compared with extracorporeal urinary diversion after robotic-assisted radical cystectomy: results from the International Robotic Cystectomy Consortium. Eur Urol 2014;65(2): 340–7.

23. Azzouni FS, Din R, Rehman S, et al. The first 100 consecutive, robotic-assisted, intracorporeal ileal conduits: evolution of technique and 90-day outcomes. Eur Urol 2013;63(4):637–43.

24. Leow JJ, Reese S, Trinh Q-D, et al. Impact of surgeon volume on the morbidity and costs of radical cystectomy in the USA: a contemporary population-based analysis. BJU Int 2015;115(5): 713–21.

25. Elting LS, Pettaway C, Bekele BN, et al. Correlation between annual volume of cystectomy, professional staffing, and outcomes: a statewide, population-based study. Cancer 2005;104(5): 975–84.

26. Hayn MH, Hussain A, Mansour AM, et al. The learning curve of robotic-assisted radical cystectomy: results from the International Robotic Cystectomy Consortium. Eur Urol 2010;58(2): 197–202.

27. Thompson JE, Egger S, Böhm M, et al. Superior quality of life and improved surgical margins are achievable with robotic radical prostatectomy after a long learning curve: a prospective single-surgeon study of 1552 consecutive cases. Eur Urol 2014;65(3):521–31.

28. Ou Y-C, Yang C-R, Wang J, et al. The learning curve for reducing complications of robotic-assisted laparoscopic radical prostatectomy by a single surgeon. BJU Int 2011;108(3):420–5.

29. Svatek RS, Hollenbeck BK, Holmäng S, et al. The economics of bladder cancer: costs and

considerations of caring for this disease. Eur Urol 2014;66(2):253–62.

30. Novara G, Catto JWF, Wilson T, et al. Systematic review and cumulative analysis of perioperative outcomes and complications after robotic-assisted radical cystectomy. Eur Urol 2015;67(3): 376–401.

31. Novara G, Catto JWF, Wilson T, et al. Systematic Review and Cumulative Analysis of Perioperative Outcomes and Complications After Robotic-assisted Radical Cystectomy. Eur Urol 2015;67(3):376–401.

32. Pruthi RS, Wallen EM. Robotic-Assisted Laparoscopic Radical Cystoprostatectomy. Eur Urol 2008; 53(2):310–22.

Robotic Nephroureterectomy

Benjamin L. Taylor, MD, Douglas S. Scherr, MD*

KEYWORDS

- Upper tract urothelial carcinoma • Nephroureterectomy • Robotic • Minimally invasive
- Distal ureterectomy

KEY POINTS

- With improved technology, robotic nephroureterectomy with excision of the bladder cuff has become a preferred approach for many institutions.
- Both single-docking and 2-docking approaches are safe and feasible; however, single-docking seems to significantly shorten the operative time.
- Perioperative outcomes for the robotic approach are comparable with laparoscopic and superior to open approaches.
- Although limited to observational studies, oncologic outcomes seem similar between all modalities.

INTRODUCTION

Among all new cancer diagnoses in 2017, upper tract urothelial carcinoma (UTUC) is estimated to account for 3% and 5% of new diagnoses in women and men, respectively.[1] Although UTUC makes up a small percent of all cancer diagnoses, there is controversy over how best to operatively manage patients, in particular when the decision to perform a nephroureterectomy (NU) is made. NU via an open approach (ONU) with bladder cuff excision has been the gold standard treatment for which all new techniques are compared.[2]

The evolution from ONU began in 1991 when laparoscopic NU (LNU) was first described.[3] Since that time, several comparative studies have demonstrated oncologic equivalence and superior perioperative results, such as length of stay, blood loss, decreased complications, convalescence, and pain with LNU.[4,5] The trend toward robotic surgery began in 2001 when the first robotic-assisted nephrectomy was described.[6] Several

years later, a robotic-assisted bilateral heminephroureterectomy was described[7]; since then the use of robotic surgery has only continued to increase.

The adoption of robotic surgery has likely been rapid and heavily marketed for various reasons. In addition to falling under the umbrella of minimally invasive surgery, compared with LNU there are extra degrees of freedom as well as technically easier isolation of the distal ureter and bladder closure with articulation of the robotic wrists.[8] When a lymph node dissection is performed, the robot can facilitate dissection around the great vessels as well as provide 3-dimensional magnified vision. There is also an improved learning curve for various surgeries. For example, the learning curve for open radical prostatectomy ranges from 250 to 1000 cases and laparoscopic radical prostatectomy ranges from 200 to 750 cases; however, the learning curve for robot-assisted laparoscopic prostatectomy has been reported to be a few as 40 cases.[9] Robot-assisted

Conflicts of Interest: D.S. Scherr and B.L. Taylor receive financial support from The Frederick J. and Theresa Dow Wallace Fund of the New York Community Trust.
Department of Urology, Weill Cornell Medical College–New York Presbyterian, 525 East 68th Street, Star Pavilion, New York, NY 10065, USA
* Corresponding author.
E-mail address: dss2001@med.cornell.edu

Urol Clin N Am 45 (2018) 189–197
https://doi.org/10.1016/j.ucl.2017.12.004

radical cystectomy has a learning curve between 16 and 30 cases.[9] There is variation in the literature on how to define proficiency and what variables constitute proficiency at each procedure[10]; however, the use of surgical simulation does seem to play a role in expediting the time to proficiency.[11]

Although high-quality evidence supporting robotic NU (RNU) over ONU or LNU are lacking, this has not prevented the rapid adoption of RNU as a treatment of UTUC. A recent study using the National Cancer Database from 2010 to 2013 found that the utilization of RNU increased from 14% to 30%, whereas ONU decreased from 42.3% to 28.6%.[12] RNU was also associated with lower positive surgical margin rates and no difference in overall survival after controlling for tumor characteristics. With widespread availability of the robotic platform, increased utilization at training centers for other genitourinary cancers, and an increased focus on minimizing surgical morbidity and hospital stay, these trends suggest urologists are able to respect oncologic principles while potentially improving patient care.

ONCOLOGIC PRINCIPLES

With the evolution in technology, there is often a natural tension between improving surgical morbidity while not violating basic oncologic principles. According to the latest iteration of the European Association of Urology's (EAU) guidelines, these principles include removing the kidney and ureter en bloc with the bladder cuff, avoiding entering the urinary tract, avoiding direct contact between instruments and tumor, avoiding morcellation of the tumor, and, because of the concern for tumor spillage, avoiding performing minimally invasive NU for invasive or large (T3/T4, N+/M+) tumors.[2] This final recommendation is largely based on 2 things: minimal long-term LNU and RNU outcomes and reports of trocar site metastasis from manipulation[13,14] or tumor seeding with pneumoperitoneum.[15] However, as longer-term data begin to mature, operating on advanced-stage UTUC via minimally invasive approaches may become a more acceptable approach.

TECHNIQUE

A variety of techniques have evolved since the advent of RNU. Early reports often used 2 different modalities whereby the nephrectomy and ureteral dissection were performed robotically and the bladder cuff was performed open or laparoscopically.[16] The development of a hybrid port technique[16] or combination of 5 to 6 ports[17] allowed for the surgeon to perform the entire procedure robotically. Some describe using a 2-dock technique whereby patients are repositioned and the robot is redocked to maximize the working space in 2 distinct parts of the body.[18] Although it has been reported that redraping and redocking the robot can add up to 50 minutes of additional operative time,[19] redocking the robot with a skilled robotics team can be done in less than 10 minutes.[20] Others have reported single-docking techniques to eliminate redocking and repositioning altogether.[21,22] Here, the authors describe their preferred method to performing RNU with excision of the bladder cuff using a single-dock approach.

Positioning

The patients are positioned with a 45° bump using 2 sandbags, one cephalad to the break in the bed and one caudal to the break. The contralateral arm is placed on an arm board extended perpendicular to the bed while the ipsilateral arm is folded over the chest on 2 folded blankets for support. An axillary role is used based on the patients' body habitus and in consultation with the anesthesiologists, and the bed is put in slight flexion. The chest and hips are secured with surgical towels, foam, and 2-in silk tape (**Fig. 1**). The bed is rotated in both directions to ensure the patients are secure on the table.

Port Placement

Pneumoperitoneum is established using a Veress needle. At the authors' institution, the Robotic Surgical System allows more versatility for single-docking

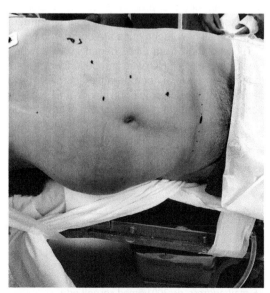

Fig. 1. Positioning for a left-sided RNU in modified flank position.

during both parts of the operation. The surgeons have experimented with various port placement configurations and found success with the linear configuration (**Fig. 2**). With this configuration, it is thought to be easier to perform both parts of the operation without changing the camera or redocking the robot[23] (**Fig. 3**). However, if the patients' body habitus is severely prohibitive (ie very tall, morbidly obese, contractures prohibiting optimal port placement), the surgeon can alternatively position patients in the modified lithotomy position, place ports similar to a robotic prostatectomy configuration, and perform the distal ureterectomy portion first. Next, patients can be repositioned and additional ports can be placed to perform the nephrectomy portion of the surgery robotically or laparoscopically. Others have described single-docking techniques whereby a port is placed lateral to the camera port below the lower pole of the kidney with only 3 robotic ports placed along the paramedian line.[24] Once the ports are placed, the robot is brought in perpendicular to patients from the ipsilateral side of the tumor. A 0° lens is used for the entirety of the case and is targeted between the kidney and the bladder to allow for maximum range of motion without needing to retarget.

Development of the Retroperitoneal Space

The first step of the operation is incising the peritoneum along the white line of Toldt from the hepatic flexure on the right or splenic flexure on the left to the iliac vessels. This incision just lateral to the colon allows reflection of the colon medially with further dissection of the renocolic ligaments (**Fig. 4**). Importantly, the lateral attachments of the Gerota fascia should remain intact so the kidney does not flop medially and lose its natural counter tension. Next, the dissection is extended cephalad to the level of the adrenal glands and caudad to the iliac vessels. Exposing the great vessels medially by mobilizing the mesocolon

aids in quickly identifying the ureter and renal hilum and facilitates the potential lymph node dissection later.

Deciding What to do Next

At the authors' institution, the distal ureterectomy and bladder cuff are performed before the nephrectomy for several reasons. First, there is a natural tension on the ureter that is lost when the kidney is mobilized, and this tension is particularly useful during the dissection of the distal ureter along the plane of the Waldeyer sheath (**Fig. 5**). Second, for ureteral and upper tract tumors, manipulation of the kidney and proximal ureter can theoretically shed tumor cells. By limiting the dissection to the distal ureter initially, a clip can be placed on the distal extent of the ureter, thus, preventing tumor spillage and seeding with manipulation. The subsequent mild hydrodistension does not prohibit range of movement or make the operation more technically challenging.

Distal Ureterectomy

Over the last several decades, and with the advent of laparoscopic and robotic surgery, many institutions have described nuanced approaches to managing the distal ureter.[25] This article focuses on minimally invasive approaches to the distal ureter. Most approaches start with extending the peritoneal incision distally deep into the pelvis. The landmarks the surgeon should aim for is the bladder medially and the medial umbilical ligament laterally. The round ligament in women, or vas deferens in men, may be ligated if needed for exposure. In women, it is often unnecessary to cut the infundibulopelvic ligament or remove the ipsilateral ovary to access the distal ureter. The ureter can be identified at the bifurcation of the common iliac or between the bladder and medial umbilical ligament. To gain better exposure of the intramural ureter, the superior vesical artery and ipsilateral

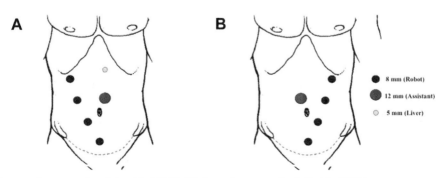

A

B

8 mm (Robot)
12 mm (Assistant)
5 mm (Liver)

Fig. 2. (*A*) Port placement for right-sided RNU. (*B*) Port placement for left-sided RNU.

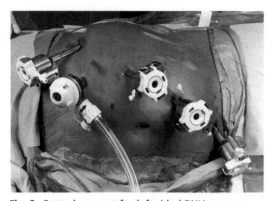

Fig. 3. Port placement for left-sided RNU.

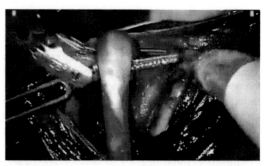

Fig. 5. Retraction of the ureter after identification.

anterior bladder pedicle can be ligated, which allows medial rotation of the bladder (**Fig. 6**). Once the ureter is completely mobilized distally (**Fig. 7**), there are numerous ways to manage the bladder cuff with each approach having its own risks and benefits[26] as well as surgeon preference. The surgeon can make a circumferential incision extravesically,[19] insert transvesical ports and laparoscopically excise the ureteral orifice,[27] staple the distal ureter and bladder cuff,[28] perform the Pluck technique by detaching the intramural ureter cystoscopically before the NU,[29] or use ureteric intussusception/ureteric stripping by splitting the ureter and removing the distal ureter via the cystoscope.[30–32] The concern with the aforementioned approaches is that they are technically challenging, not easily reproducible, require repositioning, and add more operative time, compromise oncologic principles, or do not allow for en bloc removal of the specimen while minimizing tumor seeding.

The authors' preferred technique is to combine the intravesical and extravesical approach as has been previously described.[33] This approach ensures careful identification of the contralateral ureteral orifice and complete excision of the

intramural ureter while minimizing tumor seeding. The bladder is filled with 240 mL of sterile saline, and a transverse cystotomy is made at the dome of the bladder (**Fig. 8**). The ureteral orifice is scored circumferentially with monopolar scissors (**Fig. 9**). Using a combination of blunt dissection with the fenestrated forceps and electrocautery with the scissors, the periureteral sheath is exposed until the intravesical dissection plane meets with the extravesical plane. Once freed, a Interlocking surgical clip is placed on the distal ureter to prevent tumor spillage. The ureter is then delivered into the extravesical space.

Two-Layer Closure

Closure of the ureteral hiatus and cystotomy are both performed in 2 layers. First, the ureteral hiatus is closed intravesically (**Fig. 10**). An interrupted 2-0 polyglactin 910 suture incorporating seromuscular tissue followed by a running 2-0 polyglactin 910 mucosal layer completes the closure of the hiatus. The cystotomy is closed with a running 0 polyglactin 910 suture incorporating detrusor and mucosa reinforced by a second interrupted 0 polyglactin 910 serosal layer (**Fig. 11**). A Foley catheter is placed, and the bladder is instilled with 300 mL of sterile saline to ensure a watertight closure. The catheter is removed in 7 days after a negative cystogram. One dose of mitomycin C is instilled in

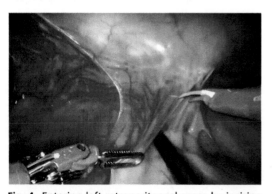

Fig. 4. Entering left retroperitoneal space by incising the white line of Toldt.

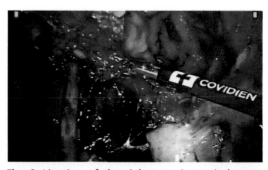

Fig. 6. Ligation of the right superior vesical artery with the Electrocautery vessel sealing device.

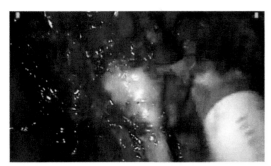

Fig. 7. Complete exposure of the distal ureter with eversion of the bladder mucosa.

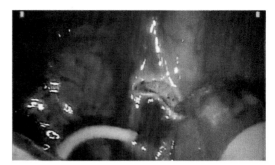

Fig. 9. Intravesical dissection of the ureteral orifice.

the bladder at the time of catheter removal, as supported by level 1 data.[34] O'Brien and colleagues[34] randomized 284 patients in a multi-institutional study to receive either a postoperative dose of intravesical mitomycin at the time of catheter removal or standard management. Patients receiving intravesical mitomycin had an absolute reduction in the risk of recurrence by 11%, and the number needed to treat to prevent one recurrence was 9. It is unclear at this time whether the use of gemcitabine intravesically (which carries significantly less toxicity) can be used in a similar fashion. However, data do support the use of an intravesical agent instilled into the bladder after catheter removal.

Nephrectomy

Right

During port placement, a 5-mm subxiphoid port is placed where a grasper can be used to gently retract the liver cephalad and hold the lateral abdominal wall. After the colon and mesentery have been medialized as described earlier, a Kocher maneuver is necessary to medially deflect the duodenum. Using a combination of sharp and blunt dissection, the duodenum is mobilized until there is exposure of the inferior vena cava (IVC).

Left

During left-sided cases, the pancreatic tail is mobilized away from the kidney. Caution should be taken with the medialized fat adjacent to the pancreas, as this is where the splenic vein or artery may be identified. More cephalad, the splenorenal ligament is divided to minimize injury to the spleen during manipulation of the kidney and upper pole.

Renal Hilum

Next, attention is directed to the lower pole of the kidney where the ureter and gonadal vein are identified. Once the ureter is isolated, attempts should be made to keep sufficient periureteral fat with the ureter if there is invasive tumor in this location. The plane between the fat of the lower pole of the kidney and the belly of the psoas muscle is developed, and the fourth robotic arm is used to elevate the kidney anterior and slightly lateral. Of note, on the right side, the ureter is elevated while the gonadal vein is dropped to minimize the risk of avulsing the gonadal vein from the IVC. On the left side, the gonadal vein is elevated and traced to its location into the left renal vein. With upward tension on the kidney, the renal hilum is identified (**Fig. 12**). The vessels are exposed using a combination of blunt and sharp dissection. If necessary, the left gonadal vein can be ligated using bipolar electrocautery or clips to allow better isolation of

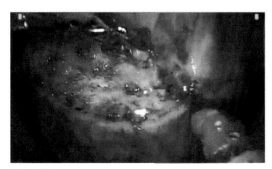

Fig. 8. Transverse cystotomy.

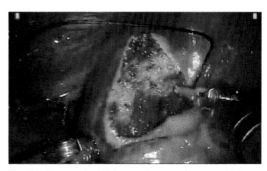

Fig. 10. Intravesical 2-layer closure of ureteral hiatus.

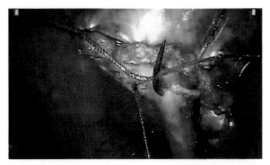

Fig. 11. Extravesical 2-layer closure of the cystotomy.

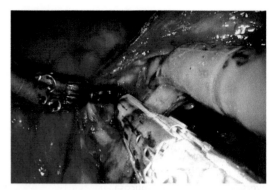

Fig. 13. Identification of left adrenal vein with distal stapling.

the renal vein. To aid in subsequent lymph node dissection, one can dissect along the renal artery and vein proximally to where they enter into the aorta and IVC, respectively. The adrenal vein can be visualized entering the left renal vein and should be preserved, as this is often an adrenal-sparing surgery (**Fig. 13**). Next, the renal artery and vein are each ligated and divided with the use of a stapling device with a vascular load.

Lymph Node Dissection

Retroperitoneal lymph node dissection is further discussed in a separate supplement. Briefly, at the authors' institution, for left renal pelvic and upper ureteral tumors, the surgeons perform a lymph node dissection that includes para-aortic and pre-aortic nodes caudally to the bifurcation of the aorta. For right renal pelvic and upper ureteral tumors, the adjacent hilar, para-caval, and interaortocaval nodal packets are removed. Although controversial, for distal ureteral tumors, the authors perform an ipsilateral pelvic lymph node dissection for prognostic and potentially therapeutic purposes. A recent systematic review demonstrated improved cancer-specific survival and risk of recurrence for subjects who underwent lymph node dissection for a pT2 or greater

UTUC,[35] and this is consistent with other studies showing a survival benefit for more extensive lymph node dissections.[36,37]

Specimen Extraction

There are many factors, including patient habitus and surgeon preference, that dictate the optimal tumor extraction location. An attempt to extract the specimen using one of the previously made skin incisions seems ideal; however, larger specimens may ultimately require a sizable incision to accommodate the kidney and ureter. At the authors' institution, if the specimen is a smaller size, the surgeons may extend the periumbilical assistant port incision caudally. For larger specimens, or for patients concerned with cosmesis, a Pfannenstiel incision is made. This technique, described by Binsaleh and colleagues,[38] includes making a transverse Pfannenstiel incision in a skin crease above the pubic symphysis. Once the dermis is dissected, a transverse incision is made in the anterior rectus fascia. The superior leaflet of the aponeurosis is held on tension and is sharply separated off the rectus bellies. Next, the rectus bellies are separated in the midline, the peritoneum is sharply entered, and the specimen is extracted intact in the bag. The investigators randomized this technique with extending a port site incision and found that there was less morbidity, pain, and shorter hospital stay with a Pfannenstiel incision without a difference in operative time. The slow adoption of this technique has likely been attributed to the concern for pain from an additional incision and increased operative time.[39]

OUTCOMES

RNU has been demonstrated for more than a decade to be a feasible method of surgical extirpation for UTUC. However, data supporting

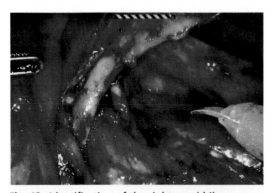

Fig. 12. Identification of the right renal hilum.

perioperative and oncologic outcomes are limited to mainly observational studies. Although robust long-term data for RNU are lacking, the current data support that perioperative outcomes are superior to ONU and oncologic outcomes seem comparable.

Perioperative

Operative time

The most commonly described perioperative outcomes for NU include operative time (OT), estimated blood loss (EBL), and hospital length of stay (LOS). Generally, LNU has shown superior perioperative outcomes compared with ONU, and this has been reinforced with RNU data. In the only randomized controlled trial (RCT) to date comparing ONU with LNU, Simone and colleagues[5] randomized 40 patients to ONU and 40 patients to LNU, which showed that EBL and LOS were significantly less for LNU.

OT can be influenced by several factors, including how the distal ureter and bladder cuff are managed, year of surgery, type of robot used, and whether patients were repositioned and the robot was redocked. The average OT reported ranges from as short as 184 minutes[21] for a single-dock approach to 326 minutes[18] for multiple positioning and docking approaches. Other investigators who redock the robot report mean operative times of 251 minutes[40] and 303 minutes.[41] For investigators who perform laparoscopic nephrectomy followed by robotic distal ureterectomy, operative times were 261 minutes on average.[33] The largest series that included both patients treated via single docking and multiple docking found an average OT of 247 minutes.[42] Although these times are comparable with the open approach, no studies to date have directly compared the 2 approaches.

Estimated blood loss

There is overlap among the reported EBL between ONU, LNU, and RNU; however, RNU seems to have a clear advantage to reported EBL over the former approaches. Reported average EBL for RNU range from 50 mL[40] to 284 mL.[43] This finding compares favorably to ONU whereby the reported average EBL is between 300 mL[44] and 700 mL[45] and EBL for LNU ranges from 104 mL[5] and in the 300-mL range.[46–51]

Length of stay

Lastly, the average LOS for RNU ranges from less than 3 days[21,41] to more than 5 days.[40,43] In an assessment of costs and perioperative outcomes for RNU and LNU using the US Healthcare Cost and Utilization Project Nationwide Inpatient Sample, Trudeau and colleagues found a mean LOS of 5.83 and 5.6 days for LNU and RNU, respectively. Compared with ONU whereby the average LOS ranges from 5 days[52] to more than 21 days,[53] LNU and RNU both consistently show superior outcomes.

Oncologic

There are comparative studies and one RCT that have demonstrated equal oncologic safety between ONU and LNU. Although there are few comparative studies that include RNU, the current body of literature suggests similar oncologic outcomes between RNU and LNU.[12,17] With a 45-month follow-up, Lim and colleagues[17] showed 2- and 5-year cancer-specific survival and recurrence-free survival of 87.3% and 75.8% and 71.5% and 68.1%, respectively. Aboumohamed and colleagues[54] described their RNU experience whereby more than a third of patients had T3 or greater disease and a median follow-up of 25.1 months. Although the 2- and 5-year cancer-specific survival rates were 92.9% and 69.5%, respectively, the advanced T stage did not seem to affect cancer-specific or recurrence-free survival. In a recent systematic review by Mullen and colleagues[55] comparing ONU versus LNU versus RNU, it was concluded that minimally invasive techniques have superior perioperative results with comparable longer-term oncologic results. However, oncologic findings must be taken with caution, as there are very few high-quality comparative studies in the literature, particularly including robotic surgery.

SUMMARY

Although there has been tremendous enthusiasm and uptake for robotic surgery in the treatment of UTUC, it is important that research standards and conclusions be held to a high standard. To date, there have been few comparative studies and no randomized controlled trials comparing RNU with the gold standard ONU or LNU. This problem is further compounded by the fact that UTUC is a rare disease; thus, most institutions report small numbers of patients. However, with the publication of numerous institutional experiences, it has become clear that RNU offers similar, if not slightly improved, perioperative outcomes compared with LNU. Robust long-term oncologic data are lacking for RNU, but observational studies to date suggest similar outcomes to its open and laparoscopic counterparts. As long-term data mature and high-quality evidence demonstrates improved safety, tolerability, and noninferior oncologic outcomes to ONU or LNU, it is expected that future guidelines will reflect this as a new gold standard. Nevertheless, similar to other urologic malignancies, robotic surgery will likely become the preferred surgical procedure for NU as more institutions adopt this approach.

REFERENCES

1. Siegel RL, Miller KD, Jemal A. Cancer statistics, 2017. CA Cancer J Clin 2017;67:7–30.
2. Rouprêt M, Babjuk M, Comperat E, et al. European Association of Urology guidelines on upper urinary tract urothelial carcinoma. Eur Urol 2018; 73(1):111–22.
3. Clayman RV, Kavoussi LR, Figenshau RS, et al. Laparoscopic nephroureterectomy: initial clinical case report. J Laparoendosc Surg 1991;1:343–9.
4. Ni S, Tao W, Chen Q, et al. Laparoscopic versus open nephroureterectomy for the treatment of upper urinary tract urothelial carcinoma: a systematic review and cumulative analysis of comparative studies. Eur Urol 2012;61:1142–53.
5. Simone G, Papalia R, Guaglianone S, et al. Laparoscopic versus open nephroureterectomy: perioperative and oncologic outcomes from a randomised prospective study. Eur Urol 2009;56: 520–6.
6. Guillonneau B, Jayet C, Tewari A, et al. Robot assisted laparoscopic nephrectomy. J Urol 2001;166: 200–1.
7. Pedraza R, Palmer L, Moss V, et al. Bilateral robotic assisted laparoscopic heminephroureterectomy. J Urol 2004;171:2394–5.
8. Autorino R, Zargar H, Kaouk JH. Robotic-assisted laparoscopic surgery: recent advances in urology. Fertil Steril 2014;102:939–49.
9. Abboudi H, Khan MS, Guru KA, et al. Learning curves for urological procedures: a systematic review. BJU Int 2014;114:617–29.
10. Cook JA, Ramsay CR, Fayers P. Statistical evaluation of learning curve effects in surgical trials. Clin Trials 2004;1:421–7.
11. Aggarwal R, Grantcharov TP, Darzi A. Framework for systematic training and assessment of technical skills. J Am Coll Surg 2007;204:697–705.
12. Rodriguez JF, Packiam VT, Boysen WR, et al. Utilization and outcomes of nephroureterectomy for upper tract urothelial carcinoma by surgical approach. J Endourol 2017;31:661–5.
13. Rouprêt M, Smyth G, Irani J, et al. Oncological risk of laparoscopic surgery in urothelial carcinomas. World J Urol 2009;27:81–8.
14. Ong AM, Bhayani SB, Pavlovich CP. Trocar site recurrence after laparoscopic nephroureterectomy. J Urol 2003;170:1301.
15. Reymond MA, Schneider C, Hohenberger W, et al. The pneumoperitoneum and its role in tumor seeding. Dig Surg 1998;15:105–9.
16. Rose K, Khan S, Godbole H, et al. Robotic assisted retroperitoneoscopic nephroureterectomy – first experience and the hybrid port technique. Int J Clin Pract 2006;60:12–4.
17. Lim SK, Shin T-Y, Kim KH, et al. Intermediate-term outcomes of robot-assisted laparoscopic nephroureterectomy in upper urinary tract urothelial carcinoma. Clin Genitourin Cancer 2013;11:515–21.
18. Eandi JA, Nelson RA, Wilson TG, et al. Oncologic outcomes for complete robot-assisted laparoscopic management of upper-tract transitional cell carcinoma. J Endourol 2010;24:969–75.
19. Park SY, Jeong W, Ham WS, et al. Initial experience of robotic nephroureterectomy: a hybrid-port technique. BJU Int 2009;104:1718–21.
20. Marshall S, Stifelman M. Robot-assisted surgery for the treatment of upper urinary tract urothelial carcinoma. Urol Clin North Am 2014;41:521–37.
21. Hemal AK, Stansel I, Babbar P, et al. Robotic-assisted nephroureterectomy and bladder cuff excision without intraoperative repositioning. Urology 2011; 78:357–64.
22. Lee Z, Cadillo-Chavez R, Lee DI, et al. The technique of single stage pure robotic nephroureterectomy. J Endourol 2013;27:189–95.
23. Zargar H, Krishnan J, Autorino R, et al. Robotic nephroureterectomy: a simplified approach requiring no patient repositioning or robot redocking. Eur Urol 2014;66:769–77.
24. Argun OB, Mourmouris P, Tufek I, et al. Radical nephroureterectomy without patient or port repositioning using the Da Vinci Xi robotic system: initial experience. Urology 2016;92:136–9.
25. Phé V, Cussenot O, Bitker M-O, et al. Does the surgical technique for management of the distal ureter influence the outcome after nephroureterectomy? BJU Int 2011;108:130–8.
26. Stravodimos KG, Komninos C, Kural AR, et al. Distal ureterectomy techniques in laparoscopic and robot-assisted nephroureterectomy: updated review. Urol Ann 2015;7:8–16.
27. Gill IS, Soble JJ, Miller SD, et al. A novel technique for management of the en bloc bladder cuff and distal ureter during laparoscopic nephroureterectomy. J Urol 1999;161:430–4.
28. Matin SF, Gill IS. Recurrence and survival following laparoscopic radical nephroureterectomy with various forms of bladder cuff control. J Urol 2005; 173:395–400.
29. Keeley FX, Tolley DA. Laparoscopic nephroureterectomy: making management of upper-tract transitional-cell carcinoma entirely minimally invasive. J Endourol 1998;12:139–41.
30. Clayman RV, Garske GL, Lange PH. Total nephroureterectomy with ureteral intussusception and transurethral ureteral detachment and pull-through. Urology 1983;21:482–6.

31. Giovansili B, Peyromaure M, Saïghi D, et al. Stripping technique for endoscopic management of distal ureter during nephroureterectomy: experience of 32 procedures. Urology 2004;64:448–52 [discussion: 452].

32. Laguna MP, la Rosette de JJ. The endoscopic approach to the distal ureter in nephroureterectomy for upper urinary tract tumor. J Urol 2001;166:2017–22.

33. Nanigian DK, Smith W, Ellison LM. Robot-assisted laparoscopic nephroureterectomy. J Endourol 2006;20:463–5 [discussion: 465–6].

34. O'Brien T, Ray E, Singh R, et al. Prevention of bladder tumours after nephroureterectomy for primary upper urinary tract urothelial carcinoma: a prospective, multicentre, randomised clinical trial of a single postoperative intravesical dose of mitomycin C (the ODMIT-C Trial). Eur Urol 2011;60:703–10.

35. Dominguez-Escrig JL, Peyronnet B, Seisen T, et al. Potential benefit of lymph node dissection during radical nephroureterectomy for upper tract urothelial carcinoma: a systematic review by the European Association of Urology guidelines panel on non-muscle-invasive bladder cancer. Eur Urol Focus 2017. [Epub ahead of print].

36. Zareba P, Rosenzweig B, Winer AG, et al. Association between lymph node yield and survival among patients undergoing radical nephroureterectomy for urothelial carcinoma of the upper tract. Cancer 2017;123:1741–50.

37. Lenis AT, Donin NM, Faiena I, et al. Role of surgical approach on lymph node dissection yield and survival in patients with upper tract urothelial carcinoma. Urol Oncol 2017. [Epub ahead of print].

38. Binsaleh S, Madbouly K, Matsumoto ED, et al. A prospective randomized study of Pfannenstiel versus expanded port site incision for intact specimen extraction in laparoscopic radical nephrectomy. J Endourol 2015;29:913–8.

39. Cadeddu JA. Re: a prospective randomized study of Pfannenstiel versus expanded port site incision for intact specimen extraction in laparoscopic radical nephrectomy. J Urol 2016;195:901–2.

40. Yang C-K, Chung S-D, Hung S-F, et al. Robot-assisted nephroureterectomy for upper tract urothelial carcinoma: the Taiwan Robot Urological Surgery Team (TRUST) experience. World J Surg Oncol 2014;12:219.

41. Hu JC, Silletti JP, Williams SB. Initial experience with robot-assisted minimally-invasive nephroureterectomy. J Endourol 2008;22:699–704.

42. Pugh J, Parekattil S, Willis D, et al. Perioperative outcomes of robot-assisted nephroureterectomy for upper urinary tract urothelial carcinoma: a multi-institutional series. BJU Int 2013;112:E295–300.

43. Lim SK, Shin T-Y, Kim KH, et al. Laparoendoscopic single-site (LESS) robot-assisted nephroureterectomy: comparison with conventional multiport technique in the management of upper urinary tract urothelial carcinoma. BJU Int 2014;114:90–7.

44. Nakashima K, Fujiyama C, Tokuda Y, et al. Oncologic assessment of hand-assisted retroperitoneoscopic nephroureterectomy for urothelial tumors of the upper tract: comparison with conventional open nephroureterectomy. J Endourol 2007;21:583–8.

45. Gill IS, Sung GT, Hobart MG, et al. Laparoscopic radical nephroureterectomy for upper tract transitional cell carcinoma: the Cleveland Clinic experience. J Urol 2000;164:1513–22.

46. Hemal AK, Kumar A, Gupta NP, et al. Retroperitoneal nephroureterectomy with excision of cuff of the bladder for upper urinary tract transitional cell carcinoma: comparison of laparoscopic and open surgery with long-term follow-up. World J Urol 2008;26:381–6.

47. Hattori R, Yoshino Y, Gotoh M, et al. Laparoscopic nephroureterectomy for transitional cell carcinoma of renal pelvis and ureter: Nagoya experience. Urology 2006;67:701–5.

48. Muntener M, Nielsen ME, Romero FR, et al. Long-term oncologic outcome after laparoscopic radical nephroureterectomy for upper tract transitional cell carcinoma. Eur Urol 2007;51:1639–44.

49. Shiong Lee L, Yip SKH, Hong Tan Y, et al. Laparoscopic nephroureterectomy for upper urinary tract transitional cell carcinoma. Scand J Urol Nephrol 2006;40:283–8.

50. Tsujihata M, Nonomura N, Tsujimura A, et al. Laparoscopic nephroureterectomy for upper tract transitional cell carcinoma: comparison of laparoscopic and open surgery. Eur Urol 2006;49:332–6.

51. Yoshino Y, Ono Y, Hattori R, et al. Retroperitoneoscopic nephroureterectomy for transitional cell carcinoma of the renal pelvis and ureter: Nagoya experience. Urology 2003;61:533–8.

52. Seifman BD, Montie JE, Wolf JS. Prospective comparison between hand-assisted laparoscopic and open surgical nephroureterectomy for urothelial cell carcinoma. Urology 2001;57:133–7.

53. Kawauchi A, Fujito A, Ukimura O, et al. Hand assisted retroperitoneoscopic nephroureterectomy: comparison with the open procedure. J Urol 2003;169:890–4 [discussion: 894].

54. Aboumohamed AA, Krane LS, Hemal AK. Oncologic outcomes following robot-assisted laparoscopic nephroureterectomy with bladder cuff excision for upper tract urothelial carcinoma. J Urol 2015;194:1561–6.

55. Mullen E, Ahmed K, Challacombe B. Systematic review of open versus laparoscopic versus robot-assisted nephroureterectomy. Rev Urol 2017;19:32–43.

Role and Indications of Organ-Sparing "Radical" Cystectomy
The Importance of Careful Patient Selection and Counseling

Svetlana Avulova, MD*, Sam S. Chang, MD, MBA

KEYWORDS

- Vaginal-sparing cystectomy • Prostate-sparing cystectomy • Sexual function • Urinary function
- Oncology • Radical cystectomy

KEY POINTS

- Possible benefits of organ-sparing cystectomy include preserving sexual function, decreasing urinary incontinence with orthotopic urinary diversion, and decreasing the postoperative complications of fistulas and pelvic organ prolapse.
- Men should undergo prostate cancer screening.
- Both men and women need to undergo careful cancer evaluation and must have ongoing surveillance for urothelial carcinoma recurrence.
- Tumor multifocality, tumor location at the trigone, bladder neck, or prostatic urethra, and/or presence of CIS should exclude patients from organ-sparing cystectomy.

INTRODUCTION

Organ-sparing cystectomy encompasses preservation of genital or pelvic organs in men and women. In men, this may refer to prostate-sparing or seminal vesicle–sparing (SVS) cystectomy and further is distinguished into apical (apex of prostate) or posterior (posterior prostate and seminal vesicles [SV]) sparing (**Fig. 1**). In women, the sparing of pelvic organs includes the uterus, fallopian tubes, ovaries, and the anterior vaginal wall (**Fig. 2**).

The concept of organ-sparing cystectomy was introduced by Spitz and colleagues[1] for management of nonurothelial neoplasms of the bladder in younger and sexually active men to preserve fertility and erectile function, and decrease rates of urinary incontinence with orthotopic urinary diversions. It was not until the early 2000s that several case series were published using this technique in select patients with urothelial malignancies.[2–7] There are several variations of prostate-sparing techniques that exist but the common goal, to preserve the neurovascular bundles, the distal sphincter complex, and the continuity of SV, vasa deferentia, and ejaculatory ducts, is accomplished by incompletely excising the entire prostate and leaving either the prostatic capsule with peripheral zone intact or the distal prostatic tissue including apex and prostatic capsule. Preservation of the posterior prostatic capsule and SV ideally would leave the cavernosal neurovascular bundles undisturbed and decrease

Disclosure: The authors have nothing to disclose.
Department of Urologic Surgery, Vanderbilt University Medical Center, A1302 Medical Center North, Nashville, TN 37203, USA
* Corresponding author.
E-mail address: svetlana.avulova@vanderbilt.edu

urologic.theclinics.com

A

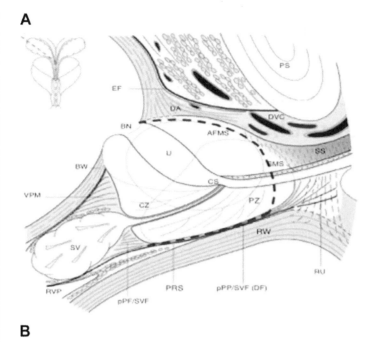

B

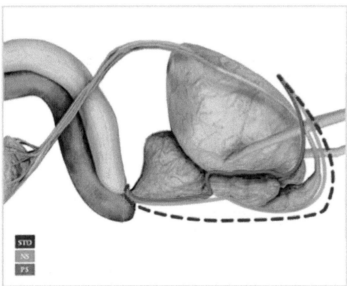

Fig. 1. (A) Midline sagittal section of prostate, bladder, urethra, and striated sphincter. The *dotted line* represents the dissection performed for apical preservation with our technique. AFMS, anterior fibromuscular stroma; BN, bladder neck; CS, colliculus seminalis (verumontanum); CZ, central zone; DA, detrusor apron; DVC, dorsal vascular complex; pPF/SVF, posterior prostatic fascia/seminal vesicle fascia (Denormillers fascia); PS, pubic symphysis; PZ, peripheral zone; RU, rectourethralis muscle; SMS, smooth muscle sphincter (lissosphincter); SS, striated sphincter (rhabdosphincter); U, urethra; VPM, vesicoprostatic muscle. (B) Dissection in standard radical (STD, *red line*), nerve-sparing radical (NS, *blue line*), and potency-sparing (PS, *green line*) cystectomy. In standard version surgical plane is developed over rectum and vascular pedicles are sectioned in proximity to anterior rectal wall. In nerve-sparing procedure same surgical plane is developed but vascular pedicles are sectioned in proximity to bladder wall, seminal vesicles, and prostate to save damage to neurovascular bundles. In potency-sparing technique surgical plane anterior to seminal vesicles is developed, which ends at ejaculatory ducts. Pelvic plexus left completely untouched behind seminal vesicles.

risk of erectile dysfunction, whereas the preservation of the distal sphincter complex would improve continence rates by leaving the external striated sphincter complex undisturbed. Most organ-sparing cystectomy literature has focused on men because correlation to the prostatectomy literature is made in regards to preservation of neurovascular bundles and sexual function outcomes. In 2005, Hautmann and Stein[8] presented a comprehensive review of prostate-sparing cystectomy with neobladder diversion and hypothesized reasons why (at that time) it was a "step in

the wrong direction." In this article, we present an update to this review and comment if and how that view has changed in the last 12 years. We excluded studies with less than 10 patients in a case series.

Organ-sparing cystectomy in women was not really reported until the early 2000s, because adoption of orthotopic urinary diversion in women was slow to catch on due to concern for urethral and local recurrence. However, as studies demonstrated that the urethra could be safely spared in women, interest in organ-sparing cystectomy

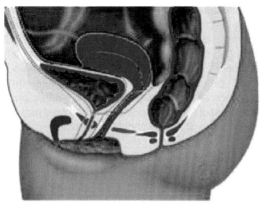

Fig. 2. Lines of resection for organ-preserving (simple; *blue line*), urethra-sparing (*green line*), and radical cystectomy (*red line*).

developed.[9,10] Horenblas and colleagues[11] was the first to prospectively evaluate the outcomes of organ-sparing cystectomy in men and women. Preservation of the anterior vaginal wall, uterus, ovaries, and fallopian tubes can provide suspensory support for an orthotopic neobladder decreasing pelvic organ descent and aiding in the prevention of angulation of the neo vesicourethral anastomosis, which has been implicated as cause of chronic urinary retention that is hypercontinence in women.[12,13] In addition, preservation of the anterior vaginal wall obviates placement of an omental flap to decrease vaginal urinary fistula rate. In sexually active women, preservation of the anterior vaginal wall can also decrease dyspareunia associated with a foreshortened vagina and decreased vaginal lubrication. In this article, we present data on all available case series of female pelvic organ-sparing radical cystectomy either identified as genital organ- or vaginal-sparing cystectomy.

PATIENT SELECTION

Patient-selection criteria for organ-sparing cystectomy in men remains variable (**Table 1**). In general, the following inclusion criteria have been used to select patients for organ sparing during cystectomy: a desire to preserve sexual function and/or fertility, tumor location distant from the bladder neck and trigone, absence of bladder cancer in the prostatic urethra, and negative screening for prostate cancer. Most studies also performed a transurethral biopsy of the prostatic urethra and/or bladder neck to exclude patients who would not be candidates for organ-sparing cystectomy.[14,15,17–21,24–33] Some groups performed a transrectal ultrasound–guided (TRUS) prostate biopsy to exclude concomitant occurrence of prostate cancer.[17,19,28,30–32] Certain studies accepted a normal prostate-specific antigen (PSA) and digital rectal examination (DRE) as a negative screen for prostate cancer.[14–16,24,25] Other studies used PSA free/total ratio of greater than 15% to 20% as a discriminating variable if the PSA was in the 4 to 10 ng/mL range to guide whether a TRUS prostate biopsy was indicated.[21,26,27] Several studies used age as an exclusion criterion.[17,18,21]

In women, the literature aimed at specifically evaluating genital- or vaginal-sparing cystectomy is sparse and all of it is retrospective reviews of case series. Selection criteria may include the

Table 1	
Patient selection criteria	
Men	**Women**
cT2 or less[14–20]	Age 55 or younger[13]
Age[17,18,21]	Performance status[22]
Performance status[21]	Premenopausal status[23]
Negative biopsies of prostatic urethra and/or bladder neck[14,15,17–21,24–33]	Preoperative sexual function[13,23]
PSA <4, normal DRE, normal TRUS and/or PSA free to total ratio >15%[18,21,27]	Manual dexterity to catheterize[22]
Absence of prostate cancer routinely confirmed by TRUS biopsy[17,19,28,30–32]	Absence of CIS[12,22,34]
Preoperative sexual function[15,17–19,21,24,29–31]	Absence of tumor at bladder neck or trigone[12,13,22,23,35]
Preoperative continence[15,19,21,29]	cT2 or less[13,23,35–37]

Abbreviations: CIS, carcinoma in situ; DRE, digital rectal examination; PSA, prostate-specific antigen; TRUS, transrectal ultrasound.

following factors: absence of multifocal disease (eg, carcinoma in situ [CIS]) or involvement of the trigone or bladder neck, organ-confined disease, manual dexterity to be able to self-catheterize (mandatory for any orthotopic diversion), premenopausal and sexually active women, good performance status, and age younger than 55 (see **Table 1**).

ONCOLOGIC FACTORS
Local and Distal Recurrence in Men

One of the main objections to organ-sparing cystectomy is possible oncologic compromise. Previously, a disproportionate increase in distal recurrence (nonregional metastases) without associated local recurrence was reported in men who underwent organ-sparing cystectomy when compared with the radical cystectomy literature.[8] One reason for such discordance is the possibility of hematologic seeding of tumor cells during preoperative transurethral debulking of prostatic adenoma or intraoperative incision of prostatic capsule during organ-sparing cystectomy that may violate tissue planes.

Muto and colleagues[18] reported on a cohort of 91 men who underwent SVS cystectomy (prostate capsule, SV, and vas deferentia are spared) with a mean follow-up of 102 months; the rate of local and distal recurrence was 2.2% and 6.6%, respectively (**Table 2**). These recurrence rates were significantly different from those demonstrated by Mertens and colleagues[28] 2014 cohort of 110 men who underwent prostate-sparing cystectomy with a mean follow-up of 77 months who experienced 10% local and 34.5% distant recurrence rates. They reported that the median time to local and distant recurrence was similar, 11 months and 10.5 months. In 2008, Rozet and colleagues[27] reported on another larger cohort of 106 men who underwent prostate-sparing cystectomy with a mean follow-up of 55 months, and reported similar recurrence rates to Mertens and colleagues[28] of local 4.7% and distant 34%. One possible reason for such discordance in oncologic outcomes is that most men in Muto and colleagues[18] cohort had pathologically low-stage disease (Ta, T1, or CIS) of 89% versus men with T2 or greater of 11%, compared with Mertens and colleagues[28] and Rozet and colleagues[27] (<pT2 37% and 20%, respectively). Muto and colleagues[18] excluded men with clinical stage greater than T2 and he argues that the reason for the higher incidence of distant recurrence compared with his series of men is a lack of rigorous patient selection criteria and clinical understaging. An additional difference between Mertens and colleagues[28] cohort and Rozet and colleagues[27] study is the surgical technique, total prostate sparing versus prostate capsule sparing (PCS) and SV sparing, that men in Rozet and colleagues[27] cohort underwent with an adenomectomy preoperatively, either with transurethral resection of the prostate or simple prostatectomy. Preservation of whole prostate tissue may provide more tissue at risk for local recurrence.

Occult Prostate Cancer

In addition to the potential for increased recurrence of bladder cancer in men, there is a concern for the detection of incidental prostate cancer in patients undergoing prostate-sparing surgery. Previous review of studies demonstrated that the rate of incidental prostate cancer detected in radical cystoprostatectomy specimens is 29% to 46% and clinically significant cancer to be around 20%.[8] In a retrospective review of whole-mount prostates from radical cystoprostatectomy specimens at one institution, Revelo and colleagues[38] demonstrated that 48% of the incidentally detected prostatic adenocarcinoma was clinically significant and that 79% of the clinically significant cancers were detected in the apex. Clinically significant prostate cancer was defined as Gleason 7 or greater, tumor volume greater than 0.5 mL, presence of extraprostatic extension, SV involvement, lymph node positivity, or positive surgical margin (PSM). However, apical cancer was only present in 25% of all detected cancers suggesting that most prostate cancer is present elsewhere.[38]

Further studies have attempted to identify features of incidentally detected prostate cancer in radical cystoprostatectomy specimens with continued attention to apical positivity. Identifying the incidence of apical positivity is paramount to safely offering men prostate-sparing cystectomy. For example, Gakis and colleagues[39] identified a 27% rate of incidental prostate cancer in radical cystoprostatectomy pathology specimens in 95 men with a mean age of 68 and apical involvement of clinically significant prostate cancer in 7.3% of men. Abdelhady and colleagues[40] demonstrated a rate of 28% of incidentally discovered prostate cancer and 12% of apical involvement in 204 men with a mean age of 67. The authors argue that all men who had apical involvement also had multifocal presence of prostate cancer in the proximal part of the prostate and therefore advocate that a prostate-sparing cystectomy is not oncologically safe.[40] However, a causal relationship between apical positivity and clinically significant prostate cancer has never been established.

Table 2
Incidence of local and distant recurrence of urothelial carcinoma and concurrent prostate cancer in prostate-sparing cystectomy series

Author, Year	n	Mean Age, y (Range)	Average/Median Follow-up (mo)	Pathologic Stage ≤T2, %	Local Recurrence, %	Distant Recurrence, %	Prostate Cancer, %
Martis et al,[26] 2005	32	59 (52–72)	32	47	0	0	0
Nieuwenhuijzen et al,[31] 2005	44	57 (NR)	40	70	6.8	29.5	2.2
Wunderlich et al,[32] 2006	31	64 (48–79)	12	84	3	0	0
Davila et al,[24] 2007	18	56 (NR)	NR	76	0	11.7	NR
Simone et al,[14] 2008	20	57 (39–66)	32.5	100	20	30	NR
Rozet et al,[27] 2008	106	62 (NR)	55	59	4.7	34	5
Puppo et al,[21] 2008	37	NR (52–66)	35	97	0	2.7	8.1
de Vries et al,[30] 2009	63	NR (NR)	56	75	8	29	3.2
Thorstenson et al,[29] 2009	25	55 (38–71)	72	88	0	20	16
Ong et al,[15] 2010	31	NR (31–77)	18	68	3	16	42
Dall'Oglio et al,[25] 2010	22	65 (44–80)	60	68	4.5	22	NR
Nour et al,[20] 2011	26	NR (42–79)	43	80	7	30	7
Basiri et al,[16] 2012	23	59 (NR)	39	74	NR	NR	7
Muto et al,[18] 2014	91	53 (34–68)	102	97	2.2	6.6	2.4
Mertens et al,[28] 2014	110	56.2 (NR)	77	76	10	34.5	2.7
Jacobs et al,[19] 2015	20	58 (NR)	12	90	NR	NR	15
Colombo et al,[17] 2015- Capsule sparing	36	48.3 (41–58)	66	89	5.5	NR	0
Colombo et al,[17] 2015- SV sparing	19	53.2 (36–64)	66	95	0	NR	15.8
Chen & Chiang,[33] 2017	14	57.5 (NR)	NR	NR	7	7	NR

Abbreviation: NR, not reported.

Age, however, is a known risk factor for incidentally discovered prostate cancer in radical cystoprostatectomy pathology specimens. For example, Pettus and colleagues[41] reported that occurrence of incidental prostate cancer (45% in a series of 235 men with a median age of 70) was associated only with age in a multivariate model. Similarly, Weizer and colleagues[42] reported that men with occult prostate cancer in the peripheral zone or prostate capsule (n = 15) were older than men without prostate cancer (n = 19) or prostate cancer detected in prostatic adenoma (n = 1; mean age 69 vs 61; P = .01).

One question that still remains is if prostate-sparing cystectomy is considered, are there accurate screening tools that can identify and locate clinically significant prostate cancer. In the past, when sextant TRUS biopsies were routinely done, there was concern that a sextant TRUS biopsy may not be sensitive enough to detect prostate cancer. In fact, a sextant biopsy detects only 12% of any prostate cancer; however, most cancer that was detected was clinically insignificant and 6% of clinically significant prostate cancer was missed.[43] Currently, a 12-core biopsy is recommended as an initial screening biopsy in men with an abnormal DRE or elevated PSA because of a higher cancer detection rate than the sextant biopsy.[44] Previous studies have demonstrated that a 12-core biopsy does not increase detection of clinically insignificant prostate cancer.[45–47] In addition to improved overall cancer detection rate, 12-core biopsies have a greater concordance rate with radical prostatectomy specimens (85.2% agreement with 12-core vs 50% with six-core), which allows for more accurate cancer risk assessment.[48] This suggests that men who are being considered for prostate-sparing cystectomy should at least be screened with a standard 12-core prostate biopsy.

Multiparametric (MP) MRI and TRUS-fusion prostate biopsy have recently been introduced to improve detection of clinically significant prostate cancer. In the recent PROMIS study comparing MP-MRI with a transperineal template prostate biopsy, MP-MRI alone has been shown to have good sensitivity (96%) in detecting clinically significant prostate cancer and high negative predictive value (92%) in ruling out presence of clinically significant prostate cancer.[49] In a different study analyzing the accuracy of MP-MRI targeted ultrasound fusion biopsy, the sensitivity of MP-MRI/ultrasound fusion targeted biopsy in detecting intermediate-/high-risk prostate cancer was 77% compared with whole-mount prostatectomy specimens. Combining MP-MRI/ultrasound fusion targeted biopsy with a standard 12-core biopsy increases the sensitivity to 85%.[50] Routine use of MP-MRI/ultrasound fusion targeted prostate biopsy has not been reported in the prostate-sparing cystectomy literature. However, in the future it may improve patient selection criteria.

The incidence of occult prostate cancer in men who have undergone prostate-sparing cystectomy is significantly lower than in the radical cystoprostatectomy specimens. From a review of recent prostate-sparing cystectomy series, the mean prevalence of occult prostate cancer was 8.4% (range, 0%–42%). The series by Ong and colleagues[15] with the highest reported rate of 42%

only screened men with PSA and DRE and a routine TRUS biopsy was not performed. An argument can be made that a high rate of occult prostate cancer is caused by less rigorous preoperative patient screening and that the reason for lower rates of occult prostate cancer in organ-sparing cystectomy specimen is incomplete resection of peripheral prostate tissue that harbors the cancer. The men in the Ong and colleagues[15] series had SV and prostatic capsule sparing with report of all prostatic tissue surgically resected. However, out of the remaining studies with a prevalence of greater than 10%, all men had preoperative screening with a 12-core TRUS biopsy and the surgical techniques were either SV sparing or prostatic capsule sparing.[17,45,46]

Urothelial Carcinoma Within the Prostate

Regardless of the incidence of occult prostate cancer, untreated prostate cancer is unlikely to impact survival as much as residual/recurrent urothelial carcinoma. Hautmann and Stein[8] reported that the incidence of urothelial carcinoma in the prostate tissue from radical cystoprostatectomy specimens ranged from 29% to 48%. Pettus and colleagues[41] reported a urothelial carcinoma incidence of 33% in 235 men with a median age of 68 whose whole-mount cystoprostatectomy specimens were analyzed. Out of the 77 men who had prostatic urothelial carcinoma, 64% had stromal invasion and 36% had CIS of the prostatic urethra and/or periurethral/peripheral prostatic ducts. On multivariable analysis, preoperative CIS and bladder neck/trigone involvement were significantly associated with occurrence of prostatic urothelial carcinoma, odds ratio (OR) of 6.3 ($P<.001$) and OR of 3.5 ($P = .001$), respectively.[41] In a more updated retrospective review of radical cystoprostatectomy specimens of 96 men with a median age of 67, a total of 25% had prostatic involvement by urothelial carcinoma. Of those men, 25% had CIS only and 75% had deep stromal invasion. On univariate analysis, preoperative presence of CIS (OR, 3.2; $P = .018$) and bladder trigonal involvement (OR, 3.3; $P = .046$) were associated with prostatic involvement by urothelial carcinoma.[51] In both of these studies, the stromal involvement rates of 64% and 75% may significantly impact patients' risk of cancer recurrence and survival.[52]

Therefore accurate screening for prostatic urothelial carcinoma remains a key consideration before performing a prostate-sparing cystectomy. To avoid missing any urothelial carcinoma, most have performed a preoperative transurethral biopsy of the prostatic urethra. A previous study demonstrated, however, that a transurethral biopsy of prostatic urethra might not be a good screening test to exclude prostatic involvement by urothelial carcinoma.[53] The authors retrospectively reviewed 246 men who underwent transurethral loop biopsies of the prostatic urethra and radical cystoprostatectomy and demonstrated that a transurethral biopsy failed to identify prostatic stromal or superficial involvement in 19% of patients. Therefore, patient selection criteria should not only be based on a negative preoperative transurethral prostate biopsy but also include absence of CIS and tumor involvement at the trigone and/or bladder neck.

In addition to recurrence in the prostatic urethra, margin status is a known risk factor for cancer recurrence in standard radical cystoprostatectomy specimens.[54,55] In a retrospective review of 4400 patients (79% men) who did not receive neoadjuvant chemotherapy, PSM was an independent predictor of cancer-specific mortality (hazard ratio, 1.51; $P<.001$).[55] Although the incidence of PSM is low (4.2%–6%), its occurrence can be lethal (5-year disease-specific survival, 26%–32% with PSM vs 69%–72% without PSM).[54,55] In a prostate-sparing cohort, Mertens and colleagues[28] reported a PSM rate of 7.2% and all PSM were present at the prostatic urethra. However, the authors reported that urothelial carcinoma recurrence in the prostate occurred in 1 out of 110 patients and the 5-year disease-specific and overall survival were 66.5% (95% confidence interval, 58.8–75.0) and 64.2% (95% confidence interval, 54.5–72.9).[28] Alternatively, Rozet and colleagues[27] performed intraoperative frozen sections of the prostatic base, distal ureters, and trigone and excluded patients with a positive frozen margin from undergoing prostate-sparing cystectomy. In their cohort, prostatic urothelial carcinoma recurrence occurred in 1 out of 108 patients and the 5-year overall survival and disease-specific survival rates were similar to those reported by Mertens and colleagues,[28] 67% and 71%, respectively. Both of these groups demonstrated low recurrence rates in the prostatic urethra, and the 5-year overall and disease-specific survival rates seem to be comparable with the radical cystoprostatectomy data.[56,57]

Comparative Studies of Prostate-Sparing Versus Radical Cystectomy

There are limited studies that actually compare prostate-sparing cystectomy with radical cystectomy. de Vries and colleagues[30] compared the oncologic results of 63 men who underwent a prostate-sparing cystectomy with a historical control of men matched by clinicopathologic characteristics who underwent a radical cystoprostatectomy during the same study period. The 5-year disease-specific survival of men in the prostate-sparing cystectomy group was not significantly different from men who had a radical cystoprostatectomy (66% vs 64%; $P = .6$). More recently, Jacobs and colleagues[19] performed a randomized controlled study of 40 men with cT2 or less urothelial carcinoma that were eligible for either prostate-sparing cystectomy or nerve-sparing (NS) radical cystoprostatectomy. All men underwent a preoperative transurethral biopsy of prostatic urethra and a 12-core TRUS biopsy and they were excluded if either was positive. The rates of occult prostate cancer and urothelial cancer in the prostatic urethra were 15% and 10%, respectively, in the prostate-sparing cystectomy group and 40% and 20% in the NS radical cystoprostatectomy group. At 12-month follow-up, there were no differences between groups in recurrence-free, metastases-free, or overall survival probabilities. Although promising, longer follow-up data are necessary to verify the oncologic safety in a carefully selected population.

Local and Distal Recurrence in Women

In women, local recurrence may occur with preservation of the anterior vaginal wall because unlike in men, there is no anatomic barrier, such as Denonvilliers fascia, between the bladder base and vaginal wall. Chang and colleagues[58] reviewed the pathology of 68 women who underwent radical cystectomy to determine the incidence of gynecologic organ involvement. Out of 68 women, the occurrence of invasive urothelial carcinoma was present in two women and the invasion was grossly evident intraoperatively.[58] Varkarakis and colleagues[59] reviewed the anterior exenteration specimens in women who underwent radical cystectomy for organ-confined urothelial carcinoma to assess the rate of involvement of the internal genital organs. The study included 52 women, 34 with muscle-invasive disease and 18 with superficial urothelial carcinoma. The authors found internal genitalia involvement was present in three women (one involving the uterus, one involving the vagina only, and one involving the vagina and cervix). The extension of tumor into the genital organ was characterized by tumor location (eg, bladder floor tumors extended into the vagina and dome tumor into the uterus).[59] Djaladat and colleagues[60] reviewed anterior pelvic exenteration specimens in 267 women (mean age, 71) who were treated for urothelial carcinoma and found gynecologic organ involvement in 7.5% of women.

Out of the 20 women that had gynecologic organ involvement, 3.8% had vaginal involvement only, 0.7% cervical involvement only, and 0.3% uterine involvement only. The clinical variables that were associated with positive pelvic organ involvement were hydronephrosis and a palpable bladder mass. Disease recurrence was 70% in the 20 women who had gynecologic organ involvement with 25% of recurrence being local and 45% with distant metastases. The 2-year overall survival and recurrence-free survival in women with gynecologic organ involvement are 29% and 15% versus 73% and 76% in women without gynecologic organ involvement. Given such poor survival rates, the authors do no advocate for gynecologic organ-sparing cystectomy.[60] However, Gregg and colleagues[61] evaluated the anterior exenteration pathology specimens of women with muscle-invasive bladder cancer and noted gynecologic organ involvement in only 23% of women who had not had a previous hysterectomy. The only preoperative clinical factor associated with positive gynecologic organ involvement and disease recurrence was the presence of a palpable posterior bladder mass. Recurrence-free survival was not associated with whether a patient had hysterectomy during anterior exenteration.[61] Further studies are necessary on the impact of reproductive organ involvement by

urothelial carcinoma on recurrence-free and overall survival.

In regards to margin status and the association on recurrence-free and overall survival in women, the data are hard to interpret for women because most patients included were men (76%–79% of men vs 20%–24% of women). The incidence of PSM has actually been reported to be higher in women than in men (6% vs 4%; $P = .04$). However, in this study in a multivariate model, female gender was not associated with disease-specific survival.[54] In a study by Novara and colleagues,[55] the margin rate was similar for men and women (6.2% vs 6.8%; $P = .536$) and female gender was also not associated with cancer-specific mortality.

Oncologic data were available for 8 out of 13 studies presented on women who underwent either vaginal- or genital-sparing cystectomy (the terms in the literature are used interchangeably) (Table 3). The rates of local recurrences ranged from 0% to 13% and of distant recurrences from 0% to 16.7%. In a retrospective review of 21 women who underwent vaginal-sparing cystectomy, all had negative margins at the posterior bladder wall and urethra even though the pattern of urothelial cancer involvement was variable, including eight with tumor in the posterior bladder floor, two involving the trigone, five involving

Table 3
Incidence of local and distant recurrence of urothelial carcinoma in genital- or vaginal-sparing cystectomy series

Author, Year	n	Mean/Median Age, y (Range)	Mean/Median Follow-up (mo)	Pathologic Stage ≤T2, %	Local Recurrence, %	Distant Recurrence, %
Hautmann et al,[62] 1996	13	48 (17–73)	55	NR	NR	NR
Chang et al,[12] 2002	21	68 (NR)	12	62	5	11
Rapp et al,[37] 2004	37	60 (52–71)	37	NR	NR	NR
Kulkarni et al,[22] 2008	14	NR (45–72)	32	64	0	14
Granberg et al,[63] 2008[a]	59	62 (20–82)	29	64	13	15
Neymeyer et al,[64] 2008	84	NR	36	NR	NR	NR
Koie et al,[65] 2010	30	71 (45–80)	35	67	3.3	16.7
Anderson et al,[35] 2012[b]	49	61 (NR)	37	76	NR	NR
Large et al,[66] 2012	94	69 (NR)	27	65	11.7	NR
Ali-El-Dein et al,[13] 2013	15	42 (25–54)	70	87	6	13
Wishahi & Elganozoury,[34] 2015	13	37 (20–54)	NR	77	NR	NR
Roshdy et al,[36] 2016	22	51 (45–60)	48	100	4.5	0
Moursy et al,[23] 2016	18	38 (NR)	70	T2	0	16.6

Abbreviation: NR, not reported.
[a] 92% vaginal sparing.
[b] 84% vaginal sparing.

bladder dome, and three with disease in the anterior bladder wall. Out of the 21 women, only one who had pT3b disease developed local recurrence, and two women died of metastatic disease.[12] One of the obvious limitations of this study is the short median follow-up time of 12 months; however, the authors argue that in the presence of a negative margin, local recurrence may be a result of tumor biology rather than surgical technique. In a study by Kulkarni and colleagues,[22] 14 women with an age range of 45 to 72, underwent genital-sparing cystectomy and after a median follow-up of 32 months, zero patients had local recurrence and 14% developed distant recurrence. Similarly, Koie and colleagues[65] retrospectively reviewed oncologic outcomes in 30 women who underwent genital-sparing cystectomy and demonstrated a local recurrence rate of 3.3% and distant recurrence of 16.7% after 35 months of follow-up. Both of these cohorts had similar follow-up and percent of patients with pT2 or less urothelial carcinoma involvement. The largest cohort of 94 women who underwent a genital-sparing cystectomy demonstrated preliminary results of a positive posterior margin rate of 8.5% and local recurrence of 11.7% after 27 months of follow-up; however, further details regarding disease-specific and overall survival are lacking.[66] Granberg and colleagues[63] retrospectively reviewed the oncologic outcomes of 59 women (median age, 62) who had a radical cystectomy with an orthotopic neobladder at a single institution. They reported local and distant recurrence rates of 13% and 15%, respectively, after a median follow-up of 29 months. Most women (80%) had a cystectomy for urothelial malignancy and most underwent a vaginal-sparing cystectomy (92%); however, the authors do not distinguish which women had a vaginal-sparing cystectomy for a urothelial malignancy and therefore recurrence rates are difficult to interpret. They do report that the 5-year disease-specific and overall survival rates for women who were treated for cancer (including urothelial, squamous, and small cell) are 87.7% and 82.9%.[63]

Ali-El-Dein and colleagues[13] report on the longest follow-up of 15 women who underwent genital-sparing cystectomy with a median follow-up of 70 months and report a local recurrence rate of 6% and distant recurrence rate of 13%. The Ali-el-Dein cohort had a mixed cohort of squamous and urothelial cell carcinomas and adenocarcinoma in the final pathology specimens; therefore, the recurrence rates may not be comparable with other series with only urothelial cell carcinoma involvement.[13] The case series

by Roshdy and colleagues[36] reported local recurrence in 1 out 22 patients who underwent a genital-sparing cystectomy. Like the Ali-El-Dein and colleagues[13] cohort, the results of the final pathology specimens contained squamous cell, urothelial cell, and adenocarcinoma.[36] Similarly, the women in the Moursy and coworkers[23] cohort had mostly squamous cell pathology (72%) and therefore local and distal recurrence rates are difficult to compare with urothelial cell carcinoma.

FUNCTIONAL OUTCOMES
Urinary Function in Men

The initial goal of prostate-sparing cystectomy was to improve incontinence rates, daytime and nighttime, which frequently occur with an orthotopic bladder substitution. Hautmann and colleagues[8] presented results from centers of excellence with their experience of neobladder substitution and the rate of daytime continence ranged from 84% to 97%, whereas nighttime continence ranged from 68% to 94%. Since that time, the rates of daytime and nighttime continence remain variable for men undergoing radical cystoprostatectomy and neobladder substitution. For example, Kretschmer and colleagues[67] reported a daytime continence rate of 54.3% and nighttime rate of 36.3% in 188 patients with a median follow-up of 61 months. Clifford and colleagues[68] reported on daytime continence rate of 92% by 12 to 18 months postoperatively and 51% of nighttime continence that occurred by 18 to 36 months postoperatively. One of the main reasons for differences in outcomes is that there is no single standard questionnaire that is used by all studies.

In Our review, daytime continence rates ranged from 50% to 100% (mean, 91%) and nighttime continence from 31% to 100% (mean, 73%) (**Table 4**). The daytime continence rates for patients who underwent prostate-sparing cystectomy are comparable with the radical cystoprostatectomy literature, with the nighttime continence rates slightly higher. In the largest cohort of 105 patients who underwent prostate-sparing cystectomy and with available urinary function data, 96% reported complete daytime continence and 82% reported complete nighttime continence. However, 11% to 15% of patients required clean intermittent catheterization for either large postvoid residual volumes or inability to have spontaneous voids.

Sexual Function in Men

In regards to potency, previous reports of 82% to 100% erectile function following prostate-sparing

Table 4
Functional outcomes of prostate-sparing cystectomy

Author, Year	n (Continence)/ n (Potency)	Daytime Continence, %	Nighttime Continence, %	Potency, %
Martis et al,[26] 2005	32	98	83	80
Nieuwenhuijzen et al,[31] 2005	43	95	74	78
Wunderlich et al,[32] 2006	31	94	94	87
Davila et al,[24] 2007	18	NR	NR	NR
Simone et al,[14] 2008	20	100	100	100
Rozet et al,[27] 2008	106	NR	NR	NR
Puppo et al,[21] 2008	37	95	92	76
de Vries et al,[30] 2009	63	NR	NR	NR
Thorstenson et al,[29] 2009	25	85	50	95
Ong et al,[15] 2010	29/19	93	66	79
Dall'Oglio et al,[25] 2010	22	94	31	68
Nour et al,[20] 2011	23/22	95	87	73
Basiri et al,[16] 2012	23	50	87	83
Muto et al,[18] 2014	91	96	37	96
Mertens et al,[28] 2014	105/87	96	82	90
Jacobs et al,[19] 2015	20	NR	NR	NR
Colombo et al,[17] 2015, capsule sparing	36	94	78	86
Colombo et al,[17] 2015, SV sparing	19	90	63	NR
Chen & Chiang,[33] 2017	14	86	64	NR

Abbreviation: NR, not reported.

cystectomy were then superseded by later case series with potency rate more variable depending on the type of technique used 20% to 100%.[8] The potency rates of this review are presented in **Table 4** and range from 68% to 100% (mean, 84%). Some have argued that if the goal is to preserve sexual function in men then NS radical cystoprostatectomy may be sufficient. Jacobs and colleagues[19] presented functional data in a randomized controlled study comparing PCS with NS radical cystectomy. At 12-month follow-up, there was no statistically significant difference in sexual function or urinary scores. However, in the prostate-sparing group the sexual function scores changed by 1 point from baseline versus 23 points for NS group. The authors contend that perhaps not reaching the accrual goal of the study contributed to variability in outcome scores.[19] Colombo and colleagues[17] presented on the evolution of "some type of nerve sparing" cystoprostatectomy, PCS, or SVS in a single institution from 1997 to 2012. At 24 months of follow-up, 28.6% of men who underwent NS reported satisfactory sexual function compared with 91.6% of men in the PCS group and 84.2% of men in the SVS group. Similar results were seen at 48 months of follow-up between NS (20%) and PCS (86%), with longer follow-up data not available for SVS because of recent adaptation of technique.[17]

Urinary Function in Women

In addition to daytime and nighttime incontinence, women develop a phenomenon of hypercontinence because of possible kinking of the neo vesicourethral anastomosis. In the largest retrospective series of 177 women with orthotopic neobladders from Egypt, Ali-el-Dein and colleagues[69] reported a hypercontinence rate of 16% with daytime and nighttime continence rates of 92% and 72%. In a more recent review, Bartsch and colleagues[70] reported a hypercontinence rate of 45% of women with an orthotopic neobladder. In our review of women who underwent a vaginal or genital organ-sparing cystectomy with a neobladder, daytime continence ranged from 31% to

100% (mean, 78%) and nighttime continence from 64% to 100% (mean, 78%). However, the hyper-continence rate ranged from 0% to 69% (mean, 26%) (**Table 5**). Unfortunately, the data heterogeneity is likely caused by variability in assessment of continence that is often performed via patient interview rather than with validated questionnaires. In addition, the definition of continence may be undefined or varies to equal one pad or less per day versus zero pads per day.

Sexual Function in Women

Although it is presumed that radical cystectomy in women affects sexual function, there are few studies available that evaluate postoperative sexual function after an orthotopic neobladder. For example, Volkmer and colleagues retrospectively reviewed sexual function in 29 women who had an orthotopic neobladder and completed the

Female Sexual Function Index (FSFI). The FSFI is a questionnaire that was validated in women with sexual arousal disorders and evaluates six domains of sexual function: desire, arousal, lubrication, orgasm, satisfaction, and pain with lower scores indicating worse sexual function.[71] In the study, women completed the questionnaire twice, once while recalling their sexual function 4 weeks before their surgery and the second time assessing their current sexual function. The responses for each question item and the domain scores were compared preoperatively and postoperatively. Although all of the domains had decreased scores postoperatively, the individual question items regarding frequency of achieving and maintaining lubrication were significantly worse postoperatively. The authors reported that resection of the upper part of the anterior vaginal wall did not affect lubrication, vaginal sensation, or ability to engage in intercourse. Although this study is

Table 5
Functional outcomes of genital- or vaginal-sparing cystectomy

Author, Year	n	Daytime Continence, %	Nighttime Continence, %	Vaginal Lubrication, %	Ability to Achieve Orgasm, %	Dyspareunia, %	NVF, %	Chronic Urinary Retention, %
Hautmann et al,[62] 1996	13	31	NR	NR	NR	8	13	69
Chang et al,[12] 2002	21	71	NR	NR	NR	NR	5	10
Rapp et al,[37] 2004	37	NR	NR	NR	NR	NR	11	NR
Kulkarni et al,[22] 2008	14	64	64	NR	NR	NR	NR	57
Granberg et al,[63] 2008[a]	49	90	57	NR	NR	NR	4	35
Neymeyer et al,[64] 2008	84	100	100	NR	NR	NR	NR	NR
Koie et al,[65] 2010	30	80	87	NR	NR	NR	0	0
Anderson et al,[35] 2012[b]	49	57	45	NR	NR	NR	6	31
Ali-El-Dein et al,[13] 2013	13	100	92	NR	NR	NR	0	0
Wishani & Elganozoury,[34] 2015	13	69	NR	NR	NR	NR	NR	31
Roshdy et al,[36] 2016	22	95	91	91	86	14	0	0
Moursy et al,[23] 2016	18	100	88	NR	72	17	0	22

Abbreviations: NR, not reported; NVF, neobladder-vaginal fistula.
[a] 92% vaginal sparing.
[b] 84% vaginal sparing.

limited by its retrospective nature and possible introduction of recall bias, it nonetheless addresses a poorly studied complication after radical cystectomy in women.[72]

As for genital organ-sparing outcome data, not all studies report uniformly on rates of dyspareunia, vaginal lubrication, ability to achieve an orgasm, or sexual desire (see **Table 5**). One study used the FSFI and compared sexual function scores of 13 women who underwent genital-sparing cystectomy with contemporary control subjects (110 women who underwent radical cystectomy). The mean FSFI scores were significantly better in women who had genital-sparing cystectomy than in women who had standard radical cystectomy. The other domains of the FSFI score, such as vaginal lubrication, pain, desire, and orgasm, were also higher in women who underwent genital-sparing cystectomy.[13] These results are difficult to compare with the percentages of sexual function reported in the other studies (see **Table 5**). Although one could reasonably assume that improved vaginal lubrication and decreased dyspareunia would lead to increased sexual desire and sexual orgasm, unfortunately these outcomes are difficult to compare among studies.

Another important consideration in women is the incidence of neobladder-vaginal fistula (NVF) that can occur with an orthotopic bladder formation and whether it is significantly decreased with sparing of the anterior vaginal wall. The reported incidence of NVF in women with an orthotopic diversion is 3% to 11%.[37,63,69,73–76] However, the literature that is cited on NVF occurrence is mixed with patients who underwent some sort of vaginal-sparing approach. When the patients who had a vaginal-sparing approach are excluded, the incidence of NVF is around 3% to 4%.[69,73,74] When patients who have had a vaginal-sparing cystectomy are included, the incidence of NVF ranges from 2.7% to 13%.[12,35,37,62,63,75,76] For example, Granberg and colleagues[63] reported that the overall NVF rate was 5% (3 out of 59 women); however, a 4% NVF rate in women who had vaginal-sparing surgery and a 20% rate in women with resection of the anterior vaginal wall was reported. However, Rapp and colleagues[37] reported a higher NVF rate of 11% in 37 women who had a vaginal-sparing radical cystectomy and orthotopic neobladder formation. The authors state that one of the major contributing factors to the formation of a fistula is injury to the vaginal wall during dissection of vagina from the posterior wall of the bladder (two out of the four patients with NVF sustained a recognized vaginal injury that was repaired intraoperatively).[37] Ali-El-Dein and Ashamallah[76] reported an NVF rate of 5% in the first 100 women

who underwent an orthotopic neobladder; however, after surgical technique modifications, such as meticulous closure of vaginal stump and omental flap interposition, the NVF rate decreased to 1.5% with an overall rate of 2.7% in the 298 women who underwent orthotopic neobladder. The authors do report that their cohort included 15 women who had anterior vaginal wall sparing and none of these women developed an NVF.[76] However, on further review of the functional data presented on these 15 women, the authors report that an omental flap was brought down and sutured to the anterior vaginal wall in all 15 women.[13] Therefore, it is unclear whether improvement in technique or interposition of omental flap prevented the occurrence of NVF.

SUMMARY

In the 2005 review, Hautmann and Stein[8] argued that pursuing sexually preserving cystectomy is a step in the wrong direction when taking into consideration the risk of worse recurrence rates, leaving behind occult prostate cancer or urothelial cancer in the prostatic urethra with not much improvement in daytime or nighttime continence and variable results when it came to sexual function. Since 2005, several modifications have been described that should be taken into consideration. For one, the prostate-sparing techniques have evolved into sparing prostate capsule and SV only so that most if not all prostatic tissue is completely removed. In addition to prostate-sparing techniques, the adaptation of robotic-assisted cystoprostatectomy can allow for NS with or without PCS or SVS, which may lead to better results than open NS radical cystoprostatectomy alone. For example, Asimakopoulos and colleagues[77] recently published on the oncologic and functional outcomes of robotic-assisted partial SV sparing and NS cystectomy in 40 men and demonstrated daytime continence of 75%, nighttime continence rate of 72.5% and return to preoperative sexual function in 72% of men by 12-month. Although follow-up was only 26 months, recurrence was demonstrated in one patient and clinically significant prostate cancer in three patients.[77]

In regards to local and distal recurrence, it seems that with longer follow-up data available, the disease-free and overall survival probabilities are comparable between organ-sparing and radical cystoprostatectomy patients in carefully selected patients; however, margin status is paramount in both. A recent systematic review of 12 eligible studies compared any sexually preserving (prostate sparing, capsule sparing, or NS) cystectomy with a standard radical cystectomy in men and found that there was no significant difference in oncologic outcomes or continence outcomes; however, sexual function was significantly better in men who had sexually preserving cystectomy than men with standard radical cystectomy.[78] Although the quality of the data was moderate and contained inherent bias, with proper patient selection, counseling, and close monitoring, the data support that organ-sparing cystectomy may be offered to these eligible men.

In women, the lack of robust studies evaluating genital-sparing cystectomy suggests that there is either a disparity in research of female subjects or women are not being offered a genital-sparing cystectomy when indicated. Pathologic studies of gynecologic organ involvement of urothelial malignancy have demonstrated low recurrence rates in the preserved pelvic organs. The most robust data comes out of the Middle East where the occurrence of squamous cell carcinoma is more commonly encountered. Therefore, it is difficult to compare oncologic outcomes because squamous cell carcinoma behaves differently than urothelial carcinoma.

Lack of standardized questionnaires to evaluate objectively patient's urinary and sexual function contributes to heterogeneity in results. The questionnaires that were validated for evaluating sexual function after prostatectomy have been historically used to evaluate sexual function following radical cystectomy. Urinary incontinence questionnaires also vary. The Bladder Cancer Index questionnaire may become analogous to the Expanded Prostate Cancer Index Composite questionnaire that is now routinely used to evaluate patient's urinary, sexual, and bowel domains after radical prostatectomy.

Improved patient selection may allow surgeons to feel more comfortable in performing organ-sparing techniques. With the advent of new screening tools for prostate cancer, such as MP-MRI and cysview technology for better diagnosis of CIS, improved patient selection will likely lead to even safer oncologic outcomes and improved functional outcomes. Oncologic precaution and safety remains paramount for these patients but should not preclude attempts to improve quality of life.

REFERENCES

1. Spitz A, Stein JP, Lieskovsky G, et al. Orthotopic urinary diversion with preservation of erectile and ejaculatory function in men requiring radical cystectomy for nonurothelial malignancy: a new technique. J Urol 1999;161:1761–4.

2. Colombo R, Bertini R, Salonia A, et al. Nerve and seminal sparing radical cystectomy with orthotopic urinary diversion for select patients with superficial bladder cancer: an innovative surgical approach. J Urol 2001;165:51–5 [discussion: 55].

3. Colombo R, Bertini R, Salonia A, et al. Overall clinical outcomes after nerve and seminal sparing radical cystectomy for the treatment of organ confined bladder cancer. J Urol 2004;171:1819–22 [discussion: 1822].

4. Muto G, Bardari F, D'Urso L, et al. Seminal sparing cystectomy and ileocapsuloplasty: long-term followup results. J Urol 2004;172:76–80.

5. Botto H, Sebe P, Molinie V, et al. Prostatic capsule- and seminal-sparing cystectomy for bladder carcinoma: initial results for selected patients. BJU Int 2004;94:1021–5.

6. Vallancien G, Abou El Fettouh H, Cathelineau X, et al. Cystectomy with prostate sparing for bladder cancer in 100 patients: 10-year experience. J Urol 2002;168:2413–7.

7. Terrone C, Cracco C, Scarpa RM, et al. Supra-ampullar cystectomy with preservation of sexual function and ileal orthotopic reservoir for bladder tumor: twenty years of experience. Eur Urol 2004;46: 264–9 [discussion: 269–70].

8. Hautmann RE, Stein JP. Neobladder with prostatic capsule and seminal-sparing cystectomy for bladder cancer: a step in the wrong direction. Urol Clin North Am 2005;32:177–85.

9. Ali-el-Dein B, el-Sobky E, Hohenfellner M, et al. Orthotopic bladder substitution in women: functional evaluation. J Urol 1999;161:1875–80.

10. Coloby PJ, Kakizoe T, Tobisu K, et al. Urethral involvement in female bladder cancer patients: mapping of 47 consecutive cysto-urethrectomy specimens. J Urol 1994;152:1438–42.

11. Horenblas S, Meinhardt W, Ijzerman W, et al. Sexuality preserving cystectomy and neobladder: initial results. J Urol 2001;166:837–40.

12. Chang SS, Cole E, Cookson MS, et al. Preservation of the anterior vaginal wall during female radical cystectomy with orthotopic urinary diversion: technique and results. J Urol 2002;168: 1442–5.

13. Ali-El-Dein B, Mosbah A, Osman Y, et al. Preservation of the internal genital organs during radical cystectomy in selected women with bladder cancer: a report on 15 cases with long term follow-up. Eur J Surg Oncol 2013;39:358–64.

14. Simone G, Papalia R, Leonardo C, et al. Prostatic capsule and seminal vesicle-sparing cystectomy: improved functional results, inferior oncologic outcome. Urology 2008;72:162–6.

15. Ong CH, Schmitt M, Thalmann GN, et al. Individualized seminal vesicle sparing cystoprostatectomy combined with ileal orthotopic bladder substitution

achieves good functional results. J Urol 2010;183: 1337–41.

16. Basiri A, Pakmanesh H, Tabibi A, et al. Overall survival and functional results of prostate-sparing cystectomy: a matched case-control study. Urol J 2012;9:678–84.

17. Colombo R, Pellucchi F, Moschini M, et al. Fifteen-year single-centre experience with three different surgical procedures of nerve-sparing cystectomy in selected organ-confined bladder cancer patients. World J Urol 2015;33:1389–95.

18. Muto G, Collura D, Rosso R, et al. Seminal-sparing cystectomy: technical evolution and results over a 20-year period. Urology 2014;83:856–61.

19. Jacobs BL, Daignault S, Lee CT, et al. Prostate capsule sparing versus nerve sparing radical cystectomy for bladder cancer: results of a randomized, controlled trial. J Urol 2015;193:64–70.

20. Nour H, Abdelrazak O, Wishahy M, et al. Prostate-sparing cystectomy: potential functional advantages and objective oncological risks; a case series and review. Arab J Urol 2011;9:107–12.

21. Puppo P, Introini C, Bertolotto F, et al. Potency preserving cystectomy with intrafascial prostatectomy for high risk superficial bladder cancer. J Urol 2008;179:1727–32 [discussion: 1732].

22. Kulkarni JN, Rizvi SJ, Acharya UP, et al. Gyneco-logic-tract sparing extra peritoneal retrograde radical cystectomy with neobladder. Int Braz J Urol 2008;34:180–7 [discussion: 187–90].

23. Moursy EES, Eldahshoursy MZ, Gamal WM, et al. Orthotopic genital sparing radical cystectomy in pre-menopausal women with muscle-invasive bladder carcinoma: a prospective study. Indian J Urol 2016;32:65–70.

24. Davila HH, Weber T, Burday D, et al. Total or partial prostate sparing cystectomy for invasive bladder cancer: long-term implications on erectile function. BJU Int 2007;100:1026–9.

25. Dall'Oglio MF, Antunes AA, Crippa A, et al. Long-term outcomes of radical cystectomy with preservation of prostatic capsule. Int Urol Nephrol 2010;42: 951–7.

26. Martis G, D'Elia G, Diana M, et al. Prostatic capsule- and nerve-sparing cystectomy in organ-confined bladder cancer: preliminary results. World J Surg 2005;29:1277–81.

27. Rozet F, Lesur G, Cathelineau X, et al. Oncological evaluation of prostate sparing cystectomy: the Montsouris long-term results. J Urol 2008;179:2170–4 [discussion: 2174–5].

28. Mertens LS, Meijer RP, de Vries RR, et al. Prostate sparing cystectomy for bladder cancer: 20-year single center experience. J Urol 2014;191: 1250–5.

29. Thorstenson A, O'connor RC, Ahonen R, et al. Clinical outcome following prostatic capsule- and

seminal-sparing cystectomy for bladder cancer in 25 men. Scand J Urol Nephrol 2009;43:127–32.

30. de Vries RR, Nieuwenhuijzen JA, van Tinteren H, et al. Prostate-sparing cystectomy: long-term oncological results. BJU Int 2009;104:1239–43.

31. Nieuwenhuijzen JA, Meinhardt W, Horenblas S. Clinical outcomes after sexuality preserving cystectomy and neobladder (prostate sparing cystectomy) in 44 patients. J Urol 2005;173:1314–7.

32. Wunderlich H, Wolf M, Reichelt O, et al. Radical cystectomy with ultrasound-guided partial prostatectomy for bladder cancer: a complication-preventing concept. Urology 2006;68:554–9.

33. Chen PY, Chiang PH. Comparisons of quality of life and functional and oncological outcomes after orthotopic neobladder reconstruction: prostate-sparing cystectomy versus conventional radical cystoprostatectomy. Biomed Res Int 2017;2017: 1983428.

34. Wishahi M, Elganozoury H. Survival up to 5-15 years in young women following genital sparing radical cystectomy and neobladder: oncological outcome and quality of life. Single-surgeon and single-institution experience. Cent European J Urol 2015;68:141–5.

35. Anderson CB, Cookson MS, Chang SS, et al. Voiding function in women with orthotopic neobladder urinary diversion. J Urol 2012;188:200–4.

36. Roshdy S, Senbel A, Khater A, et al. Genital sparing cystectomy for female bladder cancer and its functional outcome; a seven years' experience with 24 cases. Indian J Surg Oncol 2016;7:307–11.

37. Rapp DE, O'connor RC, Katz EE, et al. Neobladder-vaginal fistula after cystectomy and orthotopic neobladder construction. BJU Int 2004;94:1092–5 [discussion: 1095].

38. Revelo MP, Cookson MS, Chang SS, et al. Incidence and location of prostate and urothelial carcinoma in prostates from cystoprostatectomies: implications for possible apical sparing surgery. J Urol 2004; 171:646–51.

39. Gakis G, Schilling D, Bedke J, et al. Incidental prostate cancer at radical cystoprostatectomy: implications for apex-sparing surgery. BJU Int 2010;105: 468–71.

40. Abdelhady M, Abusamra A, Pautler SE, et al. Clinically significant prostate cancer found incidentally in radical cystoprostatectomy specimens. BJU Int 2007;99:326–9.

41. Pettus JA, Al-Ahmadie H, Barocas DA, et al. Risk assessment of prostatic pathology in patients undergoing radical cystoprostatectomy. Eur Urol 2008;53: 370–5.

42. Weizer AZ, Shah RB, Lee CT, et al. Evaluation of the prostate peripheral zone/capsule in patients undergoing radical cystoprostatectomy: defining risk with prostate capsule sparing cystectomy. Urol Oncol 2007;25:460–4.

43. Hautmann RE, de Petriconi R, Kleinschmidt K, et al. Orthotopic ileal neobladder in females: impact of the urethral resection line on functional results. Int Urogynecol J Pelvic Floor Dysfunct 2000;11:224–9 [discussion: 230].

44. Taneja, SS, Bjurlin MA, Carter HB, et al. White paper: AUA/optimal techniques of prostate biopsy and specimen handling. 2015. Available at: http://www.auanet.org/guidelines/prostate-biopsy-and-specimen-handling. Accessed October 26, 2017.

45. Chan TY, Chan DY, Stutzman KL, et al. Does increased needle biopsy sampling of the prostate detect a higher number of potentially insignificant tumors? J Urol 2001;166:2181–4.

46. Siu W, Dunn RL, Shah RB, et al. Use of extended pattern technique for initial prostate biopsy. J Urol 2005;174:505–9.

47. Meng MV, Elkin EP, DuChane J, et al. Impact of increased number of biopsies on the nature of prostate cancer identified. J Urol 2006;176:63–8 [discussion: 69].

48. Elabbady AA, Khedr MM. Extended 12-core prostate biopsy increases both the detection of prostate cancer and the accuracy of Gleason score. Eur Urol 2006;49:49–53 [discussion: 53].

49. Ahmed HU, El-Shater Bosaily A, Brown LC, et al. Diagnostic accuracy of multi-parametric MRI and TRUS biopsy in prostate cancer (PROMIS): a paired validating confirmatory study. Lancet 2017;389:815–22.

50. Siddiqui MM, Rais-Bahrami S, Turkbey B, et al. Comparison of MR/ultrasound fusion-guided biopsy with ultrasound-guided biopsy for the diagnosis of prostate cancer. JAMA 2015;313:390–7.

51. Richards KA, Parks GE, Badlani GH, et al. Developing selection criteria for prostate-sparing cystectomy: a review of cystoprostatectomy specimens. Urology 2010;75:1116–20.

52. Esrig D, Freeman JA, Elmajian DA, et al. Transitional cell carcinoma involving the prostate with a proposed staging classification for stromal invasion. J Urol 1996;156:1071–6.

53. Donat SM, Wei DC, McGuire MS, et al. The efficacy of transurethral biopsy for predicting the long-term clinical impact of prostatic invasive bladder cancer. J Urol 2001;165:1580–4.

54. Dotan ZA, Kavanagh K, Yossepowitch O, et al. Positive surgical margins in soft tissue following radical cystectomy for bladder cancer and cancer specific survival. J Urol 2007;178:2308–12 [discussion: 2313].

55. Novara G, Svatek RS, Karakiewicz PI, et al. Soft tissue surgical margin status is a powerful predictor of outcomes after radical cystectomy: a multicenter study of more than 4,400 patients. J Urol 2010;183:2165–70.

56. Manoharan M, Ayyathurai R, Soloway MS. Radical cystectomy for urothelial carcinoma of the bladder: an analysis of perioperative and survival outcome. BJU Int 2009;104:1227–32.

57. Shariat SF, Karakiewicz PI, Palapattu GS, et al. Outcomes of radical cystectomy for transitional cell carcinoma of the bladder: a contemporary series from the Bladder Cancer Research Consortium. J Urol 2006;176:2414–22 [discussion: 2422].

58. Chang SS, Cole E, Smith JA Jr, et al. Pathological findings of gynecologic organs obtained at female radical cystectomy. J Urol 2002;168:147–9.

59. Varkarakis IM, Pinggera G, Antoniou N, et al. Pathological review of internal genitalia after anterior exenteration for bladder cancer in women. Evaluating risk factors for female organ involvement. Int Urol Nephrol 2007;39:1015–21.

60. Djaladat H, Bruins HM, Miranda G, et al. Reproductive organ involvement in female patients undergoing radical cystectomy for urothelial bladder cancer. J Urol 2012;188:2134–8.

61. Gregg JR, Emeruwa C, Wong J, et al. Oncologic outcomes after anterior exenteration for muscle invasive bladder cancer in women. J Urol 2016;196:1030–5.

62. Hautmann RE, Paiss T, de Petriconi R. The ileal neobladder in women: 9 years of experience with 18 patients. J Urol 1996;155:76–81.

63. Granberg CF, Boorjian SA, Crispen PL, et al. Functional and oncological outcomes after orthotopic neobladder reconstruction in women. BJU Int 2008;102:1551–5.

64. Neymeyer J, Jungmann O, Alansari AW, et al. Preservation of sexual function, womanhood and continence by combined urological & gynecological approaches in oncologic surgery: performing nerve-sparing cystectomy with ileum neobladder and pelvic floor repair in a single session- results after 4.5 years and 86 patients. J Sex Med 2008;6(Suppl. 2) [abstract: MP–033].

65. Koie T, Hatakeyama S, Yoneyama T, et al. Uterus-, fallopian tube-, ovary-, and vagina-sparing cystectomy followed by U-shaped ileal neobladder construction for female bladder cancer patients: oncological and functional outcomes. Urology 2010;75:1499–503.

66. Large M, Prasad S, Patel A, et al. 1168 can vaginal-sparing cystectomy be safely attempted in all women undergoing radical cystectomy? A single institution study of perioperative and oncologic outcomes. J Urol 2012;187:e473–4.

67. Kretschmer A, Grimm T, Buchner A, et al. Prognostic features for objectively defined urinary continence after radical cystectomy and ileal orthotopic neobladder in a contemporary cohort. J Urol 2017;197:210–5.

68. Clifford TG, Shah SH, Bazargani ST, et al. Prospective evaluation of continence following radical cystectomy and orthotopic urinary diversion using a validated questionnaire. J Urol 2016;196:1685–91.

69. Ali-el-Dein B, Shaaban AA, Abu-Eideh RH, et al. Surgical complications following radical cystectomy and orthotopic neobladders in women. J Urol 2008;180:206–10 [discussion: 210].

70. Bartsch G, Daneshmand S, Skinner EC, et al. Urinary functional outcomes in female neobladder patients. World J Urol 2014;32:221–8.

71. Rosen R, Brown C, Heiman J, et al. The Female Sexual Function Index (FSFI): a multidimensional self-report instrument for the assessment of female sexual function. J Sex Marital Ther 2000; 26:191–208.

72. Volkmer BG, Gschwend JE, Herkommer K, et al. Cystectomy and orthotopic ileal neobladder: the impact on female sexuality. J Urol 2004;172: 2353–7.

73. Abol-Enein H, Ghoneim MA. Functional results of orthotopic ileal neobladder with serous-lined extramural ureteral reimplantation: experience with 450 patients. J Urol 2001;165:1427–32.

74. Lee CT, Hafez KS, Sheffield JH, et al. Orthotopic bladder substitution in women: nontraditional applications. J Urol 2004;171:1585–8.

75. Badawy AA, Abolyosr A, Mohamed ER, et al. Orthotopic diversion after cystectomy in women: a single-centre experience with a 10-year follow-up. Arab J Urol 2011;9:267–71.

76. Ali-El-Dein B, Ashamallah A. Vaginal repair of pouch-vaginal fistula after orthotopic bladder substitution in women. Urology 2013;81:198–202.

77. Asimakopoulos AD, Campagna A, Gakis G, et al. Nerve sparing, robot-assisted radical cystectomy with intracorporeal bladder substitution in the male. J Urol 2016;196:1549–57.

78. Hernández V, Espinos EL, Dunn J, et al. Oncological and functional outcomes of sexual function-preserving cystectomy compared with standard radical cystectomy in men: a systematic review. Urol Oncol 2017;35(9):539.e17-29.

Lymphadenectomy for Muscle-Invasive Bladder Cancer and Upper Tract Urothelial Cell Carcinoma

Niranjan J. Sathianathen, MBBS, Michael C. Risk, MD, PhD,
Badrinath R. Konety, MD, MBA*

KEYWORDS

- Cystectomy • Lymph node dissection • Transitional cell carcinoma • Urinary bladder neoplasms

KEY POINTS

- No randomized studies have been published to date examining lymph node dissection in either bladder cancer or upper tract urothelial carcinoma.
- It is estimated that one-quarter of patients undergoing radical surgery for bladder cancer or upper tract urothelial carcinoma harbor lymph node metastases.
- An extended pelvic lymph node dissection template is recommended for patients undergoing radical cystectomy to optimize prognostic and therapeutic benefit.
- Lymphadenectomy recommendations for patients with upper tract urothelial carcinoma are less clear but a complete dissection according to one of the two well-known templates seems to be required to maximize outcomes.

INTRODUCTION

Urothelial cell carcinoma is the ninth most common malignancy of which more than 95% arise in the bladder.[1] Although 15% to 25% of bladder cancers (BC) are invasive at the time of diagnosis, upper tract urothelial carcinomas (UTUC) are markedly more aggressive with approximately 60% of cancers demonstrating invasive characteristics at the time of presentation.[2] Therefore, radical surgery is widely recommended as the optimal management option in patients who do not have distant disease and can tolerate the stressors of surgery.[3–5] Although the role of surgery does not ignite much debate, there remains ongoing conjecture regarding the independent utility of lymphadenectomy for BC and UTUC. Several unanswered questions remain in this domain focused on the indications and patient selection for pelvic lymph node dissection (PLND), extent of dissection, its impact on outcome, and potential risks.

INDICATION AND PATIENT SELECTION

Considering the limitations of the available imaging modalities, accurate staging remains the primary benefit of performing a lymphadenectomy. Conventional modalities commonly used as part of the diagnostic work-up to stage BC or UTUC, such as computed tomography (CT) and MRI, are limited by their poor sensitivity, which is reported to range between 48% and 87%.[5] This is because CT and MRI rely on lymph node (LN) enlargement to discern the possibility of nodal metastases. The guidelines suggest that pelvic nodes

Disclosure: The authors have nothing to disclose.
Department of Urology, University of Minnesota, Delaware Street Southeast, Minneapolis, MN 55455, USA
* Corresponding author. University of Minnesota, 420 Delaware Street Southeast, Mayo Building, MMC 394, Minneapolis, MN 55455.
E-mail address: brkonety@umn.edu

urologic.theclinics.com

greater than 8 mm and abdominal nodes greater than 10 mm in the short-axis maximal diameter should be considered to be abnormally enlarged.[6,7] However, normal-sized nodes can harbor metastatic disease and LNs can also be enlarged as a result of benign processes. It was thus hypothesized that functional imaging techniques, such as PET, could address these shortcomings but it too has demonstrated limited utility.[8,9] Therefore, relying on imaging to inform nodal status would result in a significant proportion of patients being understaged and thus not receiving optimal management in a timely manner.[10–12]

Bladder Cancer

The burden of nodal disease in patients with BC is considerable and has prognostic implications. An early autopsy study of 98 patients found nodal disease in a quarter of the cohort.[13] A second autopsy study reported that LN disease may be the only site of metastases in up to 40% of patients.[14] These figures have been supported by modern-day cohorts that have reported the incidence of nodal involvement to be approximately 25%.[15,16] There is a correlation between tumor stage and LN involvement with the rates of nodal metastases for pTa, pTis, pT1, pT2, pT3, and pT4 patients undergoing extended PLND (ePLND) being 0%, 2%, 4%, 14%, 35%, and 52%, respectively.[15] LN disease has been associated with poor survival outcomes. The 10-year cancer-specific survival rates between N0 and N+ disease is 66.9% versus 28.8%, respectively.[17]

There are no published randomized trials that compare radical cystectomy (RC) patients with or without concomitant lymphadenectomy. Therefore, current guidelines that suggest a benefit in performing nodal dissection rely on observational data to support their recommendations. Although not addressing the question of RC plus PLND versus RC alone, the preliminary results of a randomized trial comparing standard PLND with superextended PLND (sePLND) observed a trend for improved outcomes using the latter template but this was not statistically significant.[18] Details of this trial are outlined further later but it raises important questions regarding the value of lymphadenectomy. Reanalysis of the Southwest Oncology Group (SWOG 8710, INT-0080) randomized trial on neoadjuvant chemotherapy in muscle-invasive BC (MIBC) found that the extent of nodal dissection and the number of nodes removed significantly influenced survival outcomes on multivariable analysis, which included receiving neoadjuvant chemotherapy as a covariate.[19] In contrast, an Italian cohort study reported by Brunocilla and colleagues[20] demonstrated no benefit in cancer-specific survival when performing a limited PLND compared with omitting it all together. However, there was a survival benefit in this group when an extended dissection was performed. In a propensity matched study of patients who underwent RC alone or in conjunction with PLND, the all-cause survival rate (36% vs 45%; P<.001) and cancer-specific survival rate (54% vs 65%; P<.001) was greater in the latter group.[16] Subgroup analysis based on age and Charleson comorbidity index demonstrated that the relationship between lymph node dissection (LND) and improved survival outcomes only remained significant for patients younger than 75 years or who had a comorbidity index score of 0. An analysis of the Surveillance, Epidemiology and End Results (SEER) database demonstrated that not performing lymphadenectomy significant increased overall mortality rates across all stages of BC but only lowered cancer-specific mortality in less than or equal to pT2 disease.[17] This study also showed that PLND is omitted in a quarter of all patients undergoing RC, especially those with lower stage disease when they too would benefit from lymphadenectomy. Therefore, given the available data, bilateral LND should be considered in all patients undergoing RC for MIBC as recommended by guidelines.[3–5] However, the evidence supporting this is less than ideal. Although not studied in BC, there is high-level evidence in some cancers that LND may not provide any benefit despite lower-level evidence, and intuition, suggesting it would. In fact, two recent randomized trials in patients with breast cancer and melanoma with sentinel node metastases (ie, positive sentinel node biopsy) randomized to completion LND versus no further node dissection found no overall survival benefit in performing nodal dissection.[21,22] However, the latter report did suggest that LND improved regional disease control (disease-free survival: 68% vs 63%; P = .05) and provided valuable prognostic information because nonsentinel nodal metastases acted as a significant predictor of melanoma recurrence,[22] although this did not translate into a cancer-specific survival benefit at median follow-up of 43 months. In the breast cancer study, axillary node clearance did not impact disease control in patients with breast cancer compared with sentinel node dissection only (hazard ratio [HR], 08.85; 95% confidence interval [CI], 0.62–1.17; P = .32).[21] This type of data emphasizes the need for randomized trials to examine these questions, rather than relying on low-level evidence and/or expert opinion. It should be noted that there is an ongoing randomized study comparing ePLND and sePLND (NCT01224665) that is expected to be completed in 2022, and which will provide valuable information regarding the extent of dissection but will not address the value of lymphadenectomy. If sePLND demonstrates a benefit in this study, then one could infer indirectly that lymphadenectomy in itself also confers benefit.

Upper Tract Urothelial Carcinoma

Similar to the BC literature, there is no high-quality evidence that demonstrates the benefit of lymphadenectomy in UTUC and thus the results from observational studies have been used to guide clinical practice. As a result, it is common for patients to undergo nephroureterectomy without retroperitoneal LND given the risks and the lack of data supporting its benefit. It should be noted that compared with disease in the bladder, UTUC seems to have a higher burden of nodal metastases at diagnosis. Among a large Canadian cohort of 1029 patients undergoing nephroureterectomy, 26.8% of patients underwent an LND, of whom 27.9% demonstrated LN disease.[23] A larger Japanese study reported that 10.9% of their sample displayed LN involvement; however, LND was performed more frequently.[24] Even after accounting for the degree of selection bias affecting these rates, it can still reasonably be claimed that several patients have N+ disease, even if clinically node-negative.

LND in UTUC can provide important prognostic information. The results of multi-institutional studies have demonstrated that patients with N+ disease have worse prognosis than patients classified as N0 or Nx.[23,25,26] The latter study reported the 5-year cancer-specific survival for N0, Nx, and N+ cases as 81% (95% CI, 73%–88%), 85% (95% CI, 80%–90%), and 47% (95% CI, 24%–69%), respectively. The literature provides conflicting reports on whether a difference exists between N0 and Nx patients.[27,28] These inconsistencies primarily arise from heterogeneity between studies. For example, Roscigno and colleagues[27] reported that 5-year cancer-specific survival was worse for Nx compared with N0 patients (48% vs 73%; $P = .001$) but this study only included muscle-invasive disease of which 55.5% were pT3-4. However, two studies that also included patients with non-muscle-invasive disease reported no difference in survival outcomes between N0 and Nx cases.[23,28] There have also been suggestions that lymphadenectomy only benefits patients with pT2-4 tumors but this may at least partially explain the lack of difference observed between N0 and Nx patients in studies that

included all disease stages.[27,29] It is however, challenging to identify muscle-invasive disease clinically although studies have suggested that the presence of hydronephrosis, positive urinary cytology, and high-grade disease on biopsy could be used to risk stratify patients.[30] Biomarkers and endoluminal ultrasound have demonstrated potential for providing superior T stage classification but have yet to be used in routine clinical practice.[31,32] The guidelines do agree with the concept that LND is likely unnecessary in Ta and T1 upper tract tumors,[2] although the difficulty lies in determining this preoperatively.

EXTENT OF LYMPH NODE DISSECTION
Bladder Cancer

There are three broad levels of dissection (**Fig. 1**), which have been extensively studied in the literature and have been the subject of considerable debate:

- Limited: perivesical nodes and lymphatic tissue in the obturator fossa; the lateral and medial boundaries are the external iliac vein and the obturator nerve, respectively
  - A slightly larger template, sometimes referred to as standard, is bound by the bifurcation of the common iliac artery, genitofemoral nerve, internal iliac vessels, circumflex iliac vein, and the obturator fossa
- Extended: the proximal boundary moves to the crossing of the ureter and the common iliac artery
- Superextended: the proximal boundary is the origin of the inferior mesenteric artery

It is important to consider the lymphatic drainage from UCs to determine an appropriate extent of dissection. Roth and colleagues[33] injected technetium nanocolloid into six non-tumor-bearing sites of the bladder and used single-photon emission CT combined with CT to map the primary lymphatic landing sites. Identified nodes were then verified intraoperatively using a gamma probe and then removed for histopathologic analysis, therefore enhancing the study validity. The authors observed that the lymphatic drainage of the bladder is complicated as evidenced by the median 24 primary lymphatic landing sites per bladder and up to 14 LNs per site. Furthermore, each site of the bladder demonstrated drainage to different areas of the pelvis, thus highlighting the challenge of trying to identify sentinel nodes or regions. The results of this mapping study underline that limited dissection would result in approximately half the LNs remaining in

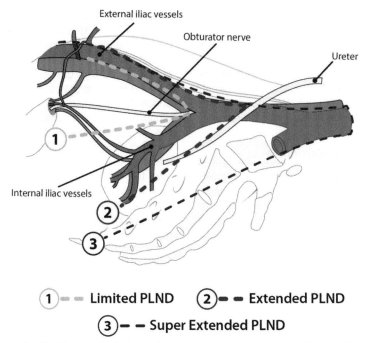

Fig. 1. Levels of PLND for bladder cancer. (*Adapted from* Ploussard G, Briganti A, de la Taille A, et al. Pelvic lymph node dissection during robot-assisted radical prostatectomy: efficacy, limitations, and complications—a systematic review of the literature. Eur Urol 2014;65(1):8; with permission.)

situ, whereas in an extended dissection only 8% of nodes would be left behind.

Similarly, pathoanatomic studies have also attempted to map the pattern of lymphatic spread from the bladder. In a comprehensive study of patients with BC undergoing PLND up to the inferior mesenteric artery where a mean of 50 nodes were harvested per case, bilateral nodal disease was observed in 39% of cases.[34] It was further reported that performing an ePLND would have a disease clearance rate of 65.6%, whereas continuing dissection up to the aortic bifurcation would have cleared disease in 79.1% of cases. This study also suggested that there were no skipped lesions. In contrast, Leissner and colleagues[35] observed that the site of a single positive node was outside the pelvis in 27% of the cohort and a limited dissection would have missed 27% of single nodal metastases. These data are supported by the findings of Dangle and colleagues,[36] where a quarter of the cohort would have been inaccurately staged if a limited dissection was undertaken. Failing to dissect the internal iliac region would result in nearly a third of metastases being missed and 1 in 10 patients being understaged as node-negative.[37] These studies, in addition to the study by Roth and colleagues,[33] outline the variability of bladder lymphatic drainage and suggest that an extended dissection is required to adequately sample nodes.

In addition to the diagnostic benefit observed, the literature also demonstrates that there is therapeutic value in extending the boundaries of dissection. A Canadian single institution matched study reported a superior recurrence-free survival for individuals who underwent an ePLND (HR, 0.63; $P = .005$) but no difference in overall survival (HR, 1.06; $P = .84$) compared with those who only had limited dissection.[38] In contrast, although a Danish cohort displayed no difference in recurrence rates, there was a significant difference in disease-specific survival in node-positive and node negative patients who underwent ePLND.[39] In addition, a retrospective comparison of outcomes between institutions that either performed limited or extended dissection demonstrated that the former template was associated with higher rates of disease recurrence.[40] The 5-year recurrence-free survival rates for pT2N0-2 cases who underwent limited or ePLND was 63% and 71%, respectively ($P<.0001$). The same rates for pT3N0-2 cases were 19% and 49%, respectively ($P<.0001$). Similar differences were also observed among node-negative patients. The staging benefits of ePLND were also apparent in the study where the node-positivity rate was 26% compared with 13% in those who had limited dissection. Furthermore, nomograms developed from contemporary series identify extent of dissection as being an independent predictor of disease-free and cancer-specific survival.[41] The outcomes from single institution studies reporting on extent of lymphadenectomy also suggest benefit for ePLND.[42,43] It should be noted that a subgroup analysis by stage in a meta-analysis examining the therapeutic benefits of extended dissection failed to demonstrate a benefit for patients with less than or equal to pT2 disease.[44] However, the analysis is contaminated by non-MIBC cases and hence it cannot be confidently concluded that limited dissection in T2 cases would not compromise outcomes. Overall, it seems that limited dissection is inadequate to confer a significant benefit and thus extended dissection is required but the evidence is based on low-quality studies and this is reflected in the grade C recommendation made by the European Association of Urology guideline panel.[2] Although we are still awaiting trial results to determine whether extended lymphadenectomy is appropriate, the American Urological Association currently recommends performing bilateral pelvic lymphadenectomy with removal of the external and internal iliac and obturator LNs at a minimum.[3]

Superextended lymphadenectomy

Although the literature suggests a benefit for extending nodal dissection to the crossing of the ureter and the external iliac artery, there is little to be gained by continuing dissection proximally to the origins of the inferior mesenteric artery. An ongoing prospective randomized trial conducted by the German Urologic Oncology Group that allocated muscle-invasive and high-grade T1 patients to either undergo PLND using a standard or superextended template was presented as an abstract recently.[18] There was no improvement in either 5-year recurrence-free (69.3% vs 62.0%; HR, 0.80; 95% CI, 0.54–1.19; $P = .28$) or cancer-specific survival (77.5% vs 66.2%; HR, 0.70; 95% CI, 0.45–1.10; $P = .13$) in patients in the superextended arm. The results of this study represent high-level evidence that sePLND does not improve outcomes. Furthermore, a Danish single institution study that compared RC outcomes between two time periods where sePLND or ePLND was performed exclusively reported that there was no difference in recurrence-free survival between the techniques.[45] This was consistent regardless of nodal status or tumor stage, although patients with non-organ-confined disease did show a nonsignificant trend to improved survival with sePLND. Additionally, among patients with BC undergoing RC at either the University of Bern or University of Southern California where ePLND and sePLND was performed, respectively, there was no difference in 5-year

recurrence-free survival rates for pT2pN0-2 (67% vs 57%; $P = .55$) or pT3pN0-2 (34% vs 32%; $P = .44$) cases.[46] However, this study only examined a highly selected group of patients, those with pT2-3 disease with negative margins and no neoadjuvant chemotherapy, which limits its utility in modern day clinical practice where neoadjuvant chemotherapy would generally be indicated in this group, and it is not possible to know the pathologic stage or margin status before surgery. The Memorial Sloan-Kettering Cancer Centre experience from 1980 to 1988 suggested that the survival benefit of sePLND is pronounced in those with organ-confined disease who had a 52.6% 5-year survival rate compared with 23.4% in patients with extravesical disease.[47] These results predate widespread use of neoadjuvant chemotherapy and hence may not be currently applicable. Therefore, there may be a group of patients whom may benefit from a superextended nodal dissection but they are yet to be clearly characterized and until such time, extended dissection is considered to be satisfactory.

Contralateral lymphadenectomy

The controversy surrounding the need for bilateral lymphadenectomy seems to be subsiding in recent times following the spate of papers that demonstrate that unilateral PLND is inadequate. The results from the mapping studies in which a single positive node was located on the contralateral side of the subset of patients with strictly unilateral tumors in 23.1% of cases strongly suggest the need to perform bilateral PLND.[35] This crossover phenomenon was also observed in 40% of the same subset by Roth and colleagues.[48] However, the latter group observed no contralateral drainage to the internal iliac region and thus proposed that contralateral dissection can be limited to the obturator fossa and external and common iliac nodes in unilateral bladder tumors. These findings were then confirmed in a subsequent pathoanatomic mapping project.[49] Given that there are no prospective studies evaluating the long-term safety of limiting contralateral dissection, the only approach that is recommended is bilateral ePLND.

Upper Tract Urothelial Carcinoma

The lymphatic drainage of UTUC has not been as extensively studied as BC but does not seem to be as complex. Two particular pathoanatomic studies have characterized the primary lymphatic landing sites of UTUC depending on the location and side of the tumor.[50,51] Compilation of the results from these studies has enabled description of anatomic dissection templates (**Fig. 2**). For

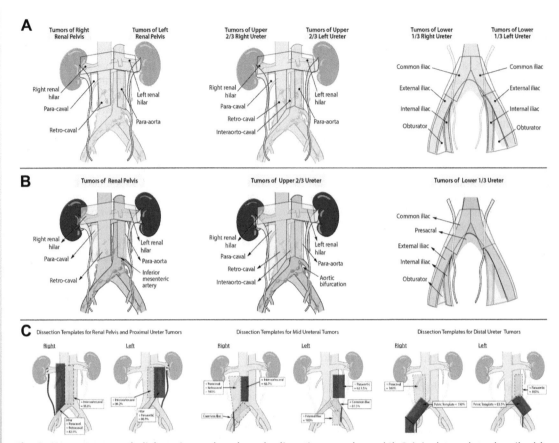

Fig. 2. Upper tract urothelial carcinoma lymph node dissection templates. (*A*) Original template described by Kondo and colleagues. (*B*) Updated template described by Kondo and colleagues. (*C*) Template described by Matin and colleagues. ([*A*] *Data from* Kondo T, Nakazawa H, Ito F, et al. Primary site and incidence of lymph node metastases in urothelial carcinoma of upper urinary tract. Urology 2007;69(2):265–9; and *Adapted from* [*B*] Kondo T, Tanabe K. Role of lymphadenectomy in the management of urothelial carcinoma of the bladder and the upper urinary tract. Int J Urol 2012;19(8):710–21, with permission; and [*C*] Matin SF, Sfakianos JP, Espiritu PN, et al. Patterns of lymphatic metastases in upper tract urothelial carcinoma and proposed dissection templates. J Urol 2015;194(6):1567–74, with permission.)

right-sided renal pelvis and proximal ureteric tumors (above the pelvic brim), removal of nodes from the hilum, paracaval, retrocaval, and interaortocaval region has been proposed to be sufficient. Only dissection of the hilar and para-aortic groups is required for left-sided tumors located in the same area. Midureteral tumors on the right side need dissection of paracaval, retrocaval, and interaortocaval nodes. The same tumors on the left side demand dissection of the para-aortic nodes in addition to the common and internal iliacs. In addition to the standard pelvic template consisting of the common, external, and internal iliac and obturator regions, for distally located disease it is necessary to remove paracaval nodes on the right and para-aortic nodes on the left. A reanalysis of the Japanese study showed positive nodes in the presacral region in 14% of the cohort.[52] The study by Matin and colleagues,[51]

which was integral in outlining the aforementioned templates, was only published recently and hence the impact of adhering to their recommendations in addition to the updated findings from the earlier study of Kondo and colleagues[52] is yet to be clearly demonstrated.

Based on the initial 2007 mapping study by Kondo and colleagues,[53] a template that included regions with more than 10% risk of metastasis demonstrated an improvement in cancer-specific survival for UTUC located in the renal pelvis (77.8% vs 51.7%; *P* = .01). There was also a trend to improved disease-free survival but the results were not statistically significant (77.8% vs 50.0%; *P* = .06). These differences were not observed for ureteral tumors. A study in patients with clinically nonmetastatic UTUC of the renal pelvis found that those who underwent complete dissection (removal of all nodal regions) according to the Tokyo

Women's and Wakayama Medical template,[50,53] used in the previously mentioned study, had a lower incidence of regional node recurrence than patients who did not have all the described nodes in the template removed or those that did not undergo a lymphadenectomy.[54] This study had important limitations that could have confounded the associations observed. The patients who did not have all the nodes in the template excised underwent surgery before 2005, whereas surgery was performed after 2005 for the other two groups. Furthermore, a degree of selection bias could be influencing outcomes because after 2005 LND was only omitted for patients with severe comorbidities and/or advanced age and a lower proportion of this group received adjuvant chemotherapy, although it only confers a minimal survival benefit.[55] Similarly, another study by the same group examining nonmetastatic, muscle-invasive ureteral tumors did demonstrate a recurrence-free and cancer-specific survival advantage for patients who had a complete dissection.[56] No difference in outcomes was evident for lower ureteral tumors. Patients in this latter group who underwent a complete dissection had a higher incidence of regional node and distant metastases. Although a small sample size may explain the insignificant result, the authors propose that diverse lymphatic spread and/or challenging dissection caused by the complex anatomy could be contributing to these results but equally lymphadenectomy may not be beneficial in this subgroup. The suboptimal outcomes experienced by patients in both studies who only had incomplete dissection suggest that removal of all nodal basins is essential to ensure the best chance of oncologic success. Therefore, it is possible that future studies based on the updated template suggested by Matin and colleagues[51] and Kondo and colleagues could improve outcomes more than currently observed, but prospective trials are required to confirm this.

PROGNOSTIC IMPLICATIONS

The therapeutic benefit of performing PLND has been well established since its benefits were originally described in 1950.[57] These observations were supported by the findings of Whitmore and Marshall[58] who demonstrated a long-term survival benefit of lymphadenectomy. Presently, the focus has turned toward using different metrics based on the LNs harvested in an attempt to predict prognosis.

Lymph Node Yield

The number of LNs obtained during PLND has been commonly used as a surrogate marker of dissection extent and quality, although it does not seem to reliably reflect either metric. It is important to recognize that factors other than the surgery influence the number of nodes, including the diligence of the pathologist and the method in which the specimen was presented to the pathologist. Meijer and colleagues[59] observed that differences in pathology department protocols between institutions can affect the number of LNs counted. This is supported by the results of a study at University of California San Francisco where a new policy was introduced that required at least 16 LNs to be examined following RC and specimens that did not meet this cutoff were required to be resubmitted. Following implementation of the aforementioned policy, median LN yield significantly increased from 15 to 20 nodes and there was also a decrease in mortality risk by 48%.[60] Furthermore, submitting specimens separately rather than en bloc also increases the LN yield.[61] A cadaveric study observed that there is considerable variation in LN count between individuals.[62] Therefore, it is now widely accepted that the anatomic boundaries of dissection are more important than the number of LNs harvested.

Although the validity of using LN yield either as a measure of surgical quality or as a prognostic marker is clearly questionable, several studies have reported an association with outcomes. A study using the SEER database observed that patients with three or fewer nodes examined had a higher risk of death than patients who had more than three nodes examined.[63] Similarly, the total number of LNs was identified as an independent predictor of recurrence-free, cancer-specific, and overall survival in a range of studies.[64–66] A large multicenter collaborative study reported that, compared with removing less than 10 nodes, removing more than 10 nodes increased 5-year survival (44% vs 61%).[67] Other studies have suggested higher thresholds to garner benefit that range from 14 to 22 nodes removed.[68,69] These findings were supported by a recent meta-analysis that pooled 25 cohort studies consisting of more than 40,000 patients in total and reported a positive correlation between the number of nodes harvested and the three previously mentioned outcomes (**Fig. 3**).[70] An updated SEER study only observed the association between LN count and survival in cases without nodal metastases, whereas nodal yield did not influence outcomes in node-positive patients.[71] This is likely explained by the Will Rogers effect: improved staging from examining a greater number of nodes would have resulted in patients being redistributed to the N1 group whose nodal metastases would have otherwise been undetected.[72]

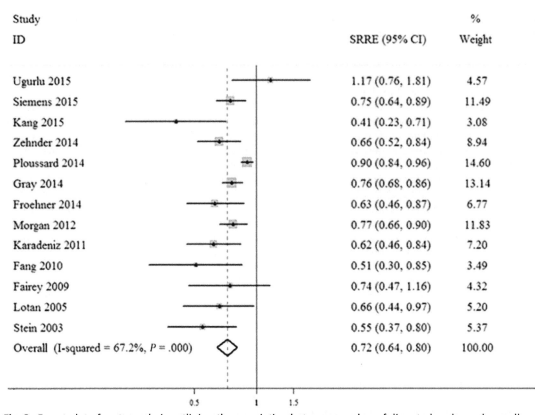

Fig. 3. Forest plot of meta-analysis outlining the association between number of dissected nodes and overall survival in bladder cancer. Values <1.0 favor extending nodal dissection. Weights are from random effects analysis. (*From* Li F, Hong X, Hou L, et al. A greater number of dissected lymph nodes is associated with more favorable outcomes in bladder cancer treated by radical cystectomy: a meta-analysis. Oncotarget 2016;7(38):61284–94; with permission.)

This reaffirms the line of thought that LN yield is confounded by several other factors, including those previously mentioned, and thus using it as a prognostic indicator is inherently flawed.

Similarly, the literature is conflicting regarding the utility of LN yield as a prognostic indicator in UTUC. A recent population-based analysis of the National Cancer Data Base found that a higher LN yield was associated with lower all-cause mortality (HR, 0.94 per five LNs removed; 95% CI, 0.89–1.00; $P = .034$).[73] Roscigno and colleagues[74,75] suggest that a minimum of eight nodes need to be removed to achieve a 75% probability of finding a positive node and also had the added benefit of prolonging survival. Conversely, a multi-institutional Canadian study reported that nodal yield did not impact survival.[23] Given the number of confounders and the inconsistency in the literature, it is challenging to specify a threshold of nodal yield as a prognostic factor, although certain centers have set a minimum number of nodes at 13 to measure adequacy of dissection.[74]

Lymph Node Density

To address the shortcomings of nodal yield as a prognostic marker, LN density was suggested to be a better indicator of outcomes. This is a ratio of positive to total number of LNs examined and is considered to reflect the burden of nodal disease in relation to the quality of LND and also accounts for anatomic variations regarding the number of nodes present.[76] In a cohort of 477 patients, nodal density greater than 20% was associated with an increased risk of cancer-specific death on multivariate analysis (HR, 1.65; 95% CI, 1.27–2.15; $P = .001$).[77] This relationship was consistent regardless of the dissection extent. Kassouf and colleagues[78] also observed an inverse relationship between LN density and disease-specific survival but their analysis categorized the former variable into quintiles. Although the literature demonstrates an association between this metric and disease-specific survival, only one study has shown a correlation to either recurrence-free or overall survival, whereas an overwhelming number of negative studies has not shown a survival advantage.[71,79,80] A meta-analysis did, however, demonstrate that LN density acts as a significant prognostic indicator of all three end points but there was considerable heterogeneity between the included studies, which limits its findings (**Fig. 4**).[81] A recent retrospective study suggests that nodal density is a better indicator of prognosis than the American Joint Committee on Cancer TNM nodal staging system in node-positive patients.[82] In patients with UTUC, an LN density less than 30% conferred a lower 5-year risk of recurrence or death.[83] It should be kept in mind that this metric is also influenced by confounders that affect LN density and hence should not be used exclusively to guide decisions.

Extranodal Extension

Similar to the previously mentioned prognostic markers, there are conflicting results regarding the value of extranodal extension (ENE) being used as a prognostic marker. Fleischmann and colleagues[79] were the first to characterize the relationship in patients with MIBC by reporting significantly decreased recurrence-free and overall survival in patients with ENE. Cases where the tumor had perforated the LN capsule had more than double the risk of recurrence. The ability of ENE to predict outcomes has been reported in several other studies and can guide decision-making post-cystectomy with regards to adjuvant treatment and follow-up schedule.[84,85] Further research in the form of prospective studies is still required in the light of reports that show no use for ENE as a prognostic marker.[78,80,86]

Fajkovic and colleagues[87] examined the prognostic value of ENE in patients with upper tract disease and concluded that it is a strong predictor of outcomes. This study found that the incidence of ENE increases with pT stage and has a significant impact on disease recurrence and cancer-specific mortality.

FEASIBILITY OF LYMPH NODE DISSECTION USING LAPAROSCOPIC OR ROBOTIC APPROACHES

With the increased use of minimally invasive approaches for RC over time, it is important to assess the feasibility and safety of performing PLND using these techniques because they possess their own challenges compared with open surgery.[88] It was initially thought that laparoscopic or robot-assisted RC and ePLND may compromise oncologic success,[89] but these concerns have subsided over time. Using LN yield as a surrogate measure for PLND quality, two randomized trials reported no significant difference between approaches.[90,91] A novel study where second-look open nodal dissection followed robotic PLND found that only a median of four extra nodes were harvested from the open portion of the case and thus robotic PLND yielded 93% of nodes.[92] Furthermore, there was less blood loss and speedier recovery among patients who underwent robotic rather than open RC.[91] Nevertheless, operating time is prolonged with the former approach.

There is paucity of data assessing the safety of performing lymphadenectomy during laparoscopic or robot-assisted nephroureterectomy but the limited reports are reassuring. A small cohort

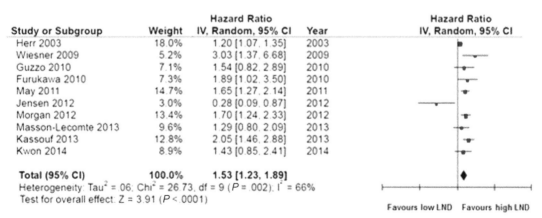

Study or Subgroup	Weight	Hazard Ratio IV, Random, 95% CI	Year	Hazard Ratio IV, Random, 95% CI
Herr 2003	18.0%	1.20 [1.07, 1.35]	2003	
Wiesner 2009	5.2%	3.03 [1.37, 6.68]	2009	
Guzzo 2010	7.1%	1.54 [0.82, 2.89]	2010	
Furukawa 2010	7.3%	1.89 [1.02, 3.50]	2010	
May 2011	14.7%	1.65 [1.27, 2.14]	2011	
Jensen 2012	3.0%	0.28 [0.09, 0.87]	2012	
Morgan 2012	13.4%	1.70 [1.24, 2.33]	2012	
Masson-Lecomte 2013	9.6%	1.29 [0.80, 2.09]	2013	
Kassouf 2013	12.8%	2.05 [1.46, 2.88]	2013	
Kwon 2014	8.9%	1.43 [0.85, 2.41]	2014	
Total (95% CI)	**100.0%**	**1.53 [1.23, 1.89]**		

Heterogeneity: Tau^2 = .06; Chi^2 = 26.73, df = 9 (P = .002); I^2 = 66%
Test for overall effect: Z = 3.91 (P < .0001)

Favours low LND   Favours high LND

Fig. 4. Forest plot of meta-analysis outlining the association between lymph node density and disease-specific survival in bladder cancer. (*From* Ku JH, Kang M, Kim HS, et al. Lymph node density as a prognostic variable in node-positive bladder cancer: a meta-analysis. BMC Cancer 2015;15:447; and *Data from* under a creative commons 4.0 attribution license. Available at: https://bmccancer.biomedcentral.com/articles/10.1186/s12885-015-1448-x.)

study examining the safety of RPLND reported no difference in nodal yield or complications between open, laparoscopic, or robot-assisted surgery.[93] Similar to RC, minimally invasive approaches had lower blood loss at the expense of prolonged operating time. Median length of hospital stay was identical for all groups. Although larger, prospective studies are required to confirm the safety and feasibility of minimally invasive nephroureterectomy and LND, current evidence suggests it is a safe procedure.

SAFETY OF LYMPHADENECTOMY

Among a cohort of octogenarians undergoing RC, there was no difference in perioperative (7% vs 5%; $P = .75$) or postoperative complications (58% vs 43%; $P = .186$) between those who had PLND and those who only had RC.[94] A heterogeneous cohort of 187 patients undergoing bilateral PLND for prostate or BC reported a 4.7% incidence of lymphocele.[95] This rate is dependent on the definition of lymphocele and the method of evaluation because using ultrasound or CT increased the incidence to 22% and 54%, respectively, after prostatectomy.[96,97] The extent of dissection was associated with the incidence of lymphoceles.[98] Likewise, a meta-analysis of the literature demonstrated that the addition of a PLND to radical prostatectomy more than doubled the risk of venous thromboembolism (relative risk, 2.15; 95% CI, 1.14–4.04; $P = .018$).[99] Despite being variable between studies, the absolute risk still remains low and is further mitigated with appropriate prophylaxis. Other complications of PLND include ureteral, neurologic, and vascular injury, but they are rare.[98]

Compared with a limited template, there seems to be minimal risk difference in performing PLND using an extended template. A single surgeon series comparing limited with extended dissection found no increase in complication in the latter group.[100] This study was not randomized and consisted of patients from two different time periods; limited dissection was performed before 1993 and extended after this time point, therefore surgical experience could confound these results. A study of well-matched patients undergoing standard or extended dissection observed that there was no increase in either intraoperative or postoperative complications nor was there a difference in the length of hospital stay in the latter group.[38] There was, however, an increase in blood loss and subsequently the rate of blood transfusions and the mean total units transfused. ePLND is feasibly performed laparoscopically or robotically but does increase operative time.[101,102]

A similar relationship is observed for UTUC cases. A comparison of patients undergoing template-based lymphadenectomy and those not having any nodal dissection demonstrated that although there was a greater number of complications across all Clavien grades in the former group, the difference was not significant.[103] This is the same for estimated blood loss, operative time, and length of hospital stay.[52] This data is based on nodal dissection being performed through a retroperitoneal approach and thus may not be generalizable to patients undergoing transperitoneal lymphadenectomy. Patients undergoing radical nephrectomy and LND for renal carcinoma using the latter approach did not experience a greater number of complications compared with those who did not have a nodal dissection.[104]

SUMMARY

This review highlights the lack of high-quality, randomized trials to guide clinical practice in terms of LND in either BC or UTUC. Therefore, clinicians are relying on observational data that is subject to confounders. Despite this, the current literature does indicate a therapeutic benefit of performing an ePLND for muscle-invasive disease as reflected in the guidelines. The benefit of ePLND (as opposed to sePLND) seems to exist for lower and upper tract urothelial tumors. Template-based node dissections are more important than pure node counts because they are subject to the diligence of the pathologist and anatomic variability. The downside risk of performing such ePLND seems to be low.

REFERENCES

1. Siegel RL, Miller KD, Jemal A. Cancer statistics, 2017. CA Cancer J Clin 2017;67(1):7–30.
2. Rouprêt M, Babjuk M, Compérat E, et al. European Association of Urology guidelines on upper urinary tract urothelial cell carcinoma: 2015 update. Eur Urol 2015;68(5):868–79.
3. Chang SS, Bochner BH, Chou R, et al. Treatment of non-metastatic muscle-invasive bladder cancer: AUA/ASCO/ASTRO/SUO guideline. J Urol 2017; 198(3):552–9.
4. Clark PE, Spiess PE, Agarwal N, et al. NCCN guidelines insights: bladder cancer, version 2.2016. J Natl Compr Canc Netw 2016;14(10): 1213–24.
5. Witjes JA, Lebret T, Compérat EM, et al. Updated 2016 EAU guidelines on muscle-invasive and metastatic bladder cancer. Eur Urol 2017;71(3): 462–75.

6. Dorfman RE, Alpern MB, Gross BH, et al. Upper abdominal lymph nodes: criteria for normal size determined with CT. Radiology 1991;180(2):319–22.

7. Einstein DM, Singer AA, Chilcote WA, et al. Abdominal lymphadenopathy: spectrum of CT findings. Radiographics 1991;11(3):457–72.

8. Maurer T, Souvatzoglou M, Kubler H, et al. Diagnostic efficacy of [11C]choline positron emission tomography/computed tomography compared with conventional computed tomography in lymph node staging of patients with bladder cancer prior to radical cystectomy. Eur Urol 2012;61(5):1031–8.

9. Swinnen G, Maes A, Pottel H, et al. FDG-PET/CT for the preoperative lymph node staging of invasive bladder cancer. Eur Urol 2010;57(4):641–7.

10. Paik ML, Scolieri MJ, Brown SL, et al. Limitations of computerized tomography in staging invasive bladder cancer before radical cystectomy. J Urol 2000;163(6):1693–6.

11. Ficarra V, Dalpiaz O, Alrabi N, et al. Correlation between clinical and pathological staging in a series of radical cystectomies for bladder carcinoma. BJU Int 2005;95(6):786–90.

12. Tritschler S, Mosler C, Straub J, et al. Staging of muscle-invasive bladder cancer: can computerized tomography help us to decide on local treatment? World J Urol 2012;30(6):827–31.

13. Colston JAC, Leadbetter WF. Infiltrating carcinoma of the bladder[1]. J Urol 1936;36(6):669–83.

14. Jewett HJ, Strong GH. Infiltrating carcinoma of the bladder; relation of depth of penetration of the bladder wall to incidence of local extension and metastases. J Urol 1946;55:366–72.

15. Shariat SF, Karakiewicz PI, Palapattu GS, et al. Outcomes of radical cystectomy for transitional cell carcinoma of the bladder: a contemporary series from the Bladder Cancer Research Consortium. J Urol 2006;176(6 Pt 1):2414–22 [discussion: 2422].

16. Larcher A, Sun M, Schiffmann J, et al. Differential effect on survival of pelvic lymph node dissection at radical cystectomy for muscle invasive bladder cancer. Eur J Surg Oncol 2015;41(3):353–60.

17. Abdollah F, Sun M, Schmitges J, et al. Stage-specific impact of pelvic lymph node dissection on survival in patients with non-metastatic bladder cancer treated with radical cystectomy. BJU Int 2012;109(8):1147–54.

18. Gschwend JE, Heck MM, Lehmann J, et al. Limited versus extended pelvic lymphadenectomy in patients with bladder cancer undergoing radical cystectomy: survival results from a prospective, randomized trial (LEA AUO AB 25/02). J Clin Oncol 2016;34(15_suppl):4503.

19. Herr HW, Faulkner JR, Grossman HB, et al. Surgical factors influence bladder cancer outcomes: a cooperative group report. J Clin Oncol 2004; 22(14):2781–9.

20. Brunocilla E, Pernetti R, Schiavina R, et al. The number of nodes removed as well as the template of the dissection is independently correlated to cancer-specific survival after radical cystectomy for muscle-invasive bladder cancer. Int Urol Nephrol 2013;45(3):711–9.

21. Giuliano AE, Ballman KV, McCall L, et al. Effect of axillary dissection vs no axillary dissection on 10-year overall survival among women with invasive breast cancer and sentinel node metastasis: the ACOSOG Z0011 (Alliance) randomized clinical trial. JAMA 2017;318(10):918–26.

22. Faries MB, Thompson JF, Cochran AJ, et al. Completion dissection or observation for sentinel-node metastasis in melanoma. N Engl J Med 2017;376(23):2211–22.

23. Mason RJ, Kassouf W, Bell DG, et al. The contemporary role of lymph node dissection during nephroureterectomy in the management of upper urinary tract urothelial carcinoma: the Canadian experience. Urology 2012;79(4):840–5.

24. Inokuchi J, Kuroiwa K, Kakehi Y, et al. Role of lymph node dissection during radical nephroureterectomy for upper urinary tract urothelial cancer: multi-institutional large retrospective study JCOG1110A. World J Urol 2017;35(11):1737–44.

25. Abe T, Shinohara N, Harabayashi T, et al. The role of lymph-node dissection in the treatment of upper urinary tract cancer: a multi-institutional study. BJU Int 2008;102(5):576–80.

26. Ouzzane A, Colin P, Ghoneim TP, et al. The impact of lymph node status and features on oncological outcomes in urothelial carcinoma of the upper urinary tract (UTUC) treated by nephroureterectomy. World J Urol 2013;31(1):189–97.

27. Roscigno M, Cozzarini C, Bertini R, et al. Prognostic value of lymph node dissection in patients with muscle-invasive transitional cell carcinoma of the upper urinary tract. Eur Urol 2008;53(4):794–802.

28. Lughezzani G, Jeldres C, Isbarn H, et al. A critical appraisal of the value of lymph node dissection at nephroureterectomy for upper tract urothelial carcinoma. Urology 2010;75(1):118–24.

29. Burger M, Shariat SF, Fritsche H-M, et al. No overt influence of lymphadenectomy on cancer-specific survival in organ-confined versus locally advanced upper urinary tract urothelial carcinoma undergoing radical nephroureterectomy: a retrospective international, multi-institutional study. World J Urol 2011;29(4):465–72.

30. Brien JC, Shariat SF, Herman MP, et al. Preoperative hydronephrosis, ureteroscopic biopsy grade and urinary cytology can improve prediction of advanced upper tract urothelial carcinoma. J Urol 2010;184(1):69–73.

31. Bagrodia A, Krabbe LM, Gayed BA, et al. Evaluation of the prognostic significance of altered mammalian target of rapamycin pathway biomarkers in upper tract urothelial carcinoma. Urology 2014;84(5):1134–40.

32. Matin SF, Kamat AM, Grossman HB. High-frequency endoluminal ultrasonography as an aid to the staging of upper tract urothelial carcinoma: imaging findings and pathologic correlation. J Ultrasound Med 2010;29(9):1277–84.

33. Roth B, Wissmeyer MP, Zehnder P, et al. A new multimodality technique accurately maps the primary lymphatic landing sites of the bladder. Eur Urol 2010;57(2):205–11.

34. Abol-Enein H, El-Baz M, Abd El-Hameed MA, et al. Lymph node involvement in patients with bladder cancer treated with radical cystectomy: a pathoanatomical study—a single center experience. J Urol 2004;172(5):1818–21.

35. Leissner J, Ghoneim MA, Abol-Enein H, et al. Extended radical lymphadenectomy in patients with urothelial bladder cancer: results of a prospective multicenter study. J Urol 2004;171(1): 139–44.

36. Dangle PP, Gong MC, Bahnson RR, et al. How do commonly performed lymphadenectomy templates influence bladder cancer nodal stage? J Urol 2010; 183(2):499–504.

37. Seiler R, von Gunten M, Thalmann GN, et al. Pelvic lymph nodes: distribution and nodal tumour burden of urothelial bladder cancer. J Clin Pathol 2010; 63(6):504–7.

38. Abdi H, Pourmalek F, Gleave ME, et al. Balancing risk and benefit of extended pelvic lymph node dissection in patients undergoing radical cystectomy. World J Urol 2016;34(1):41–8.

39. Jensen JB, Ulhoi BP, Jensen KM. Extended versus limited lymph node dissection in radical cystectomy: impact on recurrence pattern and survival. Int J Urol 2012;19(1):39–47.

40. Dhar NB, Klein EA, Reuther AM, et al. Outcome after radical cystectomy with limited or extended pelvic lymph node dissection. J Urol 2008;179(3):873–8.

41. Simone G, Bianchi M, Giannarelli D, et al. Development and external validation of nomograms predicting disease-free and cancer-specific survival after radical cystectomy. World J Urol 2015; 33(10):1419–28.

42. Stein JP, Quek ML, Skinner DG. Lymphadenectomy for invasive bladder cancer: I. Historical perspective and contemporary rationale. BJU Int 2006; 97(2):227–31.

43. Stein JP, Quek ML, Skinner DG. Lymphadenectomy for invasive bladder cancer. II. Technical aspects and prognostic factors. BJU Int 2006;97(2):232–7.

44. Bi L, Huang H, Fan X, et al. Extended vs non-extended pelvic lymph node dissection and their influence on recurrence-free survival in patients undergoing radical cystectomy for bladder cancer: a systematic review and meta-analysis of comparative studies. BJU Int 2014;113(5b):E39–48.

45. Møller MK, Høyer S, Jensen JB. Extended versus superextended lymph-node dissection in radical cystectomy: subgroup analysis of possible recurrence-free survival benefit. Scand J Urol 2016;50(3):175–80.

46. Zehnder P, Studer UE, Skinner EC, et al. Super extended versus extended pelvic lymph node dissection in patients undergoing radical cystectomy for bladder cancer: a comparative study. J Urol 2011;186(4):1261–8.

47. Vieweg J, Whitmore WF, Herr HW, et al. The role of pelvic lymphadenectomy and radical cystectomy for lymph node positive bladder cancer. The Memorial Sloan-Kettering Cancer Center experience. Cancer 1994;73(12):3020–8.

48. Roth B, Zehnder P, Birkhauser FD, et al. Is bilateral extended pelvic lymphadenectomy necessary for strictly unilateral invasive bladder cancer? J Urol 2012;187(5):1577–82.

49. Kiss B, Paerli M, Schondorf D, et al. Pelvic lymph node dissection may be limited on the contralateral side in strictly unilateral bladder cancer without compromising oncological radicality. Bladder Cancer 2016;2(1):53–9.

50. Kondo T, Nakazawa H, Ito F, et al. Primary site and incidence of lymph node metastases in urothelial carcinoma of upper urinary tract. Urology 2007; 69(2):265–9.

51. Matin SF, Sfakianos JP, Espiritu PN, et al. Patterns of lymphatic metastases in upper tract urothelial carcinoma and proposed dissection templates. J Urol 2015;194(6):1567–74.

52. Kondo T, Tanabe K. Role of lymphadenectomy in the management of urothelial carcinoma of the bladder and the upper urinary tract. Int J Urol 2012;19(8):710–21.

53. Kondo T, Hara I, Takagi T, et al. Template-based lymphadenectomy in urothelial carcinoma of the renal pelvis: a prospective study. Int J Urol 2014; 21(5):453–9.

54. Kondo T, Hara I, Takagi T, et al. Possible role of template-based lymphadenectomy in reducing the risk of regional node recurrence after nephroureterectomy in patients with renal pelvic cancer. Jpn J Clin Oncol 2014;44(12):1233–8.

55. Hellenthal NJ, Shariat SF, Margulis V, et al. Adjuvant chemotherapy for high risk upper tract urothelial carcinoma: results from the Upper Tract Urothelial Carcinoma Collaboration. J Urol 2009;182(3): 900–6.

56. Kondo T, Hara I, Takagi T, et al. Template-based lymphadenectomy reduces the risk of regional lymph node recurrence among patients with

upper/middle ureteral cancer. Int J Clin Oncol 2017;22(1):145–52.

57. Kerr WS, Colby FH. Pelvic lymph node dissection and total cystectomy in the treatment of carcinoma of the bladder. J Urol 1950;63:842–51.

58. Whitmore WF Jr, Marshall VF. Radical total cystectomy for cancer of the bladder: 230 consecutive cases five years later. J Urol 1962;87:853–68.

59. Meijer RP, Nunnink CJ, Wassenaar AE, et al. Standard lymph node dissection for bladder cancer: significant variability in the number of reported lymph nodes. J Urol 2012;187(2):446–50.

60. Fang AC, Ahmad AE, Whitson JM, et al. Effect of a minimum lymph node policy in radical cystectomy and pelvic lymphadenectomy on lymph node yields, lymph node positivity rates, lymph node density, and survivorship in patients with bladder cancer. Cancer 2010;116(8):1901–8.

61. Bochner BH, Herr HW, Reuter VE. Impact of separate versus en bloc pelvic lymph node dissection on the number of lymph nodes retrieved in cystectomy specimens. J Urol 2001;166(6):2295–6.

62. Davies JD, Simons CM, Ruhotina N, et al. Anatomic basis for lymph node counts as measure of lymph node dissection extent: a cadaveric study. Urology 2013;81(2):358–63.

63. Konety BR, Joslyn SA, O'Donnell MA. Extent of pelvic lymphadenectomy and its impact on outcome in patients diagnosed with bladder cancer: analysis of data from the surveillance, epidemiology and end results program data base. J Urol 2003; 169(3):946–50.

64. Zehnder P, Studer UE, Daneshmand S, et al. Outcomes of radical cystectomy with extended lymphadenectomy alone in patients with lymph node-positive bladder cancer who are unfit for or who decline adjuvant chemotherapy. BJU Int 2014; 113(4):554–60.

65. Karadeniz T, Baran C, Topsakal M, et al. Importance of the number of retrieved lymph nodes during cystectomy. Urol J 2011;8(3):197–202.

66. Siemens DR, Mackillop WJ, Peng Y, et al. Lymph node counts are valid indicators of the quality of surgical care in bladder cancer: a population-based study. Urol Oncol 2015;33(10):425.e15-23.

67. Herr H, Lee C, Chang S, et al. Standardization of radical cystectomy and pelvic lymph node dissection for bladder cancer: a collaborative group report. J Urol 2004;171(5):1823–8 [discussion: 1827–8].

68. Koppie TM, Vickers AJ, Vora K, et al. Standardization of pelvic lymphadenectomy performed at radical cystectomy: can we establish a minimum number of lymph nodes that should be removed? Cancer 2006;107(10):2368–74.

69. Vazina A, Dugi D, Shariat SF, et al. Stage specific lymph node metastasis mapping in radical cystectomy specimens. J Urol 2004;171(5):1830–4.

70. Li F, Hong X, Hou L, et al. A greater number of dissected lymph nodes is associated with more favorable outcomes in bladder cancer treated by radical cystectomy: a meta-analysis. Oncotarget 2016;7(38):61284–94.

71. Morgan TM, Barocas DA, Penson DF, et al. Lymph node yield at radical cystectomy predicts mortality in node-negative and not node-positive patients. Urology 2012;80(3):632–40.

72. Feinstein AR, Sosin DM, Wells CK. The Will Rogers phenomenon. Stage migration and new diagnostic techniques as a source of misleading statistics for survival in cancer. N Engl J Med 1985;312(25): 1604–8.

73. Zareba P, Rosenzweig B, Winer AG, et al. Association between lymph node yield and survival among patients undergoing radical nephroureterectomy for urothelial carcinoma of the upper tract. Cancer 2017;123(10):1741–50.

74. Roscigno M, Shariat SF, Freschi M, et al. Assessment of the minimum number of lymph nodes needed to detect lymph node invasion at radical nephroureterectomy in patients with upper tract urothelial cancer. Urology 2009;74(5):1070–4.

75. Roscigno M, Shariat SF, Margulis V, et al. The extent of lymphadenectomy seems to be associated with better survival in patients with nonmetastatic upper-tract urothelial carcinoma: how many lymph nodes should be removed? Eur Urol 2009; 56(3):512–8.

76. Herr HW. Superiority of ratio based lymph node staging for bladder cancer. J Urol 2003;169(3): 943–5.

77. May M, Herrmann E, Bolenz C, et al. Lymph node density affects cancer-specific survival in patients with lymph node–positive urothelial bladder cancer following radical cystectomy. Eur Urol 2011;59(5): 712–8.

78. Kassouf W, Svatek RS, Shariat SF, et al. Critical analysis and validation of lymph node density as prognostic variable in urothelial carcinoma of bladder. Urol Oncol 2013;31(4):480–6.

79. Fleischmann A, Thalmann GN, Markwalder R, et al. Extracapsular extension of pelvic lymph node metastases from urothelial carcinoma of the bladder is an independent prognostic factor. J Clin Oncol 2005;23(10):2358–65.

80. Stephenson AJ, Gong MC, Campbell SC, et al. Aggregate lymph node metastasis diameter and survival after radical cystectomy for invasive bladder cancer. Urology 2010;75(2):382–6.

81. Ku JH, Kang M, Kim HS, et al. Lymph node density as a prognostic variable in node-positive bladder cancer: a meta-analysis. BMC Cancer 2015;15:447.

82. Lee D, Yoo S, You D, et al. Lymph node density vs. the American Joint Committee on Cancer TNM nodal staging system in node-positive bladder

cancer in patients undergoing extended or super-extended pelvic lymphadenectomy. Urol Oncol 2017;35(4):151.e1-7.

83. Bolenz C, Shariat SF, Fernandez MI, et al. Risk stratification of patients with nodal involvement in upper tract urothelial carcinoma: value of lymph-node density. BJU Int 2009;103(3):302–6.

84. Seiler R, von Gunten M, Thalmann GN, et al. Extracapsular extension but not the tumour burden of lymph node metastases is an independent adverse risk factor in lymph node-positive bladder cancer. Histopathology 2011;58(4):571–8.

85. Fajkovic H, Cha EK, Jeldres C, et al. Extranodal extension is a powerful prognostic factor in bladder cancer patients with lymph node metastasis. Eur Urol 2013;64(5):837–45.

86. Jeong IG, Ro JY, Kim SC, et al. Extranodal extension in node-positive bladder cancer: the continuing controversy. BJU Int 2011;108(1):38–43.

87. Fajkovic H, Cha EK, Jeldres C, et al. Prognostic value of extranodal extension and other lymph node parameters in patients with upper tract urothelial carcinoma. J Urol 2012;187(3):845–51.

88. Pak JS, Lee JJ, Bilal K, et al. Utilization trends and short-term outcomes of robotic versus open radical cystectomy for bladder cancer. Urology 2017;103:117–23.

89. Schumacher MC, Jonsson MN, Wiklund NP. Does extended lymphadenectomy preclude laparoscopic or robot-assisted radical cystectomy in advanced bladder cancer? Curr Opin Urol 2009;19(5):527–32.

90. Parekh DJ, Messer J, Fitzgerald J, et al. Perioperative outcomes and oncologic efficacy from a pilot prospective randomized clinical trial of open versus robotic assisted radical cystectomy. J Urol 2013;189(2):474–9.

91. Nix J, Smith A, Kurpad R, et al. Prospective randomized controlled trial of robotic versus open radical cystectomy for bladder cancer: perioperative and pathologic results. Eur Urol 2010;57(2):196–201.

92. Davis JW, Gaston K, Anderson R, et al. Robot assisted extended pelvic lymphadenectomy at radical cystectomy: lymph node yield compared with second look open dissection. J Urol 2011;185(1):79–83.

93. Rao SR, Correa JJ, Sexton WJ, et al. Prospective clinical trial of the feasibility and safety of modified retroperitoneal lymph node dissection at time of nephroureterectomy for upper tract urothelial carcinoma. BJU Int 2012;110(11b):E475–80.

94. Grabbert M, Grimm T, Buchner A, et al. Risks and benefits of pelvic lymphadenectomy in octogenarians undergoing radical cystectomy due to urothelial carcinoma of the bladder. Int Urol Nephrol 2017;49(12):2137–42.

95. Sogani PC, Watson RC, Whitmore WF Jr. Lymphocele after pelvic lymphadenectomy for urologic cancer. Urology 1981;17(1):39–43.

96. Spring DB, Schroeder D, Babu S, et al. Ultrasonic evaluation of lymphocele formation after staging lymphadenectomy for prostatic carcinoma. Radiology 1981;141(2):479–83.

97. Solberg A, Angelsen A, Bergan U, et al. Frequency of lymphoceles after open and laparoscopic pelvic lymph node dissection in patients with prostate cancer. Scand J Urol Nephrol 2003;37(3):218–21.

98. Loeb S, Partin AW, Schaeffer EM. Complications of pelvic lymphadenectomy: do the risks outweigh the benefits? Rev Urol 2010;12(1):20–4.

99. Eifler JB, Levinson AW, Hyndman ME, et al. Pelvic lymph node dissection is associated with symptomatic venous thromboembolism risk during laparoscopic radical prostatectomy. J Urol 2011;185(5):1661–5.

100. Poulsen AL, Horn T, Steven K. Radical cystectomy: extending the limits of pelvic lymph node dissection improves survival for patients with bladder cancer confined to the bladder wall. J Urol 1998;160(6 Pt 1):2015–9 [discussion: 2020].

101. Finelli A, Gill IS, Desai MM, et al. Laparoscopic extended pelvic lymphadenectomy for bladder cancer: technique and initial outcomes. J Urol 2004;172(5):1809–12.

102. Brossner C, Pycha A, Toth A, et al. Does extended lymphadenectomy increase the morbidity of radical cystectomy? BJU Int 2004;93(1):64–6.

103. Kondo T, Takagi T, Tanabe K. Therapeutic role of template-based lymphadenectomy in urothelial carcinoma of the upper urinary tract. World J Clin Oncol 2015;6(6):237–51.

104. Blom JH, van Poppel H, Marechal JM, et al. Radical nephrectomy with and without lymph-node dissection: final results of European Organization for Research and Treatment of Cancer (EORTC) randomized phase 3 trial 30881. Eur Urol 2009;55(1):28–34.

Enhanced Recovery After Surgery Pathways
Role and Outcomes in the Management of Muscle Invasive Bladder Cancer

Daniel Zainfeld, MD, Ankeet Shah, MD,
Siamak Daneshmand, MD*

KEYWORDS

• Bladder cancer • Cystectomy • Enhanced recovery • ERAS • Fast track

KEY POINTS

• Radical cystectomy is an important therapeutic procedure in the management of muscle-invasive urothelial carcinoma but is accompanied by significant morbidity.
• Enhanced recovery protocols represent focused multidisciplinary care plans that aim to optimize patient outcomes through use of evidence-based interventions at all phases of care.
• In the setting of radical cystectomy, enhanced recovery after surgery (ERAS) decreases the incidence of gastrointestinal complications and shortens the length of postoperative hospitalization.
• Continued refinement of ERAS pathways and identification of meaningful interventions will allow further improvements in patient care and outcomes from radical cystectomy.

INTRODUCTION

Coordinated multidisciplinary care pathways aimed at optimizing patient recovery from complex surgeries have deservedly received significant attention in recent years. Most commonly termed enhanced recovery after surgery (ERAS) protocols, these multidisciplinary efforts to improve perioperative care across a wide spectrum of patients have been implemented within many surgical disciplines. Benefits have been most demonstrable among patients undergoing complex surgical interventions wherein multiple care teams are involved, perioperative morbidity is significant, and extended postoperative hospitalization is typical. Although often difficult to study and directly analyze, a growing body of evidence indicates that structured application of evidence-based principles and standardization of perioperative care significantly improve clinical outcomes.

Among urologic surgeons, radical cystectomy has been especially targeted for application of ERAS pathways because of the complexity of care and frequency of perioperative complications. The authors examine the history of radical cystectomy in the management of urothelial carcinoma, introduction of ERAS pathways, and reported outcomes of radical cystectomy in the setting of ERAS.

RADICAL CYSTECTOMY

Urothelial carcinoma is a common malignancy expected to account for almost 80,000 new cases of cancer in the United States in 2017.[1] Most new cases represent non–muscle-invasive disease, which is generally managed successfully through endoscopic techniques.[2] Even among this cohort, however, close surveillance due to high rates of recurrence and progression make bladder cancer

Disclosure Statement: The authors have nothing to disclose.
Department of Urology, USC Keck/Norris Comprehensive Cancer Center, 1441 Eastlake Avenue, Suite 7416, Los Angeles, CA 90089, USA
* Corresponding author. 1441 Eastlake Avenue, Suite 7416, Los Angeles, CA 90089.
E-mail address: daneshma@med.usc.edu

Urol Clin N Am 45 (2018) 229–239
https://doi.org/10.1016/j.ucl.2017.12.007

among the most costly malignancies to manage.[3] For those patients with muscle-invasive disease as well as some high risk non–muscle-invasive patients, surgical excision of the bladder (radical cystectomy) remains the gold standard therapy often preceded by neoadjuvant chemotherapy.

Radical cystectomy is among the most technically demanding procedures performed by urologists. Adding complexity is the generally older age at diagnosis of many patients and significant medical comorbidities, which commonly coexist in this cohort.[4] In addition, the recommended administration of neoadjuvant chemotherapy due to a known survival benefit among eligible patients with muscle-invasive disease exacerbates the physiologic stress of an already demanding procedure, though it is overall well tolerated.[5] Along with excision of the bladder, concomitant urinary diversion is necessarily performed with resultant physiologic, lifestyle, body image, and psychosocial adjustments required of patients.

When performed with curative intent, however, oncologic outcomes from radical cystectomy are quite good.[6] Indeed, recent studies indicate radical cystectomy is generally underutilized in the management of advanced urothelial carcinoma, particularly among older patients in whom concerns regarding stress and recovery from radical cystectomy may detract providers and patients alike from pursuing surgical intervention regardless of potential benefits.[7] Therefore, methods to limit perioperative morbidity and increase patients' ability to tolerate and recover from the procedure are essential. Application of ERAS to radical cystectomy aims to address this critical need through optimization of patient care at all levels of care from the time of diagnosis to postoperative settings.

ESTABLISHED OUTCOMES FOLLOWING RADICAL CYSTECTOMY

As noted, radical cystectomy is an extremely complex procedure. Performance of radical cystectomy requires isolation and division of ureters, mobilization of the bladder, ligation of vascular pedicles, and division of the urethra while preventing tumor spillage or damage to surrounding structures, including the rectum. In addition, the prostate in men and the uterus, ovaries, fallopian tubes, and anterior vagina in women are removed en bloc. Pelvic lymph node dissection is mandatory for staging as well as for therapeutic benefit.[8] Continent diversions, including orthotopic neobladders and continent cutaneous reservoirs, are constructed through a variety of techniques. The most commonly performed urinary diversion is the ileal conduit, an incontinent diversion. Virtually all reconstructive options require division of small or large bowel with primary reanastomosis contributing significantly to the morbidity of these procedures.

Several large series have been published examining clinical, pathologic, and oncologic outcomes from radical cystectomy performed for bladder cancer.[6,9,10] Although perioperative mortality is generally reported in fewer than 5% of patients, perioperative complications are extremely common. Multiple series consistently note the incidence of complications among patients undergoing radical cystectomy in the range of 30% to 60%.[6,10,11] Length of stay is highly variable and often impacted by factors beyond clinical preparedness for discharge but generally range from 10 to 11 days. Analyses of complications related to cystectomy, such as subsequent readmissions or surgical interventions, are limited in part by the fragmentation of care between providers and institutions. This limitation is especially relevant in the comparison of historical data with contemporary practice. Indeed, the manner in which clinical follow-up is completed, recorded, and analyzed directly impacts any direct conclusions that can be made. Chappidi and colleagues[12] recently demonstrated that fragmentation of care and non-index hospitalizations may result in underestimation of 30-day and 90-day readmission rates by 18.5% and 23.0%, respectively. These underestimations very likely apply to historical series as well as more recent reports. Theoretically, appropriate history taking may mitigate contemporary underestimation of complications and readmissions; but care fragmentation remains a pertinent issue, as oncologic care is increasingly delivered regionally in high-volume centers.[13] The authors have noted within their own prospectively maintained database that attentive monitoring of outcomes has identified more frequent low-grade complications in comparison with older patient cohorts (Daneshmand, unpublished data, 2016). Although the possibility of increasing complications must be entertained, the more probable explanation is the careful attention to data collection and monitoring that has been used in recent years. Similar results have been noted at other centers of excellence where modern reported complications may exceed those reported in historical series.[14] Therefore, comparison with prior studies is difficult, yet the significant morbidity and extensive recovery period from radical cystectomy is evident, even if undercaptured. When strict definitions are used and complications are categorized by major and minor severity, the complication rates associated with radical cystectomy at referral centers have been noted to be closer to 50% to 60% over a 90-day postoperative period with most composed of minor complications.[15]

Surgical techniques evolve with time and modifications in the performance and care of patients undergoing radical cystectomy have been significant (**Fig. 1**). Historically, radical cystectomy often required preoperative admission for bowel preparation and incisions frequently extended supraumbilically allowing for extensive mobilization of the large and small bowel mesenteries. Stein and colleagues[6] reported a single-center technique and experience wherein performance of radical cystectomy included routine placement of a gastrostomy tube at the time of surgery. Older patients often received digoxin perioperatively, and admission to the intensive care unit was standard. Alterations in surgical techniques, that is, smaller incisions, limited mobilization of bowel, and even minimally invasive techniques, have certainly been impactful in improving some patient outcomes. Increasingly appreciated, however, is the role of patient factors, additional intraoperative components, and variations in postoperative management that drive clinical outcomes. Recognizing venues for optimization in the care of surgical patients, colorectal surgeons were among the first to introduce and popularize the ERAS concept as a means of standardizing and improving surgical quality.[16,17]

ENHANCED RECOVERY AFTER SURGERY OVERVIEW

Inspired by an appreciation of the physiologic stress caused by many surgical procedures and a recognition of significant variability in clinical outcomes for similar procedures among European centers, researchers sought to determine those interventions that improve and accelerate recovery following invasive surgeries. The ERAS study group was formed in 2001 with the intent of evaluating techniques to improve and standardize perioperative care with an emphasis on evidence-based principles.[18]

The ERAS approach has received occasional criticism for a focus on discharging patients quickly following surgical procedures. These concerns often relate in part to previous fast-track protocols and a perception that patients may be discharged too quickly in efforts to limit the length of stay. Determining optimal length of hospitalization following surgery is difficult. Relevant factors are myriad and variable even between patients. Among patients undergoing radical cystectomy in particular, determination of patient readiness for discharge is essential, as readmission rates are quite high. A recent analysis of the National Surgical Quality Improvement Program's database revealed a trend toward shorter length of stay but slightly increased rate of readmission highlighting the importance of this issue.[18]

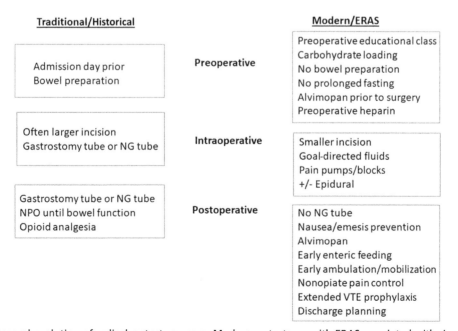

Fig. 1. General evolution of radical cystectomy care. Modern cystectomy with ERAS associated with significantly decreased time to return of bowel function, tolerance of regular diet, and length of hospitalization. NG, nasogastric; NPO, nothing by mouth; VTE, venous thromboembolic event.

Shortened length of stay, however, is not a specific target of ERAS. Instead, length of stay represents an easily quantifiable metric that often serves as a surrogate for recovery from surgery and, therefore, has been central to many ERAS publications. Enhancing overall perioperative quality is and must remain the foremost goal of all ERAS protocols.[19]

The ERAS Society (www.erassociety.org) has established specialty-specific guidelines for implementation of ERAS based on the current available data. The most recent guideline for colonic resections, for instance, specifies 24 discrete elements.[20] In the area of colorectal surgery, ERAS principles have been demonstrated to decrease postoperative morbidity and length of hospitalization.[21–23] No detrimental effects of ERAS use or these outcomes have been identified, though further study is needed to verify the role of ERAS on outcomes, such as patient quality of life, patient satisfaction, and economic ramifications.[24,25]

Although sometimes necessarily reliant on clinical principles and practice, many of the care components endorsed in ERAS protocols represent a departure from dogmatic surgical processes through adoption of evidence-based practices. Representative of this is the avoidance of nasogastric (NG) tubes and adoption of early enteric feeding of patients following bowel resections. Despite objective data demonstrating improved outcomes, this remains a somewhat controversial practice among many surgeons, as it represents a significant deviation from established practice and historical teaching. In the era of evidence-based medicine, however, it is essential that health care practitioners, while adhering to established clinical principles, remain open to assessment and adoption of novel practices when justified by rigorous objective evaluations. In this way, ERAS formalizes a surgical transition to evidence-based practice that aligns closely with current medical practice and encourages intentional analysis and modification of care delivered to the benefit of patients.

ENHANCED RECOVERY FOLLOWING RADICAL CYSTECTOMY

Urologists have made great progress in implementing evidence-based ERAS principles in the setting of radical cystectomy, and the ERAS Society has published recommendations for radical cystectomy as well.[26] Despite obvious need and great interest, however, only limited prospective studies have been completed. Given the complexity of care involved in completing radical cystectomies as well as the tremendous variability in individual patient characteristics, institutional

policies, and even health care delivery systems, objective evaluations often prove difficult. Further, limited consistency of care patterns between providers and institutions prevents generalizability of many findings to widespread practice. Therefore, many ERAS principles have been adopted to the care of patients undergoing radical cystectomy based on evidence demonstrated in other surgical procedures.

Although somewhat limited, practices that have been directly investigated with regard to their impact on clinical outcomes following radical cystectomy represent best techniques that should be incorporated into standard clinical practice because of the established safety and efficacy. Interventions targeted toward improved recovery of bowel function and the role of anticoagulation have been best studied.

Gastrointestinal Complications

Methods to address gastrointestinal (GI) complications are among the most closely studied interventions and are highly relevant given the well-reported frequency of GI complications associated with radical cystectomy and urinary diversion.[27] Where previous interventions, including bowel preparations, intraoperative placement of gastrostomy tubes, or prolonged NG drainage were commonplace, bowel preps and prolonged use of NG tubes are no longer recommended. Multiple evaluations have shown bowel preparation can be safely excluded and maintenance of NG tubes fails to prevent ileus while contributing to patient discomfort.[28–32] Also relevant in accelerating recovery of bowel function is the simple use of chewing gum, which has been demonstrated to decrease the time to flatus and the return of bowel function in multiple studies without negative consequences.[33,34] Perhaps of greatest value in hastening the return of bowel function following cystectomy is the use of the peripherally acting μ-opioid antagonist alvimopan. This medication has been objectively evaluated and demonstrated to accelerate GI recovery in multiple studies.[35] A multicenter randomized trial evaluated the use of alvimopan versus placebo among patients undergoing radical cystectomy and found the use of the medication resulted not only in quicker return of GI function but also shorter postoperative hospitalization and decreased GI complications. In addition, no change in opioid use for pain control was noted.[36] Hamilton and colleagues[37] evaluated the effects of adding alvimopan to an existing enhanced recovery protocol and found the use of the medication resulted in decreased time to regular diet (5.3 vs 4.1 days, $P < .01$) and decreased length of hospitalization (6.9 vs 5.7 days, $P = .01$) among 34 patients receiving alvimopan and 46 receiving standard care.

Pain Management

The impact of narcotic pain medications on slowing bowel function are well known. However, adequate pain control following any surgical intervention is essential to appropriate recovery. Optimal pain control following radical cystectomy has not yet been well defined. Many published series have used epidural anesthesia in accordance with traditional ERAS protocols for colorectal surgery. Others have instead eschewed the use of epidurals and instead recommended avoidance of narcotics through the use of non-narcotic pain medications, including ketorolac and intravenous acetaminophen acetate, with regional anesthetics.[38–40] Cost, patient satisfaction, and comparative outcomes between various pain management approaches remain to be explored, though minimizing opioid use remains an important focus while limiting postoperative pain.

Venous Thromboembolism Prophylaxis

The final aspect of perioperative care that has been carefully evaluated among patients undergoing radical cystectomy is the role of anticoagulation for prophylaxis against venous thromboembolic events (VTEs). Patients undergoing radical cystectomy are at an increased risk for VTE because of numerous factors, including presence of malignancy, pelvic surgery of significant length, and generally older patient age. In a review of the authors' own experience following radical cystectomy, VTEs were noted to occur in nearly 5% of patients with greater than half (57.8%) occurring after discharge at a median of 20 days postoperatively.[41] A single-center study by Pariser and colleagues[42] found a significant decrease in VTE occurrence following initiation of extended duration enoxaparin to postoperative day 28. Although significant work remains to objectively assess the role of various care techniques and refine implementation, the measures noted earlier merit inclusion in any care protocol for patients undergoing radical cystectomy.

PUBLISHED SERIES WITH ENHANCED RECOVERY AFTER SURGERY FOR RADICAL CYSTECTOMY

As noted earlier, published series evaluating the outcomes of ERAS among patients undergoing radical cystectomy are sparse and difficult to fully assess because of the highly variable institutional protocols and end points. **Table 1** lists many of the proposed or used ERAS components to date. It is evident in the body of published series and experiences, however, that the application of ERAS protocols to patients undergoing radical cystectomy is feasible and can be accomplished without deleterious consequences regardless of potential clinical benefits of which many have been reported.

Among the benefits consistently reported by various groups regarding experiences with individual ERAS protocols and radical cystectomy are decreased time to regular diet, shorter time to return of bowel function, and shorter length of hospitalization.[38–40,43–45] The protocols used within each series are unique but often emphasize early oral nutrition, early mobilization, avoidance of bowel preps or NG drainage, and limitation of opioid use. Because of the fashion in which individual protocols are implemented as well as a paucity of randomized studies, the relative value or impact of individual components cannot be assessed beyond those noted previously. A meta-analysis of the effect of ERAS pathways on perioperative outcomes following radical cystectomy in comparison with standard care found a lower rate of complications among patients in whom ERAS pathways were used (39.6% vs 51.5%). In addition, the return of bowel function occurred 1 day earlier and the mean length of stay was decreased 5 days for patients in the ERAS group.[46] The authors' own series of 113 consecutive patients receiving care in the context of an ERAS pathway found significantly shorter length of stay (4 vs 8 days, $P <.001$), but complications and readmissions remained stable at 30 and 90 days in comparison with matched controls, results that the authors have found subsequently sustained.[40] Patients had decreased opioid use but slightly greater pain than those who received standard care.[47] An updated analysis specifically evaluating the incidence of GI complications demonstrated similar results among 292 ERAS patients with a significant decrease in 30-day GI complications in comparison with a matched cohort.[48] Other ERAS series have similarly demonstrated a shorter length of stay with variable impacts on complication and readmission rates.[37,44,49,50] Criteria for discharge following cystectomy are not altered in the context of an ERAS protocol and include return of bowel function, satisfactory pain control with oral medications, sufficient oral intake, appropriate patient mobility, and comfort with managing urinary diversion. The capacity to decrease length of stay following radical cystectomy is clear and has not been

Table 1
Potential enhanced recovery after surgery components

Reported and Potential ERAS Components	Comment
Preoperative	
Counseling/education	Informs patient expectations and perioperative planning
[a]Medical optimization	Smoking cessation, additional medical evaluation if needed
[a]Carbohydrate loading	Nutritional optimization
[a]Elimination of bowel preparation	
[a]Alvimopan	Administered before surgery
Epidural	No well-described efficacy in cystectomy setting
Intraoperative	
Opioid-sparing analgesia	
[a]Restrictive transfusion protocol	Demonstrated safe in cystectomy setting
[a]Goal-directed fluid management	Improves perioperative outcomes, decreases GI complications
Postoperative	
[a]Avoidance of NG tube use	No worsening of GI complications, increased patient comfort
Antimicrobial prophylaxis	Unclear optimal antibiotic or timing
[a]Ileus prevention: chewing gum	
Early mobilization	No objective evaluation of clinical results in cystectomy population
Early enteric feeding	
[a]Alvimopan	Accelerates return of bowel function and time to discharge
Nausea and vomiting prophylaxis	
Neostigmine	
Home IV hydration	Helps to prevent readmission secondary to dehydration
Sodium bicarbonate (as needed)	
[a]Extended VTE prophylaxis	Decreases incidence of VTE when extended 28 d postoperative

Abbreviation: IV, intravenous.
[a] Objectively evaluated in radical cystectomy setting.

consistently associated with increased incidence of readmission. Optimal length of stay postoperatively is uncertain and likely unique to individual patients. Cost constraints and risks of extended hospitalizations favor earlier discharge, yet patient experience and satisfaction must also be considered. In one of the few prospective randomized studies of ERAS use in the cystectomy population, Karl and colleagues[50] compared standard radical cystectomy care with an ERAS pathway including high-calorie protein drinks before surgery, avoidance of bowel prep and NG tube, early enteral feeding, early mobilization, and early drain removal. Uniquely among outcome measures was a focus on objective early quality-of-life measures obtained through the European Organization for the Research and Treatment of Cancer's Quality of Life Questionnaire (QLQ-30). In addition to various improved clinical outcomes, researchers noted significant early improvements in quality of life among patients in the ERAS protocol as determined by the QLQ-30, particularly with regard to the emotional functioning score, which was noted to improve over the course of hospitalization among patients on the ERAS protocol.

Although not directly related to clinical outcomes, evaluation of the associated costs of ERAS implementation is important. Shorter length of stay postoperatively has been demonstrated to translate to decreased overall expenditures among patients undergoing other major surgeries.[51] Chipollini and colleagues[52] described in-hospital charges for patients undergoing radical cystectomy with ERAS in comparison with a group receiving standard care. Although a median length of stay of 6 days was similar between the groups, those on the ERAS protocol had less miscellaneous, supply, and treatment charges as well as decreased variability in billed charges, overall. The authors analyzed 30-day global costs among patients undergoing radical cystectomy and found an average savings of $4488 per procedure when comparing those receiving care through their ERAS pathway versus those immediately preceding ERAS implementation.[53] Recently, Semerjian and colleagues[54] reported single-center outcomes from implementation of an ERAS protocol and found a median charge for index hospitalization of $31,090 for ERAS patients versus $35,489 for patients before ERAS use as well as a similar incidence of complication and readmission. Further study is needed to define the overall impact of ERAS on costs. Although costs alone should not drive clinical practices, limited current evidence of decreased costs and improved standardization suggests enhanced quality in this regard as well.

FUTURE DIRECTIONS

ERAS pathways continue to evolve as comprehensive multidisciplinary approaches to the care of complex surgical patients. Therefore, exciting work remains to be completed at all phases of perioperative care. Many topics/interventions, such as fluid management and pain control, are relevant at multiple levels of care and require involvement and communication of all providers involved in the care of these patients.

Preoperative

The preoperative setting is among the most exciting avenue for ERAS development and application. Currently, ERAS protocols are applied uniformly to virtually all patients; standardization of perioperative care seems to greatly improve the care of patients. Improved risk stratification through better understanding of the role of independent patient factors, including age, social support system, financial factors, medical comorbidities, and others, may allow modification and personalization of ERAS protocols to better match individual patients and prove beneficial. Further, concepts such as prehabilitation and nutritional interventions, wherein patient medical and functional status are optimized before surgery, continue to be examined.[55] In the setting of bladder cancer, the window of available time in which patient health or functional status may be modified is quite limited because of the urgency of surgical intervention, yet attempts have been made to improve patient outcomes through simple interventions in the preoperative timeframe with mixed results.[56] Further development of educational platforms may enable patients to better anticipate and prepare for operative interventions physically and emotionally. Preoperative nutritional status has been linked to perioperative outcomes, including wound healing and infectious complications, with a high incidence of malnutrition noted in the cystectomy population.[57–59] Carbohydrate loading is encouraged for patients undergoing radical cystectomy because of the evidence for improved patient comfort following surgery and the suggestion of improved clinical outcomes.[60] The effects of various nutritional interventions have not been well described in urologic literature; however, research into the capacity for immuno-nutrition supplements to improve clinical outcomes has produced promising initial results and will continue to be developed offering additional avenues through which perioperative care may be optimized.[61]

Intraoperative

Modifications in the performance of radical cystectomy have occurred gradually over time. Perhaps the most dramatic recent change has been the introduction of minimally invasive and robotic-assisted surgeries. Robotic-assisted radical cystectomy is now performed with some frequency and promising initial results.[9] A randomized trial comparing an open versus robotic approach for radical cystectomy found decreased blood loss coupled with increased operative time for robotic cystectomy. Postoperative length of stay, complication rates, and quality-of-life outcomes were not significantly different between open or robotic groups.[62] At this time, no high-level evidence suggests that minimally invasive approaches for radical cystectomy enhances recovery in terms of length of hospitalization or rates of complications when compared with modern open series applying ERAS care pathways.[63] Further study will verify oncologic efficacy of minimally invasive cystectomy as well as identify other potential patient benefits. Current data seem to indicate that clinical outcomes are impacted most by perioperative care patterns (ie, ERAS) than by surgical approach. Indeed, ERAS principles are easily applicable regardless of surgical approach. The European Association of Urology Robotic Urology Section Scientific Working Group has endorsed enhanced recovery protocols as standard perioperative care in the setting of robotic-assisted radical cystectomy.[63] Beyond surgical approach, a growing appreciation of the importance of intraoperative fluid management has emphasized the multidisciplinary nature of comprehensive ERAS pathways and the role of anesthesiologists in enhancing patient care and outcomes. Optimization of fluid management through goal-directed therapy is essential as is careful use of blood products for both oncologic and fluid management reasons. Several studies have highlighted an association between perioperative blood transfusion and worsened oncologic outcomes, including increased cancer-specific mortality and cancer recurrence, among patients receiving intraoperative blood transfusion.[64,65] The authors have shown that a restrictive transfusion protocol wherein transfusions are limited to single units and depend on hemoglobin parameters per the guidelines from the American College of Cardiology/American Heart Association and the American Society of Anesthesiologists is safe in the radical cystectomy population and can significantly decrease the use of blood products.[66] In a more aggressive restrictive protocol, Wuethrich and colleagues[67] reported outcomes from a prospective study in which continuous norepinephrine infusions and restricted hydration were used until excision of the bladder, thereby limiting the need for both blood transfusion and intravenous fluid resuscitation. They found significantly less blood loss and incidence of transfusion when using this restrictive protocol in comparison with a standard protocol. Follow-up studies with the use of this protocol showed restricted hydration contributed to decreased incidence of GI complications, blood loss, and even some functional outcomes.[68–70] Although further study is required to determine the best practices in terms of intraoperative fluid management, technological advances continue to enhance the ability of anesthesiologists to accurately monitor patients' status. Devices which simply connect to an arterial catheter as well as other devices that use easily applied superficial sensor pads are among a growing number of technologies designed to provide safe and accurate monitoring of hemodynamic parameters and will allow continued refinement of perioperative fluid management approaches. Finally, optimal approaches to pain control continue to be examined, including the role of epidurals, local blocks, local anesthetics, and others. Each of these intraoperative issues will contribute to bettering overall patient care and outcomes.

Postoperative

The postoperative setting encompasses an extended period of time in which opportunities to enhance patient care and recovery are virtually limitless. Among the most obvious areas for further study and improvement are the determination of methods for preventing infectious complications and optimization of pain control.

Infectious complications represent among the most common causes of readmission following radical cystectomy.[14] Although single-dose antibiotic prophylaxis before surgical incision is recommended, optimal perioperative antibiotic coverage is unknown.[64] The indications for and role of suppressive antibiotics beyond 24 hours postoperatively must be better defined. Perioperative antibiotic management is highly variable between centers. Efforts toward improved risk stratification and early identification of complications may prevent readmissions and progression to more severe issues. New technologies may enable improved patient monitoring following discharge and help to improve patient adherence to care recommendations and prevent postoperative complications and readmission. Other factors, including postoperative rehabilitation programs and optimal dietary modifications, may prove clinically significant in enhancing the care of patients undergoing radical cystectomy and will be incorporated into future ERAS pathways. Among the exciting studies underway is SWOG S1600, a multiinstitutional trial intended to examine the impact of various nutritional factors on recovery from radical cystectomy.

SUMMARY

ERAS is firmly established as a valuable component of perioperative care for patients undergoing radical cystectomy. Ongoing research and future studies will continue to refine care pathways and reveal the best methods for improving the care of these patients. ERAS is both safe and effective in improving surgical quality and clinical outcomes. In a recent editorial, McGrath and Pruthi note[71] "the ERAS culture of consistency, performance measurement, and continual adoption of best practice are also crucial" to improving patient outcomes. Implementation of individual intervention is important for enhancing patient care, but the intentional analysis and multidisciplinary care coordination required to create and implement ERAS pathways are demonstrative of appropriate modern medical practice. ERAS represents a patient-centered and evidence-based approach to provide high-quality care to surgical patients and should be embraced at all levels of care. Although the American Urological Association's current guidelines do not expressly recommend ERAS pathways, it is hoped that, with continued evaluation and refinement of ERAS pathways, these will become the standard of care for patients undergoing radical cystectomy.

REFERENCES

1. Siegel RL, Miller KD, Jemal A. Cancer statistics, 2017. CA Cancer J Clin 2017;67(1):7–30.
2. Burger M, Catto JWF, Dalbagni G, et al. Epidemiology and risk factors of urothelial bladder cancer. Eur Urol 2013b;63(2):234–41.
3. Svatek RS, Hollenbeck BK, Holmäng S, et al. The economics of bladder cancer: costs and considerations of caring for this disease. Eur Urol 2014; 66(2):253–62.
4. Chappidi MR, Kates M, Patel HD, et al. Frailty as a marker of adverse outcomes in patients with bladder cancer undergoing radical cystectomy. Urol Oncol 2016;34(6):256.e1-6.
5. Gandaglia G, Popa I, Abdollah F, et al. The effect of neoadjuvant chemotherapy on perioperative outcomes in patients who have bladder cancer treated with radical cystectomy: a population-based study. Eur Urol 2014;66(3):561–8.
6. Stein JP, Lieskovsky G, Cote R, et al. Radical cystectomy in the treatment of invasive bladder cancer: long-term results in 1,054 patients. J Clin Oncol 2001;19(3):666–75.
7. Williams SB, Huo J, Chamie K, et al. Underutilization of radical cystectomy among patients diagnosed with clinical stage t2 muscle-invasive bladder cancer. Eur Urol Focus 2017;3(2–3): 258–64.
8. American Urological Association - Treatment of non-metastatic muscle-invasive bladder cancer: AUA/ASCO/ASTRO/SUO guideline. Available at: http://www.auanet.org/guidelines/muscle-invasive-bladder-cancer-new-(2017). Accessed Jun 16, 2017.
9. Yuh B, Wilson T, Bochner B, et al. Systematic review and cumulative analysis of oncologic and functional outcomes after robot-assisted radical cystectomy. Eur Urol 2015;67(3):402–22.
10. Ghoneim MA, el-Mekresh MM, el-Baz MA, et al. Radical cystectomy for carcinoma of the bladder: critical evaluation of the results in 1,026 cases. J Urol 1997;158(2):393–9.
11. Thalmann GN, Stein JP. Outcomes of radical cystectomy. BJU Int 2008;102(9 Pt B):1279–88.
12. Chappidi MR, Kates M, Stimson CJ, et al. Quantifying nonindex hospital readmissions and care fragmentation after major urological oncology surgeries in a nationally representative sample. J Urol 2017; 197(1):235–40.
13. Pak JS, Lascano D, Kabat DH, et al. Patterns of care for readmission after radical cystectomy in New York State and the effect of care fragmentation. Urol Oncol 2015;33(10):426.e13-19.
14. Altobelli E, Buscarini M, Gill HS, et al. Readmission rate and causes at 90-day after radical cystectomy in patients on early recovery after surgery protocol. Bladder Cancer 2017;3(1):51–6.
15. Shabsigh A, Korets R, Vora KC, et al. Defining early morbidity of radical cystectomy for patients with bladder cancer using a standardized reporting methodology. Eur Urol 2009;55(1):164–74.
16. Bardram L, Funch-Jensen P, Jensen P, et al. Recovery after laparoscopic colonic surgery with epidural analgesia, and early oral nutrition and mobilisation. Lancet 1995;345(8952):763–4.
17. Kehlet H, Wilmore DW. Multimodal strategies to improve surgical outcome. Am J Surg 2002;183(6): 630–41.
18. Johnson SC, Smith ZL, Golan S, et al. Temporal trends in perioperative morbidity for radical cystectomy using the National Surgical Quality Improvement Program database. Urol Oncol 2017;35(11): 659.e13–9.
19. Ljungqvist O, Scott M, Fearon KC. Enhanced recovery after surgery: a review. JAMA Surg 2017;152(3): 292–8.
20. Gustafsson UO, Scott MJ, Schwenk W, et al. Guidelines for perioperative care in elective colonic surgery: Enhanced Recovery After Surgery (ERAS(®)) Society recommendations. World J Surg 2013; 37(2):259–84.
21. Varadhan KK, Neal KR, Dejong CHC, et al. The enhanced recovery after surgery (ERAS) pathway for patients undergoing major elective open colorectal surgery: a meta-analysis of randomized controlled trials. Clin Nutr 2010;29(4):434–40.
22. Spanjersberg WR, Reurings J, Keus F, et al. Fast track surgery versus conventional recovery strategies for colorectal surgery. Cochrane Database Syst Rev 2011;(2):CD007635.
23. Adamina M, Kehlet H, Tomlinson GA, et al. Enhanced recovery pathways optimize health outcomes and resource utilization: a meta-analysis of randomized controlled trials in colorectal surgery. Surgery 2011;149(6):830–40.
24. Sammour T, Zargar-Shoshtari K, Bhat A, et al. A programme of enhanced recovery after surgery (ERAS) is a cost-effective intervention in elective colonic surgery. N Z Med J 2010;123(1319): 61–70.
25. Khan S, Wilson T, Ahmed J, et al. Quality of life and patient satisfaction with enhanced recovery protocols. Colorectal Dis 2010;12(12):1175–82.
26. Cerantola Y, Valerio M, Persson B, et al. Guidelines for perioperative care after radical cystectomy for bladder cancer: Enhanced Recovery After Surgery (ERAS®) Society recommendations. Clin Nutr 2013;32(6):879–87.
27. Novotny V, Hakenberg OW, Wiessner D, et al. Perioperative complications of radical cystectomy in a contemporary series. Eur Urol 2007;51(2):397–401 [discussion: 401–2].
28. Large MC, Kiriluk KJ, DeCastro GJ, et al. The impact of mechanical bowel preparation on postoperative

complications for patients undergoing cystectomy and urinary diversion. J Urol 2012;188(5):1801–5.

29. Xu R, Zhao X, Zhong Z, et al. No advantage is gained by preoperative bowel preparation in radical cystectomy and ileal conduit: a randomized controlled trial of 86 patients. Int Urol Nephrol 2010;42(4):947–50.

30. Park HK, Kwak C, Byun SS, et al. Early removal of nasogastric tube after cystectomy with urinary diversion: does postoperative ileus risk increase? Urology 2005;65(5):905–8.

31. Adamakis I, Tyritzis SI, Koutalellis G, et al. Early removal of nasogastric tube is beneficial for patients undergoing radical cystectomy with urinary diversion. Int Braz J Urol 2011;37(1):42–8.

32. Nelson R, Edwards S, Tse B. Prophylactic nasogastric decompression after abdominal surgery. Cochrane Database Syst Rev 2007;(3):CD004929.

33. Choi H, Kang SH, Yoon DK, et al. Chewing gum has a stimulatory effect on bowel motility in patients after open or robotic radical cystectomy for bladder cancer: a prospective randomized comparative study. Urology 2011;77(4):884–90.

34. Kouba EJ, Wallen EM, Pruthi RS. Gum chewing stimulates bowel motility in patients undergoing radical cystectomy with urinary diversion. Urology 2007; 70(6):1053–6.

35. Cui Y, Chen H, Qi L, et al. Effect of alvimopan on accelerates gastrointestinal recovery after radical cystectomy: a systematic review and meta-analysis. Int J Surg 2016;25:1–6.

36. Lee CT, Chang SS, Kamat AM, et al. Alvimopan accelerates gastrointestinal recovery after radical cystectomy: a multicenter randomized placebo-controlled trial. Eur Urol 2014;66(2):265–72.

37. Hamilton Z, Parker W, Griffin J, et al. Alvimopan in an enhanced recovery program following radical cystectomy. Bladder Cancer Amst Neth 2015;1(2): 137–42.

38. Brodner G, Van Aken H, Hertle L, et al. Multimodal perioperative management–combining thoracic epidural analgesia, forced mobilization, and oral nutrition–reduces hormonal and metabolic stress and improves convalescence after major urologic surgery. Anesth Analg 2001;92(6):1594–600.

39. Mukhtar S, Ayres BE, Issa R, et al. Challenging boundaries: an enhanced recovery programme for radical cystectomy. Ann R Coll Surg Engl 2013; 95(3):200–6.

40. Daneshmand S, Ahmadi H, Schuckman AK, et al. Enhanced recovery protocol after radical cystectomy for bladder cancer. J Urol 2014;192(1):50–5.

41. Sun AJ, Djaladat H, Schuckman A, et al. Venous thromboembolism following radical cystectomy: significant predictors, comparison of different anticoagulants and timing of events. J Urol 2015;193(2): 565–9.

42. Pariser JJ, Pearce SM, Anderson BB, et al. Extended duration enoxaparin decreases the rate of venous thromboembolic events after radical cystectomy compared to inpatient only subcutaneous heparin. J Urol 2017;197(2):302–7.

43. Saar M, Ohlmann CH, Siemer S, et al. Fast-track rehabilitation after robot-assisted laparoscopic cystectomy accelerates postoperative recovery. BJU Int 2013;112(2):E99–106.

44. Collins JW, Adding C, Hosseini A, et al. Introducing an enhanced recovery programme to an established totally intracorporeal robot-assisted radical cystectomy service. Scand J Urol 2016;50(1):39–46.

45. Pang KH, Groves R, Venugopal S, et al. Prospective implementation of enhanced recovery after surgery protocols to radical cystectomy. Eur Urol 2017. [Epub ahead of print].

46. Tyson MD, Chang SS. Enhanced recovery pathways versus standard care after cystectomy: a meta-analysis of the effect on perioperative outcomes. Eur Urol 2016;70(6):995–1003.

47. Xu W, Daneshmand S, Bazargani ST, et al. Postoperative pain management after radical cystectomy: comparing traditional versus enhanced recovery protocol pathway. J Urol 2015;194(5): 1209–13.

48. Djaladat H, Katebian B, Bazargani ST, et al. 90-Day complication rate in patients undergoing radical cystectomy with enhanced recovery protocol: a prospective cohort study. World J Urol 2017;35(6): 907–11.

49. Djaladat H, Daneshmand S. Gastrointestinal complications in patients who undergo radical cystectomy with enhanced recovery protocol. Curr Urol Rep 2016;17(7):50.

50. Karl A, Buchner A, Becker A, et al. A new concept for early recovery after surgery for patients undergoing radical cystectomy for bladder cancer: results of a prospective randomized study. J Urol 2014;191(2): 335–40.

51. Regenbogen SE, Cain-Nielsen AH, Norton EC, et al. Costs and consequences of early hospital discharge after major inpatient surgery in older adults. JAMA Surg 2017;152(5):e170123.

52. Chipollini J, Tang DH, Hussein K, et al. Does implementing an enhanced recovery after surgery protocol increase hospital charges? Comparisons from a radical cystectomy program at a specialty cancer center. Urology 2017;105:108–12.

53. Nabhani J, Ahmadi H, Schuckman AK, et al. Cost analysis of the enhanced recovery after surgery protocol in patients undergoing radical cystectomy for bladder cancer. Eur Urol Focus 2016;2(1):92–6.

54. Semerjian A, Milbar N, Kates M, et al. Hospital charges and length of stay following radical cystectomy in the enhanced recovery after surgery era. Urology 2017;111:86–91.

55. Le Roy B, Selvy M, Slim K. The concept of prehabilitation: what the surgeon needs to know? J Visc Surg 2016;153(2):109–12.

56. Jensen BT, Petersen AK, Jensen JB, et al. Efficacy of a multiprofessional rehabilitation programme in radical cystectomy pathways: a prospective randomized controlled trial. Scand J Urol 2015;49(2): 133–41.

57. Tobert CM, Hamilton-Reeves JM, Norian LA, et al. Emerging impact of malnutrition on surgical patients: literature review and potential implications for cystectomy in bladder cancer. J Urol 2017; 198(3):511–9.

58. Barrass BJR, Thurairaja R, Collins JW, et al. Optimal nutrition should improve the outcome and costs of radical cystectomy. Urol Int 2006;77(2):139–42.

59. Karl A, Staehler M, Bauer R, et al. Malnutrition and clinical outcome in urological patients. Eur J Med Res 2011;16(10):469–72.

60. Bilku DK, Dennison AR, Hall TC, et al. Role of preoperative carbohydrate loading: a systematic review. Ann R Coll Surg Engl 2014;96(1):15–22.

61. Hamilton-Reeves JM, Bechtel MD, Hand LK, et al. Effects of immunonutrition for cystectomy on immune response and infection rates: a pilot randomized controlled clinical trial. Eur Urol 2016;69(3): 389–92.

62. Bochner BH, Dalbagni G, Sjoberg DD, et al. Comparing open radical cystectomy and robot-assisted laparoscopic radical cystectomy: a randomized clinical trial. Eur Urol 2015;67(6):1042–50.

63. Collins JW, Patel H, Adding C, et al. Enhanced recovery after robot-assisted radical cystectomy: EAU robotic urology section scientific working group consensus view. Eur Urol 2016;70(4):649–60.

64. Wang YL, Jiang B, Yin FF, et al. Perioperative blood transfusion promotes worse outcomes of bladder cancer after radical cystectomy: a systematic review and meta-analysis. PLoS One 2015;10(6):e0130122.

65. Abel EJ, Linder BJ, Bauman TM, et al. Perioperative blood transfusion and radical cystectomy: does timing of transfusion affect bladder cancer mortality? Eur Urol 2014;66(6):1139–47.

66. Syan-Bhanvadia S, Drangsholt S, Shah S, et al. Restrictive transfusion in radical cystectomy is safe. Urol Oncol 2017;35(8):528.e15–21.

67. Wuethrich PY, Studer UE, Thalmann GN, et al. Intraoperative continuous norepinephrine infusion combined with restrictive deferred hydration significantly reduces the need for blood transfusion in patients undergoing open radical cystectomy: results of a prospective randomised trial. Eur Urol 2014; 66(2):352–60.

68. Pillai P, McEleavy I, Gaughan M, et al. A double-blind randomized controlled clinical trial to assess the effect of Doppler optimized intraoperative fluid management on outcome following radical cystectomy. J Urol 2011;186(6):2201–6.

69. Wuethrich PY, Burkhard FC, Thalmann GN, et al. Restrictive deferred hydration combined with preemptive norepinephrine infusion during radical cystectomy reduces postoperative complications and hospitalization time: a randomized clinical trial. Anesthesiology 2014;120(2):365–77.

70. Burkhard FC, Studer UE, Wuethrich PY. Superior functional outcome after radical cystectomy and orthotopic bladder substitution with restrictive intraoperative fluid management: a follow-up study of a randomized clinical trial. J Urol 2015;193(1):173–8.

71. McGrath JS, Pruthi RS. Surgery: enhanced recovery after cystectomy: cocktails, culture, or consistency? Nat Rev Urol 2017;14(11):648–9.

Follow-up Management of Cystectomy Patients

Madhumitha Reddy, DO, Karim Kader, MD, PhD*

KEYWORDS

- Cystectomy • Functional outcomes • Follow-up • Recurrence • Muscle-invasive bladder cancer

KEY POINTS

- After cystectomy, follow-up with laboratory assessment and imaging is critical in diagnosing recurrence and preventing functional complications.
- Recurrence after cystectomy occurs in 35% of patients.
- Distant metastases are the most common sites of recurrence; however, local, upper tract, and urethral recurrence can also occur.
- Functional complications after urinary diversion can include bowel dysfunction, vitamin B12 deficiency, acidosis, electrolyte abnormalities, osteopenia, nephrolithiasis, urinary tract infections, renal functional decline, and urinary obstruction.
- These complications can be reversed when diagnosed early.

INTRODUCTION

Bladder cancer is the 6th most commonly diagnosed cancer in the United States. An estimated 79,000 new cases of bladder cancer will be diagnosed in 2017, with a median age at diagnosis of 73 years.[1] Of these patients, 25% to 30% will have muscle-invasive bladder cancer (MIBC) at diagnosis. In addition, 15% to 20% of patients with non-MIBC (NMIBC) will progress to muscle invasion. Of all the patients with MIBC, only 39% will undergo cystectomy.[2] Anywhere from 8000 to 10,000 cystectomies are performed every year in the United States. Although cystectomy is the gold standard for the treatment of MIBC, a significant number of patients will have recurrence and functional complications after cystectomy and, therefore, long-term follow-up is mandatory.

RECURRENCE

Recurrence after cystectomy and bladder cancer–specific mortality can occur in up to 35% and 28% of the patients, respectively. Higher stage pathologic stage T3 or T4 grade, lymphovascular invasion, and presence of lymph node (LN) metastases have been shown to be poor prognosticators for recurrence.[3]

Distant Metastasis

Of all the patients with recurrence, more than 50% are with distant metastases. Risk factors for distant metastases are higher stage, Lymphovascular invasion (LVI), positive margins, smaller extent of LN dissection, and lack of neoadjuvant chemotherapy. Of the distant metastases, 80% to 90% will occur in the first 3 years. The most common sites of metastases are bone (11%–13%), liver (10.7%), and lungs (9.9%–11%). Prognosis after the development of distant metastases is poor, with a median survival of 13.8 to 14.8 months.[4] Primary treatment of distant metastases consists of chemotherapy or immunotherapy. However, there may be a role for metastasectomy in carefully selected patients.[5,6]

Disclosure: The authors have nothing to disclose.
Moores Cancer Center, UC San Diego, 3855 Health Sciences Drive, La Jolla, CA 92093, USA
* Corresponding author.
E-mail address: kkader@ucsd.edu

Urol Clin N Am 45 (2018) 241–247
https://doi.org/10.1016/j.ucl.2018.01.001
0094-0143/18/© 2018 Elsevier Inc. All rights reserved.

urologic.theclinics.com

Pelvic (Local) Recurrence

Contemporary literature has shown local recurrence in 5% to 15% of the cases. Higher stage, LN-positive disease, positive margins, lesser extent of LN dissection, and lack of neoadjuvant chemotherapy are some of the risk factors for local recurrence. Most of these cases are diagnosed in the first 2 years after surgery. Local recurrence results in a poor prognosis with associated systemic recurrence in 36% to 64% of the patients, and survival is generally less than a year.[4] Sites of local resection are the original surgical site, including the prerectal space and incompletely resected pelvic LNs. Treatment most commonly consists of chemotherapy, radiotherapy, surgical resection in select cases, or any combination of these.

Upper Tract Recurrence

Upper tract recurrence is generally diagnosed later (median time >3 years) and has an incidence of 2% to 6%. Some of the risk factors are presence of tumor in the distal ureter, multifocal or recurrent urothelial carcinoma (UC), NMIBC, and presence of carcinoma in situ (CIS). Patients who had none of these risk factors had an upper tract recurrence rate of only 0.8% at 15 years, whereas those with greater than 3 of these risk factors had a 13.5% risk of recurrence in the same time frame.[7] Greater than 50% of these recurrences are diagnosed after the onset of symptoms, and about 70% are diagnosed at an advanced stage. Urine cytology results in primary detection of 7% of these recurrences, whereas upper urinary tract imaging primarily diagnoses 29.6%.[8] Symptoms of upper tract recurrence include flank pain and hematuria. Unfortunately, the prognosis is poor with 18% to 33% of the patients having metastases at diagnosis.[4] Unlike other types of recurrence, the risk of upper tract recurrence is lifelong.

Urethral Recurrence

The incidence of urethral recurrence has been reported to be approximately 1.5% to 6% in male patients and 0.83% to 4.3% in female patients who underwent urethral-sparing cystectomy.[9] Most of these cases are diagnosed in the first 3 years. The incidence of urethral recurrence is lower in patients undergoing orthotopic bladder replacements, likely secondary to patient selection. Symptoms of urethral recurrence include hematuria, change in urinary stream in patients with orthotopic neobladders, urethral bleeding, and induration of periurethral tissue in those with a cutaneous diversion. Some of the risk factors for urethral recurrence are presence of prostatic urethral involvement by the UC (especially stromal involvement), multifocal UC, NMIBC, and presence of CIS.[4] Patients diagnosed with urethral recurrence by surveillance have a significant survival advantage when compared with those who are diagnosed symptomatically.[10] Hence, follow-up of the male urethra is indicated in patients who are at an increased risk of urethral recurrence. Treatment of urethral recurrence consists of transurethral resection, Bacillus Calmette-Guerin (BCG) in cases of CIS, and urethrectomy in patients with invasive disease localized to the urethra.[11]

SURVEILLANCE FOR RECURRENCE OR METASTASES

The NCCN guidelines recommend the following surveillance for patients who underwent cystectomy for NMIBC: 1) CT Urogram (CTU) or MR Urogram (MRU) at 3 and 12 months and then annually for 5 years. Beyond 5 years they recommend renal imaging annually and, 2) Urine cytology with urethral washings every 6–12 months for the first 2 years for high risk pts (Positive urethral margin, multifocal CIS, prostatic urethral involvement). For MIBC, they recommend CTU/MRU, CXR every 3–6 months for 2 years and then annually for 3–5 years. Beyond 5 years they recommend renal imaging annually and, 2) Urine cytology with urethral washings every 6–12 months for the first 2 years for high risk percentages.[12] It should be noted that the follow-up for urethral recurrence in men using urethral washings for cytology is controversial. A retrospective study of 85 male subjects with urethral recurrence showed an improved cancer-specific rate in men diagnosed before the onset of symptoms (P<.0001).[10] However, another retrospective study of 24 subjects who had undergone urethrectomy did not find a statistical difference in overall survival in these groups when controlling for original bladder tumor stage (P = .769).[13] With the limited data present and the lack of consensus, cytology of urethral washings and urethroscopy should be performed in symptomatic patients, and cytology of urethral washings in asymptomatic patients should be performed at the discretion of the clinician, bearing in mind the aforementioned risk factors.

Even with the high incidence of recurrence and progression after cystectomy, there is debate regarding the role of surveillance imaging in improving survival in patients who have recurrence. An observational study of 1270 subjects in Germany who underwent cystectomy showed that, of the 444 recurrences noted, 154 were detected in asymptomatic subjects with imaging and 290 were symptom-driven detections. Some of the symptoms of recurrence were pain, hematuria, urinary retention, hydronephrosis with flank pain, neurologic symptoms, palpable mass, priapism, or ileus. The prognosis following recurrence was poor, with 80% of the subjects dying within 1 year. Overall survival after the diagnosis of recurrence did not differ significantly between the asymptomatic or symptom-driven groups at 1, 2, or 5 years (18.9% vs 22.5%, 8.2% vs 10.1%, 2.9% vs 5.5%, respectively).[14] Although this study does raise important questions regarding the benefits of surveillance imaging, it is not known if the findings are still relevant in the era of the immunotherapy, which has shown a modest improved survival in the setting of metastatic bladder cancer.

In contrast, another retrospective study of 479 subjects did show improved overall (HR 0.66, 95% CI 0.48–0.92, $P = .015$) and cancer-specific survival (HR 0.65, 95% CI 0.46–0.91, $P = .013$) in subjects diagnosed with asymptomatic recurrence. This study excluded subjects who received neoadjuvant therapy. The 87 asymptomatic subjects diagnosed with recurrence mostly had lung metastases or urethral recurrence, whereas the 87 symptomatic recurrence subjects predominantly had bone and concomitant pelvic or distant recurrence. Because soft tissue metastases respond better to chemotherapy, the pattern of recurrence in the 2 groups may have contributed to the survival difference.[15]

The disadvantages of routine surveillance include the monetary cost and psychological distress for the subject. Symptomatic recurrence was noted in 61% to 80% of the subjects who were followed up with regular imaging and laboratory protocols.[14,16,17] With the current literature being inconclusive regarding the survival benefit of the diagnosis of asymptomatic recurrence, it is not known if a symptom-driven follow-up protocol will have similar outcomes to routine follow-up.

Because most recurrences occur within the first 3 to 5 years, the concept of conditional survival applies. Patient prognosis improves significantly with each additional year survived after surgery. After the initial 5 years of survival, additional 5-year conditional overall survival improved to 72.9% compared with 55.1% immediately after surgery and cancer-specific survival improved to 90.8% compared with 65.9% immediately after surgery.[18] Hence surveillance for recurrence with imaging is not recommended after 5 years. Late recurrences tend to be predominantly in the upper urinary tract and thus the renal imaging recommended annually after 5 years should be able to diagnose these.

FUNCTIONAL COMPLICATIONS

Long-term functional complications after cystectomy are common. A study of subjects who underwent ileal conduit diversion showed that 45% of these subjects had a functional complication at 5-year follow-up. This rate increased to 50%, 54%, and 94% in those surviving 10, 15, or greater than 15 years, respectively.[19] Patients should be educated about these complications before cystectomy and monitored closely for the same after cystectomy. When these complications are diagnosed and treated early, long-term sequelae can be minimized. The NCCN guidelines recommend the following for monitoring of functional complications. Creatinine, electrolytes and LFTS every 3–6 months for the first year and then annually for 5 years. They also recommend monitoring Vitamin B12 levels annually from 2 to 5 years. Beyond 5 years they recommend monitoring as clinically indicated.[12,20]

Urinary reconstruction after a cystectomy permanently alters the storage and voiding of urine, which can result in long-term functional complications. Most of these complications are reversible or manageable if caught early and can be devastating if diagnosed late. Any surveillance protocols should include monitoring for these complications.

The principal forms of reconstruction can be classified into incontinent ileal diversions and continent ileal or colonic diversions (which include neobladder and continent cutaneous diversions). Incontinent ileal conduits are made from 15 to 25 cm of preterminal ileum, whereas continent diversions typically use 40 to 80 cm of preterminal ileum or colon, which predisposes them to longer urinary dwell time. A recent study using a random sample of about 27,500 patients from the Healthcare Cost and Utilization Project Nationwide Impatient Sample found that 83.5% of the patients had undergone an ileal conduit creation, whereas 16.5% underwent a continent cutaneous diversion.[21] This finding, in keeping with several other studies, shows that most urinary diversions performed in the United States are ileal conduits. Discussion of the metabolic and functional abnormalities that can arise follows.

Bowel Dysfunction and Vitamin B12 Deficiency

The terminal ileum is the site of the reabsorption of bile salts initially secreted into the duodenum. The resection of large segments of ileum or the ileocecal valve results in the possibility of these bile salts reaching the colon and causing irritative diarrhea and steatorrhea. Ultimately, this may cause dehydration and acidosis. Patients who undergo resection of large segments of ileum or the terminal ileum (neobladder or Indiana pouch) should be monitored for diarrhea. Persistent diarrhea can be treated with cholestyramine, a bile salt–binding resin, and high-fiber diet. The terminal ileum is also the site of vitamin B12 absorption. The body has reserves of up to 3 to 5 years of vitamin B12, hence any malabsorption of the same will not be evident during that time. However, the deficiency can result in irreversible neurologic damage and megaloblastic macrocytic anemia. Patients should be closely monitored with periodic B12 levels and intramuscular supplementation of vitamin B12 should be started if B12 deficiency is suspected.[22]

Acidosis

When distal ileum is used in urinary reconstruction, a hyperchloremic, hypokalemic, metabolic acidosis may develop. The bowel wall reabsorbs ammonia, hydrogen, and chloride from the urine that is in contact with it, causing this acidosis. Patients with good renal function can compensate for this acidosis and are not typically affected. Other risk factors include prolonged urine contact time and a large bowel surface area (eg, neobladders or continent cutaneous conduits). Patients with ileal conduits have been shown to have a 10% risk of clinically important metabolic acidosis at 1-year follow-up.[23] Those who undergo a continent diversion have much higher rates of up to 26% to 45%.[22] A basic metabolic panel should be obtained every 3 to 6 months during the first year after cystectomy, annually from year 2 to 5, and longer as needed to monitor for acidosis. Some of the symptoms of significant acidosis are lethargy, anorexia, and vomiting. In severe cases, it can lead to bone demineralization, which can be avoided or treated with alkalinizing therapies such as sodium bicarbonate, sodium citrate, or potassium citrate. These therapies can have profound effects on serum electrolytes (eg, hyperkalemia after potassium citrate) and response to the same should be closely monitored.

Electrolyte Abnormalities

Hypokalemia, hypocalcemia, and hypomagnesemia can occur because of intestinal urinary diversion. The potassium and magnesium ions are lost in the intestinal segment and by renal wasting. The BMP schedule previously recommended for monitoring of acidosis can also help in the monitoring of these abnormalities. Special consideration of surveillance schedule, including possible consultation with a nephrologist, should be performed in patients with preexisting or emerging renal insufficiency. Care should be taken when correcting the acidosis because it can significantly

worsen this hypokalemia. The ongoing acidosis prevents renal calcium reabsorption and results in hypocalcemia.[24] Calcium, magnesium supplements, and potassium citrate can be used to correct these abnormalities.

Bone Loss

Chronic acidosis is buffered by bone minerals. The acidosis also impairs renal activation of vitamin D and activates osteoclasts. The net effect is bone demineralization. Patients with renal insufficiency are particularly prone to this. Affected patients may present with pain in weightbearing bones. A recent SEER analysis found that cystectomy was associated with a 21% increased risk of fracture.[25] Treatment of the acidosis, along with supplementation of vitamin D, C, and calcium, may help improve bone remineralization.[22,24] There is no consensus regarding the indication, if any, for bone dual-energy X-ray absorptiometry (DEXA) scans for monitoring bone health in these patients.

Calculi

About 20% of patients with an ileal conduit will develop renal calculi and about 10% of patients with a continent diversion will develop pouch calculi in long-term follow-up.[26,27] The systemic acidosis that develops increases the risk of calcium phosphate stones. Loss of bile salts in the intestine can result in binding of calcium to these salts, increased oxalate absorption, and increased risk of calcium oxalate stones. Intestinal mucous and any foreign objects (eg, staples) can serve as nidus for stone formations. Chronic urinary tract infections (UTIs) with urease-splitting organisms can increase the risk of struvite stones. The imaging obtained to monitor for recurrence should help in the diagnosis of renal and pouch calculi. Surgical treatment of renal and pouch calculi can be challenging secondary to the alternations in anatomy with urinary reconstruction.

Urinary Tract Infections

UTIs are the most common complication after urinary diversions. Asymptomatic bacteriuria is very common after urinary diversions because the bowel epithelium lacks the inhibitory properties against bacterial adherence that the urothelium has.[28] Symptoms of a UTI after a urinary diversion can be atypical and can include diffuse abdominal pain, fevers, explosive incontinence, or upper tract symptoms such as flank pain. About 25% of patients with urinary diversions have a symptomatic UTI every year.[29–31] Patients with continent urinary diversions have a higher incidence of UTIs compared with those with ileal conduits.[32]

Symptomatic UTIs should be treated with culture-specific antibiotics when possible.

Recurrent UTIs are a significant concern secondary to increased risk of urosepsis and upper tract deterioration. The presence of recurrent UTIs should prompt a thorough evaluation of the urinary tract for obstruction, reflux, or incomplete emptying of the reservoir or stoma. Recurrent UTIs are a significant risk factor for urosepsis and, hence, antibiotic prophylaxis can be considered in some patients.[30]

One unique, yet potentially lethal, complication in these patients is hyperammonemic encephalopathy secondary to UTIs from urease-producing organisms. This complication typically occurs in patients with preexisting liver dysfunction. The ammonia produced by bacterial splitting of uric acid is readily absorbed by the intestinal segment of the urinary diversion and enters the systemic circulation. The increased ammonia loads are not able to be processed by the already dysfunctional liver and cause encephalopathy. Patients usually present with somnolence, behavior alterations, and seizures, which can be confused for the more common urosepsis and, when left untreated, can lead to death.[33,34] These symptoms can be reversed acutely by treating the hyperammonemia and the UTI.

Renal Function

Advancing age is a risk factor for renal insufficiency. Starting at the age of 40 years, the glomerular filtration rate (GFR) decreases at a rate of 1 mL/min/1.73 m^2 per year.[35] With bladder cancer generally being a disease of advanced age, most patients start out with a lower GFR than their younger counterparts. However, urinary diversions can result in complications such as ureteral obstruction, recurrent infections, and urolithiasis, which can further impair renal function. GFR has been reported to decrease up to 15% to 25% after urinary diversion with long-term follow-up.[36] Any preservation of GFR by diagnosing and treating reversible causes is important. Long-term follow-up with renal ultrasound and serum creatinine can help diagnose these complications early and allow early intervention.

Urinary Obstruction

Urinary obstruction after cystectomy can be secondary to stomal stenosis, parastomal hernias, inadequate emptying of the neobladder or pouch, ureteroileal anastomotic strictures, calculi, or recurrence of tumor.

Ureteroenteric stricture (UES) remains the most common cause of reoperation after a cystectomy.[37] UES has been found to occur in anywhere from 13% to 19% of the patients on long-term follow-up.[38–40] These strictures may be benign or malignant. Most of the benign strictures are diagnosed in the first year and are asymptomatic on presentation. Benign strictures are more common on the left side, likely related to the need to bring the left ureter under the sigmoid mesentery.[41,42] Because most are asymptomatic, delayed diagnosis and management can compromise renal function. Hence, a strict follow-up regimen with imaging and serum creatinine testing is crucial. Short (<1 cm) benign strictures can occasionally be managed with stenting or balloon dilation initially to avoid the morbidity of an open revision. However, endoscopic management does not have long-term durability. Open surgical revision, though challenging, has a long-term success rate of 93%.[41]

Parastomal hernias remain a common complication after cystectomy, with reports of about 20% to 30% incidence on long-term follow-up. Most patients with these hernias are asymptomatic. However, bowel may herniate and strangulate, requiring prompt surgical attention.[43] These parastomal hernias, when large enough, can distort the conduit, resulting in urinary retention. Stomal stenosis is thought to be secondary to poor vascular supply to the bowel segment. Short-segment stenosis at the skin level can initially be managed with catheter or digital dilation but this is associated with a risk of perforation or false passages.[44] Retrograde studies are required to evaluate the extent of stenosis and associated anatomic abnormalities such as false passage or conduit elongation.[45] Surgical revision has the best long-term results for treatment of stomal stenosis.

Patients with orthotopic urinary diversions can have difficulty emptying their bladder substitute. Educating the patient regarding the need for timed voiding and technique of clean intermittent catheterization is crucial in the setting of chronic urinary retention. Any incontinence with orthotopic diversions should be evaluated with a Post void residual to rule out overflow incontinence. Difficulty emptying orthotopic neobladders is particularly true in female patients. A recent survey of patients from the University of Southern California Bladder Cancer Database showed that 44.6% of the patients depended on catheterization to empty their neobladders.[46] This retention can sometimes be severe and lead to reservoir rupture. Symptoms of rupture include diffuse abdominal pain, ileus, fevers, or signs of peritonitis. Although there are case reports of conservative management with Foley catheter drainage and antibiotics, signs of peritonitis or worsening symptoms while on conservative management should prompt emergent laparotomy.[47]

SUMMARY

Follow-up is a critical component of patient care following radical cystectomy. Periodic upper tract or chest imaging, assessment of renal function and electrolyte abnormalities, together with select cytologic analyses should be obtained to monitor for recurrence and functional complications. Attention should be paid to the increased risk of bone loss, calculi, UTIs, urosepsis, and urinary obstruction. Although controversial, it is thought that timely treatment of recurrent disease and functional complications may lead to improved outcomes. The optimal follow-up schedule needs to balance risk with morbidity and cost.

REFERENCES

1. Surveillance, Epidemiology, and End Results (SEER) Program. SEER*stat database: incidence-SEER 18 regs research data + hurricane Katrina impacted Louisiana cases, Nov 2014 sub (1973-2012 varying)-linked to county attributes-total US, 1969–2013 counties. Bethesda (MD): National Cancer Institute, Department of Cancer Control and Population Sciences, Surveillance Research Program, Surveillance Systems Branch; 2015. Available at: https://seer.cancer.gov/statfacts/html/urinb.html.

2. Miller KD, Siegel RL, Lin CC, et al. Cancer treatment and survivorship statistics, 2016. CA Cancer J Clin 2016;66:271–89.

3. Shariat SF, Karakiewicz PI, Palapattu GS, et al. Outcomes of radical cystectomy for transitional cell carcinoma of the bladder: a contemporary series from the Bladder Cancer Research Consortium. J Urol 2006;176(6 Pt 1):2414–22 [discussion: 2422].

4. Huguet J. Follow-up after radical cystectomy based on patterns of tumour recurrence and its risk factors. Actas Urol Esp 2013;37(6):376–82.

5. Siefker-Radtke AO, Walsh GL, Pisters LL, et al. Is there a role for surgery in the management of metastatic urothelial cancer? The M. D. Anderson experience. J Urol 2004;171(1):145–8.

6. Lehmann J, Suttmann H, Albers P, et al. Surgery for metastatic urothelial carcinoma with curative intent: the German experience (AUO AB 30/05). Eur Urol 2009;55(6):1293–9.

7. Volkmer BG, Schnoeller T, Kuefer R, et al. Upper urinary tract recurrence after radical cystectomy for bladder cancer – who is at risk? J Urol 2009;182:2632–7.

8. Picozzi S, Ricci C, Gaeta M, et al. Upper urinary tract recurrence following radical cystectomy for bladder cancer: a meta-analysis on 13,185 patients. J Urol 2012;188(6):2046–54.

9. Soukup V, Babjuk M, Bellmunt J, et al. Follow-up after surgical treatment of bladder cancer: a critical analysis of the literature. Eur Urol 2012;62(2):290–302.

10. Boorjian SA, Kim SP, Weight CJ, et al. Risk factors and outcomes of urethral recurrence following radical cystectomy. Eur Urol 2011;60(6):1266–72.

11. Alfred Witjes J, Lebret T, Compérat EM, et al. Updated 2016 EAU Guidelines on Muscle-invasive and Metastatic Bladder Cancer. Eur Urol 2017; 71(3):462–75.

12. Ehdaie B, Atoria CL, Lowrance WT, et al. Adherence to surveillance guidelines after radical cystectomy: a population-based analysis. Urol Oncol 2014;32(6):779–84.

13. Lin DW, Herr HW, Dalbagni G. Value of urethral wash cytology in the retained male urethra after radical cystoprostatectomy. J Urol 2003;169(3):961–3.

14. Volkmer BG, Kuefer R, Bartsch GC Jr, et al. Oncological followup after radical cystectomy for bladder cancer-is there any benefit? J Urol 2009;181(4):1587–93 [discussion: 1593].

15. Giannarini G, Kessler TM, Thoeny HC, et al. Do patients benefit from routine follow-up to detect recurrences after radical cystectomy and ileal orthotopic bladder substitution? Eur Urol 2010; 58(4):486–94.

16. Umbreit EC, Crispen PL, Shimko MS, et al. Multifactorial, site specific recurrence model after radical cystectomy for urothelial cancer. Cancer 2010;116:3399–407.

17. Dhar NB, Jones JS, Reuther AM, et al. Presentation, location and overall survival of pelvic recurrence after radical cystectomy for transitional cell carcinoma of the bladder. BJU Int 2008;101:969–72.

18. Ploussard G, Shariat SF, Dragomir A, et al. Conditional survival after radical cystectomy for bladder cancer: evidence for a patient changing risk profile over time. Eur Urol 2014;66(2):361–70.

19. Madersbacher S, Schmidt J, Eberle JM, et al. Long-term outcome of ileal conduit diversion. J Urol 2003; 169(3):985–90.

20. Spiess PE, Agarwal N, Bangs R, et al. NCCN Clinical Practice Guidelines in Oncology. J Natl Compr Canc Netw 2017;15(10):1240–67.

21. Gore JL, Yu H-Y, Setodji C, et al. Urinary diversion and morbidity after radical cystectomy for bladder cancer. Cancer 2010;116(2):331–9.

22. Van der Aa F, Joniau S, Van Den Branden M, et al. Metabolic changes after urinary diversion. Adv Urol 2011;2011:764325.

23. Kamidono S, Oda Y, Ogawa T. Clinical study of urinary diversion. II: Review of 41 ileocolic conduit cases, their complications and long term (6-9 years) follow-up. Nishinihon J Urol 1985;47:415–20.

24. Vasdev N, Moon A, Thorpe AC. Metabolic complications of urinary intestinal diversion. Indian J Urol 2013;29(4):310–5.

25. Gupta A, Atoria CL, Ehdaie B, et al. Risk of fracture after radical cystectomy and urinary diversion for bladder cancer. J Clin Oncol 2014;32(29):3291–8.

26. McDougal WS, Koch MO. Impaired growth and development and urinary intestinal interposition. The American Association of Genitourinary Surgeons 1991;105:3.

27. Terai A, Ueda T, Kakehi Y, et al. Urinary calculi as a late complication of the Indiana continent urinary diversion: comparison with the kock pouch procedure. J Urol 1996;155(1):66–8.

28. Suriano F, Gallucci M, Flammia GP, et al. Bacteriuria in patients with an orthotopic ileal neobladder: urinary tract infection or asymptomatic bacteriuria? BJU Int 2008;101(12):1576–9.

29. Henningsohn L, Wijkström H, Dickman PW, et al. Distressful symptoms after radical cystectomy with urinary diversion for urinary bladder cancer: a Swedish population-based study. Eur Urol 2001;40(2):151–62.

30. Wood DP Jr, Bianco FJ Jr, Pontes JE, et al. Incidence and significance of positive urine cultures in patients with an orthotopic neobladder. J Urol 2003;169(6):2196–9.

31. Wullt B, Holst E, Steven K, et al. Microbial flora in ileal and colonic neobladders. Eur Urol 2004;45(2):233–9.

32. Nieuwenhuijzen JA, de Vries RR, Bex A, et al. Urinary diversions after cystectomy: the association of clinical factors, complications and functional results of four different diversions. Eur Urol 2008;53(4):834–42 [discussion: 842–4].

33. Jäger W, Viertmann A-O, Janßen C, et al. Intermittent hyperammonemic encephalopathy after ureterosigmoidostomy: spontaneous onset in the absence of hepatic failure. Cent European J Urol 2015;68(1):121–4.

34. Kaveggia FF, Thompson JS, Schafer EC, et al. Hyperammonemic encephalopathy in urinary diversion with urea-splitting urinary tract infection. Arch Intern Med 1990;150(11):2389–92.

35. Bakke A, Jensen KM, Jonsson O, et al. The rationale behind recommendations for follow-up after urinary diversion: an evidence-based approach. Scand J Urol Nephrol 2007;41(4):261–9.

36. Kristjansson A, Wallin L, Mansson W. Renal function up to 16 years after conduit (refluxing or anti-reflux anastomosis) or continent urinary diversion. 1.

Glomerular filtration rate and patency of ureterointestinal anastomosis. Br J Urol 1995;76:539–45.

37. Hussein AA, Hashmi Z, Dibaj S, et al. Reoperations following robot-assisted radical cystectomy: a decade of experience. J Urol 2016;195(5):1368–76.

38. Hautmann RE, de Petriconi RC, Volkmer BG. 25 Years of experience with 1,000 neobladders: long-term complications. J Urol 2011;185:2207.

39. Shah SH, Movassaghi K, Skinner D, et al. Ureteroenteric strictures after open radical cystectomy and urinary diversion: the University of Southern California experience. Urology 2015;86:87–91.

40. Anderson CB, Morgan TM, Kappa S, et al. Ureteroenteric anastomotic strictures after radical cystectomy—does operative approach matter? J Urol 2013;189:541.

41. Tal R, Sivan B, Kedar D, et al. Management of benign ureteral strictures following radical cystectomy and urinary diversion for bladder cancer. J Urol 2007;178(2):538–42.

42. Nassar OA, Alsafa ME. Experience with ureteroenteric strictures after radical cystectomy and diversion: open surgical revision. Urology 2011;78(2):459–65.

43. Hussein AA, Ahmed YE, May P, et al. Natural history and predictors of parastomal hernia after robot-assisted radical cystectomy and ileal conduit urinary diversion. J Urol 2017. https://doi.org/10.1016/j.juro.2017.08.112.

44. Szymanski KM, St-Cyr D, Alam T, et al. External stoma and peristomal complications following radical cystectomy and ileal conduit diversion: a systematic review. Ostomy Wound Manage 2010;56(1):28–35.

45. Lawrentschuk N, Colombo R, Hakenberg OW, et al. Prevention and management of complications following radical cystectomy for bladder cancer. Eur Urol 2010;57(6):983–1001.

46. Bartsch G, Daneshmand S, Skinner EC, et al. Urinary functional outcomes in female neobladder patients. World J Urol 2014;32(1):221–8.

47. Hosseini SY, Dehghani M, Afsharimoghaddam A, et al. Spontaneous rupture of continent cutaneous urinary diversion after 25 years. J Renal Inj Prev 2017;6(2):80–2.

Quality of Life After Radical Cystectomy

Mark D. Tyson II, MD[a],*, Daniel A. Barocas, MD, MPH[b]

KEYWORDS

- Cystectomy • Ileal conduit • Neobladder • Quality of life • Bladder cancer

KEY POINTS

- Studies comparing quality of life across diversion types have demonstrated similar patient-reported outcomes regardless of diversion type except in recent years, where a trend in favor of neobladder diversions has been observed.
- Cystectomy is associated with well-known declines in sexual function for both men and women, but these declines can be mitigated with nerve-sparing and organ-sparing approaches.
- Body image changes that often accompany external urinary drainage devices and emotional and psychosocial stress endured by the patient with cancer can significantly impair sexual relationships.
- The neurovascular bundles, located on the lateral walls of the vagina, are usually removed or damaged during surgery. Significant devascularization of the clitoris can also occur during the removal of the distal urethra.
- There are bladder-sparing alternatives to radical cystectomy, including radiation protocols, for which the effect on quality of life is largely unknown.

INTRODUCTION

Bladder cancer is the second most common genitourinary malignancy in the United States with an estimated incidence of approximately 11.6 cases per 100,000 per year.[1] Approximately 1 in 5 new bladder cancer cases are muscle invasive for which the current standard of care is neoadjuvant chemotherapy followed by radical cystectomy.[2] The main options for urinary tract reconstruction are incontinent conduit diversions, continent cutaneous diversions, and orthotopic neobladders. Although these treatments are associated with well-known short-term effects on patient well-being and quality of life,[3] long-term quality-of-life impairments in functional independence, urinary and sexual function, social and emotional health, body image, and psychosocial stress are often attributed to the urinary diversion. Therefore, understanding how the different options for urinary diversion influence these important quality-of-life parameters is paramount for informed consent and should be rooted in data acquired from rigorous scientific investigation.

Compared with the literature on other malignancies like breast or prostate cancer,[4,5] high-quality studies evaluating the effect of bladder cancer treatment on quality of life are lacking. Although the number of studies in this space has dramatically increased in recent years, strong conclusions from these studies are mitigated by methodological limitations, such as cross-sectional designs, small sample sizes, and inadequate confounding control.

In this article, the authors (1) provide an overview of the most commonly used quality-of-life instruments in patients with bladder cancer, including general, cancer-specific, and bladder

Disclosure: The authors have nothing to disclose.
[a] Department of Urology, Mayo Clinic Arizona, Mayo Clinic Hospital, 5777 East Mayo Boulevard, Phoenix, AZ 85054, USA; [b] Department of Urologic Surgery, Vanderbilt University Medical Center, A1302 Medical Center North, Nashville, TN 37203, USA
* Corresponding author.
E-mail address: tyson.mark@mayo.edu

cancer–specific quality-of-life instruments and (2) summarize the effect of cystectomy and urinary diversion on general quality-of-life outcomes as well as disease-specific outcomes, such as sexual, urinary, and bowel function.

OVERVIEW OF QUALITY-OF-LIFE INSTRUMENTS

"Quality of life" is a construct that encompasses physical, psychosocial, and functional health and reflects a patient's satisfaction with various aspects of his or her life.[6,7] More broadly speaking, quality of life is essentially a person's satisfaction with his or her life in the context of the current health circumstances. To minimize bias, quality of life is most commonly assessed by standardized patient-reported survey instruments or questionnaires. Valid, reliable, longitudinal measurement of quality of life has important implications for research comparing treatment options as well as for delivery of patient-centered clinical care.

Because measurements of quality of life can be general or specific to the disease under study, quality-of-life instruments for patients with bladder cancer fall into 1 of 3 broad categories: general, cancer specific, and bladder cancer specific.[8]

General Quality-of-Life Outcomes

Many different psychometrically validated survey instruments assessing general quality of life exist and can be used for patients with cancer. The most established and perhaps most widely used general quality-of-life instrument is the RAND Medical Outcomes Study 36-Item Health Survey (SF-36). This survey comprises 36 questions across 8 distinct functional domains, including vitality, physical function, bodily pain, general health perceptions, physical role functioning, emotional role functioning, social role functioning, and mental health.[9] Although the SF-36 does not contain specific items related to cancer, it has been used to assess general quality of life in patients with bladder cancer undergoing cystectomy.[10–13] Although the SF-36 is among the most validated and responsive general quality-of-life instrument, it lacks the specificity to gauge cancer-specific issues.[14–16]

Cancer-Specific Instruments

Quality-of-life instruments have also been developed to assess general quality-of-life outcomes for patients with cancer, such as The European Organization for Research and Treatment of Cancer Quality of Life Core Questionnaire (EORTC QLQ-C30) and the Functional Assessment of

Cancer Therapy (FACT-G).[17,18] However, similar to the general quality-of-life instruments, these surveys only address cancer-related issues in broad terms and are not bladder cancer specific. Although these types of instruments are needed to assess general cancer-related issues such as nausea, vomiting, pain, or insomnia, this broad applicability across the cancer spectrum detracts from their ability to capture key quality-of-life issues that are most important to patients with bladder cancer, such as urinary, bowel, and sexual function.[14]

Bladder Cancer-Specific Instruments

Several bladder cancer–specific quality-of-life instruments have been validated for use in patients undergoing radical cystectomy and urinary diversion. Bladder cancer–specific instruments assess important endpoints pertaining to urinary, bowel, and sexual dysfunction as well as body image and practical issues pertaining to their specific urinary diversion type. These instruments fall into 1 of 2 categories: treatment-neutral instruments such as the Bladder Cancer Index (BCI) and the FACT-BI and treatment-specific instruments such as the FACT-VCI and EORTC-QLQ-BLM30, which pertain specifically to patients who have undergone a cystectomy with urinary diversion. Although these instruments capture more disease-specific information, they should be coadministered with general quality-of-life instruments so as not to miss important information regarding their overall health.

The European Organization for Research and Treatment of Cancer Quality of Life Core Questionnaire–bladder cancer muscle invasive

The EORTC-QLQ-BLM30 is a 30-item supplementary questionnaire module that is specifically designed for use in those with muscle-invasive bladder cancer.[19] The instrument is intended to be administered in conjunction with the EORTC-QLQ-C30, which contains items within 15 domains pertaining to physical, role, emotional, cognitive, and social functioning as well as items related to fatigue, nausea, vomiting, pain, dyspnea, insomnia, appetite loss, constipation, diarrhea, and financial difficulties.[20] The QLQ-BLM30 is the bladder cancer–specific module that incorporates multi-item scales that assess urinary symptoms, urostomy problems, future perspectives, abdominal bloating, body image, sexual function, and catheter use problems. The scoring methods for the QLQ-BLM30 are similar, in principle, to the scoring methods for the symptom and function scales of the QLQ-C30. All of the scales and single-item measures range from 0 to 100, and whereas higher scores for the symptom domains indicate a higher level of symptoms, a higher score for the functional domain represents a higher level of functioning.[21]

Functional Assessment of Cancer Therapy–Vanderbilt Cystectomy Index

The FACT-VCI is a questionnaire for patients undergoing cystectomy and urinary diversion.[22] It centers on urinary, bowel, and sexual symptoms following cystectomy and is designed to be administered with the FACT-G core. The 17 questions are adapted from 3 previously validated instruments (the FACT-Bladder Cancer, FACT-Colorectal, and the Functional Assessment of Incontinence Therapy-Urinary).[22,23] Each of the 17 items is scored on a 5-point Likert scale and added to form a single score without domains. Importantly, it has been validated for use in cystectomy patients and has demonstrated consistent ability to discriminate quality of life between ileal conduit and orthotopic neobladder patients.[23] Because it is limited in its scope with respect to diversion management, it may not be best suited to answer quality-of-life questions within particular diversion types.

Functional Assessment of Cancer Therapy–bladder cancer

The FACT-BI is a questionnaire that was designed for use across a range of bladder cancer treatment and stages.[24–26] It consists of 27-item FACT-G core that evaluates the physical, social and family, emotional, and functional well-being as well as a condition-specific component that assesses issues related to bladder cancer, such as urinary, bowel, and sexual function, with 2 more items for those with a stoma.[18] The disease-specific questions are generic enough that patients with non-muscle-invasive or muscle-invasive bladder cancer can be compared, making this a "treatment-neutral" instrument. Treatment-neutral instrument differs from "treatment-specific" instruments like the FACT-VCI and QLQ-BLM30, which were designed for patients undergoing treatment of muscle-invasive bladder cancer. However, the versatility of treatment-neutral instruments allows investigators to compare 2 different urinary diversion types, 2 intravesical treatments, or bladder-sparing protocols on equal scales. The advantage of the FACT-BI over the BCI, which is discussed in the next section, is the seamless incorporation of the FACT-G core to measure general quality of life. However, the principal disadvantage of the FACT-BI compared with the BCI is that the FACT-BI lacks the ability to discriminate which symptoms are most bothersome because it does not offer separate function and bother subscales.[8,27]

Bladder Cancer Index

The University of Michigan's BCI is a gender-neutral, treatment-indifferent, condition-specific, quality-of-life instrument established using conventional psychometric methodology and has demonstrated test-retest validity, internal consistency, and divergent/convergent validity in several performance phases. The survey was designed to be inclusive of patients from all stages of bladder cancer and consists of 34 items within 3 domains that measure urinary, sexual, and bowel function with 2 subdomains (bother and function) for each main domain. For ileal conduit patients, the BCI measures stoma and appliance function as well as leakage and skin irritation. Item responses are based on a Likert scale with the composite score standardized on a scale from 0 to 100 with higher scores indicating better function. The bother subscale offers the ability to measure severity of bother for urinary, sexual, and bowel dysfunction, which is unparalleled among bladder cancer–specific quality-of-life instruments. The principal limitations of the BCI are the lack of a core module to measure general quality of life as well as the lack of gender-specific, urinary diversion–specific, and body image–specific items.

Sexual function instruments

In additional to the disease-specific quality-of-life instruments summarized above, 2 general quality-of-life instruments have been used to measure sexual function after cystectomy in men: the International Index of Erectile Function (IIEF)[28] and the Sexual Health Inventory for Men (SHIM).[29] Although both scales give a composite score on a continuous scale, cutoffs such as 26 for the IIEF and 21 for the SHIM have been commonly used in the literature to simplify the identification of abnormal erectile function. Among women, the instrument most commonly used to assess sexual dysfunction after cystectomy is the Female Sexual Function Index (FSFI).[30]

GENERAL AND DISEASE-SPECIFIC QUALITY-OF-LIFE OUTCOMES

In general, studies comparing quality of life across diversion types have demonstrated similar patient-reported outcomes regardless of diversion type. Of course, these studies are not randomized, and the lack of an effect may be due to success in matching patients to the appropriate diversion type, management of patient expectations, or patient's acceptance of the diversion they selected.

In the largest study to date, investigators from Germany studied general quality-of-life outcomes among 823 patients treated for bladder cancer. Using commonly accepted thresholds for clinical significance on the EORTC-QLQ-C30, cystectomy was associated with a negative effect on role function, fatigue, and appetite compared with controls without bladder cancer after adjusting for age, sex, tumor invasiveness, and time since surgery.[31] With respect to outcomes by diversion type, patients with neobladders had more problems with diarrhea, financial difficulties, and worse social functioning, and patients with conduits reported more problems with constipation. Somewhat surprisingly, neobladder patients did not report more problems with sleep; rather, it was elderly patients (age >70) with conduits who reported the most insomnia. Importantly, however, the difference according to type of urinary diversion was mostly small and did not meet the thresholds for clinical significance.

In a registry-based population analysis, Allareddy and colleagues[32] reported the effect of cystectomy on quality of life (FACT-BI) by comparing 82 patients who underwent cystectomy to 177 patients who still had their bladder intact, mostly because of noninvasive disease. Unlike the German study, there were no major differences in general or disease-specific quality of life in patients undergoing a cystectomy (compared with controls). In the secondary analysis comparing ileal conduits to continent diversion, there were again no differences in the general quality-of-life outcomes. However, given the cross-sectional nature of this study, there are several threats to the validity of the findings, including recall bias, response bias, and inability to control for baseline function.

Several other studies have examined general quality of life after cystectomy, and the results are relatively consistent, with little variation by diversion type. Recognizing that the nonrandomized allocation of treatment makes definitive causal inferences more difficult, in general, neobladder patients in some studies report a slightly higher global health status, better physical functioning, but more diarrhea.[33] In a separate study of 41 women treated with cystectomy, no significant differences were noted on any of the domains on FACT-BL and EORTC-QLQ-BLM30.[34] Even among different types of neobladder (sigmoid vs ileal), very little variation is observed.[13]

Recent Trends in Quality-of-Life Outcomes

Although there is little variation in general or disease-specific quality-of-life outcomes by urinary diversion type from these historical series, emerging evidence from publications in recent years has suggested that some important differences may exist. Although several systematic reviews have failed to demonstrate superiority of one form of diversion over the others,[15,35–37] Ghosh and Somani[38] noted a trend in favor of neobladder diversion when one only considers studies from the last 5 years. This observation is important because the quality-of-life studies in this space have been relatively poor quality historically, and differences may emerge as higher-quality studies get published. For example, only 3 of the 16 studies performed between 1998 and 2010 showed outcomes in favor of the neobladder,[10,39,40] but 4 of the 6 studies published since 2011 showed superior quality-of-life outcomes with neobladder compared with the comparator diversion type.[33,41–43] Furthermore, of the 5 prospective comparisons published to date, 3 have favored neobladder over the comparator diversion type.[41–43]

SEXUAL FUNCTION OUTCOMES

Not unlike other surgeries of the pelvis, cystectomy is associated with well-known declines in sexual function for both men and women. In addition to body image changes that often accompany external urinary drainage devices, emotional and psychosocial stress endured by the patient with cancer can significantly impair sexual relationships as well.[44] When these factors are considered in the context of anatomic changes during surgery, such as cavernous nerve damage and partial vaginectomy, it is not surprising that upwards of 80% of cystectomy patients complain of sexual dysfunction after surgery.[45]

Although the association between sexual dysfunction and prostate cancer surgery is well studied,[4,46] sexual dysfunction is not well characterized after cystectomy owing to the lack of high-quality, appropriately powered, longitudinal cohort studies. In the State Health Registry of Iowa study referenced earlier,[32] 21% of respondents whose bladder was preserved were not interested in sex compared with 39% of radical cystectomy patients. For erectile dysfunction, the results were even more dramatic with 89% of respondents in the cystectomy group reporting the inability to get and keep an erection compared with only 32% in the bladder-preserved group. In the Michigan study, patients who had a cystectomy scored approximately 20 points lower on the BCI than patients undergoing intravesical therapy (42.2 vs 20.0 for ileal conduits and 25.5 for neobladders).[47] Although the causal relationship between cystectomy and poor sexual function remains somewhat ill defined, these findings have been corroborated in several other studies,[24,48–50] and the biological mechanism is plausible. How sexual function varies over time after cystectomy remains unknown.

Sexual Function Outcomes by Diversion Type

The effect of diversion type on sexual function outcomes is still largely unknown, but a few head-to-head comparisons have been published. Recognizing the conclusions in these studies are limited by small sample sizes and the lack of baseline assessment, 2 studies have suggested improved sexual function outcomes with neobladder compared with ileal conduits.[26,51] In a retrospective, single-institution, cross-sectional study, only 3% of ileal conduit patients could maintain an erection compared with 23% of neobladder patients, despite similar interest in sex.[26] A separate study suggested that sexual function worsened over time for men with ileal conduits, but improved over time for neobladder patients. However, the mean age in the 2 groups in this study was quite different (61 vs 71 years), and age is known to impact sexual function recovery after pelvic surgery.[51] Several other studies have failed to show meaningful differences in sexual function between diversion choices, but in any case, the chance of a significant sexual function recovery is low for a man undergoing radical cystectomy.[24,32,47,52]

Nerve-sparing techniques have been shown to improve sexual function after cystectomy. In a study of 21 patients managed with nerve-sparing cystectomy, 12 (57.8%) demonstrated return of complete penile tumescence.[53] The other 9 patients reported return of erections with use of medical therapy. A separate study of sexually active men who had undergone nerve-sparing cystectomy reported that 8 of the 9 patients recovered erections firm enough for penetration.[54] There is at least some evidence to suggest that age and precystectomy erectile function explain a large amount of the variation in outcome between nerve-sparing and non-nerve-sparing techniques.[55] The effect of nerve-sparing approaches in women seems to have similar beneficial effects on sexual function.[56]

Sexual Function in Women

Sexual function is a major concern among sexually active women with invasive bladder cancer. The neurovascular bundles, which are located on the lateral walls of the vagina, are usually removed or damaged during surgery as well as significant devascularization of the clitoris that can occur during the removal of the distal urethra.[57–59]

Moreover, the anterior vaginal wall is commonly removed en bloc with the bladder, resulting in a foreshortened or narrowed vagina. In a small study of 27 patients, the most common complaints after surgery included diminished ability to achieve orgasm in 45%, decreased lubrication in 41%, decreased sexual desire in 37%, and dyspareunia in 22%.[60] Significant declines were also observed in total FSFI scores, and only 48% were able to have successful vaginal intercourse. No significant differences were noted between patients who underwent neobladders and Indiana pouches, but ileal conduit patients scored substantially lower after cystectomy.

In an effort to preserve sexual function after cystectomy in women, several modifications to the surgical technique have been proposed.[60] First, the clitoral neurovasculature can be preserved by sparing the distal urethra in selected cases. Second, in an effort to maintain vaginal lubrication and neurovascular innervations, the anterior vaginal wall can be preserved in selected cases where the tumor is not involving the bladder neck and trigone. Third, tubular reconstruction of the vagina preserves vaginal depth and may facilitate pain-free intercourse. Last, transection of the urethra at the level of the bladder neck with retrograde dissection of the bladder off the anterior vaginal wall has been suggested as a way of preserving the blood supply to the clitoris.[61] Whether any of these modifications compromises oncologic efficacy remains unknown, and comparative studies to validate the impact of these modifications are lacking. Indeed, much more comparative data are needed to identify the optimal methods for preserving sexual function in both men and women.

SUMMARY

Despite a litany of studies, quality-of-life outcomes after radical cystectomy are not well characterized. However, with the development of psychometrically validated survey instruments, high-quality, prospective, longitudinal studies are a critical need in the urologic literature. These data will undoubtedly serve to improve the state of evidence for informed consent and quality-of-life expectations for patients undergoing bladder cancer surgery with significant quality-of-life implications.

REFERENCES

1. Ferlay J, Soerjomataram I, Ervik M, et al. GLOBO-CAN 2012 v1.1, Cancer incidence and mortality worldwide: IARC cancerbase No. 11. Lyon (France): Int Agency Res Cancer; 2014. p. 2014. Available at: http://globocan.iarc.fr.

2. Chang SS, Bochner BH, Chou R, et al. Treatment of non-metastatic muscle-invasive bladder cancer: AUA/ASCO/ASTRO/SUO guideline. J Urol 2017; 198(3):552–9.

3. Stein JP, Lieskovsky G, Cote R, et al. Radical cystectomy in the treatment of invasive bladder cancer: long-term results in 1,054 patients. J Clin Oncol 2001;19:666–75.

4. Barocas DA, Alvarez J, Resnick MJ, et al. Association between radiation therapy, surgery, or observation for localized prostate cancer and patient-reported outcomes after 3 years. JAMA 2017;317:1126.

5. Resnick MJ, Barocas DA, Morgans AK, et al. Contemporary prevalence of pretreatment urinary, sexual, hormonal, and bowel dysfunction: defining the population at risk for harms of prostate cancer treatment. Cancer 2014;120:1263–71.

6. WHO. WHOQOL: measuring quality of life. Psychol Med 1998;28:551–8.

7. Dolan P. The measurement of health-related quality of life for use in resource allocation decisions in health care. Handb Heal Econ 2000;1: 1723–60.

8. Danna BJ, Metcalfe MJ, Wood EL, et al. Assessing symptom burden in bladder cancer: an overview of bladder cancer specific health-related quality of life instruments. Bladder Cancer 2016;2:329–40.

9. Ware JJ, Sherbourne C. The MOS 36-item Short-Form Health Survey (SF-36). I. Conceptual framework and item selection. Med Care 1992;30:473–83.

10. Philip J, Manikandan R, Venugopal S, et al. Orthotopic neobladder versus ileal conduit urinary diversion after cystectomy - a quality-of-life based comparison. Ann R Coll Surg Engl 2009;91:565–9.

11. Autorino R, Quarto G, Di Lorenzo G, et al. Health related quality of life after radical cystectomy: comparison of ileal conduit to continent orthotopic neobladder. Eur J Surg Oncol 2009;35: 858–64.

12. Hara I, Miyake H, Hara S, et al. Health-related quality of life after radical cystectomy for bladder cancer: a comparison of ileal conduit and orthotopic bladder replacement. BJU Int 2002;89:10–3.

13. Miyake H, Furukawa J, Muramaki M, et al. Health related quality of life after radical cystectomy: comparative study between orthotopic sigmoid versus ileal neobladders. Eur J Surg Oncol 2012; 38:1089–94.

14. Wright JL, Porter MP. Quality-of-life assessment in patients with bladder cancer. Nat Clin Pract Urol 2007;4:147–54.

15. Porter MP, Penson DF. Health related quality of life after radical cystectomy and urinary diversion for bladder cancer: a systematic review and critical analysis of the literature. J Urol 2005;173: 1318–22.

16. Parkinson JP, Konety BR. Health related quality of life assessments for patients with bladder cancer. J Urol 2004;172:2130–6.

17. Aaronson NK, Ahmedzai S, Bergman B, et al. The European Organisation for Research and Treatment of Cancer QLQ-C30: a quality-of-life instrument for use in international clinical trials in oncology. J Natl Cancer Inst 1993;85:365–76.

18. Cella D, Tulsky D, Gray G. The functional assessment of cancer therapy scale: development and validation of the general measure. J Clin Oncol 1993;11:570–9.

19. Imbimbo C, Mirone V, Siracusano S, et al. Quality of life assessment with orthotopic ileal neobladder reconstruction after radical cystectomy: results from a prospective italian multicenter observational study. Urology 2015;86:974–9.

20. Scott NW, Fayers PM, Aaronson NK, et al. EORTC QLQ-C30 reference values. 2008.p. 1–427. Available at: www.groupsEORTC.be. Accessed January 17, 2017.

21. Fayers P, Aaronson N, Bjordal K. EORTC QLQ-C30 scoring manual. Eortc; 2001. p. 1–77.

22. Cookson MS, Dutta S, Chang SS, et al. Health related quality of life in patients treated with radical cystectomy and urinary diversion for urothelial carcinoma of the bladder: development and validation of a new disease specific questionnaire. J Urol 2003; 170:1926–30.

23. Anderson CB, Feurer ID, Large MC, et al. Psychometric characteristics of a condition-specific, health-related quality-of-life survey: the FACT-Vanderbilt Cystectomy Index. Urology 2012;80:77–83.

24. Karvinen KH, Courneya KS, North S, et al. Associations between exercise and quality of life in bladder cancer survivors: a population-based study. Cancer Epidemiol Biomarkers Prev 2007;16:984–90.

25. Botteman MF, Pashos CL, Hauser RS, et al. Quality of life aspects of bladder cancer: a review of the literature. Qual Life Res 2003;12:675–88.

26. Månsson Å, Davidsson T, Hunt S, et al. The quality of life in men after radical cystectomy with a continent cutaneous diversion or orthotopic bladder substitution: is there a difference? BJU Int 2002; 90:386–90.

27. Gilbert SM, Dunn RL, Hollenbeck BK, et al. Development and validation of the Bladder Cancer Index: a comprehensive, disease specific measure of health related quality of life in patients with localized bladder cancer. J Urol 2010;183:1764–70.

28. Rosen RC, Riley A, Wagner G, et al. The International Index of Erectile Function (IIEF): a multidimensional scale for assessment of erectile dysfunction. Urology 1997;49:822–30.

29. Rhoden EL, Telöken C, Sogari PR, et al. The use of the simplified International Index of Erectile Function (IIEF-5) as a diagnostic tool to study the prevalence

of erectile dysfunction. Int J Impot Res 2002;14:245–50.

30. Rosen R, Brown C, Heiman J, et al. The Female Sexual Function Index (FSFI): a multidimensional self-report instrument for the assessment of female sexual function. J Sex Marital Ther 2000;26:191–208.

31. Singer S, Ziegler C, Schwalenberg T, et al. Quality of life in patients with muscle invasive and non-muscle invasive bladder cancer. Support Care Cancer 2013;21:1383–93.

32. Allareddy V, Kennedy J, West MM, et al. Quality of life in long-term survivors of bladder cancer. Cancer 2006;106:2355–62.

33. Erber B, Schrader M, Miller K, et al. Morbidity and quality of life in bladder cancer patients following cystectomy and urinary diversion: a single-institution comparison of ileal conduit versus orthotopic neobladder. ISRN Urol 2012;2012:1–8.

34. Gacci M, Saleh O, Cai T, et al. Quality of life in women undergoing urinary diversion for bladder cancer: results of a multicenter study among long-term disease-free survivors. Health Qual Life Outcomes 2013;11:43.

35. Gerharz EW, Månsson A, Hunt S, et al. Quality of life after cystectomy and urinary diversion: an evidence based analysis. J Urol 2005;174:1729–36.

36. Ali AS, Hayes MC, Birch B, et al. Health related quality of life (HRQoL) after cystectomy: comparison between orthotopic neobladder and ileal conduit diversion. Eur J Surg Oncol 2015;41:295–9.

37. Yang LS, Shan BL, Shan LL, et al. A systematic review and meta-analysis of quality of life outcomes after radical cystectomy for bladder cancer. Surg Oncol 2016;25:281–97.

38. Ghosh A, Somani BK. Recent trends in postcystectomy health-related quality of life (QoL) favors neobladder diversion: systematic review of the literature. Urology 2016;93:22–6.

39. Hobisch A, Tosun K, Kinzl J, et al. Quality of life after cystectomy and orthotopic neobladder versus ileal conduit urinary diversion. World J Urol 2000;18:338–44.

40. Dutta SC, Chang SC, Coffey CS, et al. Health related quality of life assessment after radical cystectomy: comparison of ileal conduit with continent orthotopic neobladder. J Urol 2002;168:164–7.

41. Yang M, Wang H, Wang J, et al. Impact of invasive bladder cancer and orthotopic urinary diversion on general health-related quality of life: an SF-36 survey. Mol Clin Oncol 2013;1:758–62.

42. Prcic A, Aganovic D, Hadziosmanovic O. Sickness impact profile (SIP) score, a good alternative instrument for measuring quality of life in patients with ileal urinary diversions. Acta Inform Med 2013;21:160–5.

43. Singh V, Yadav R, Sinha RJ, et al. Prospective comparison of quality-of-life outcomes between ileal conduit urinary diversion and orthotopic neobladder reconstruction after radical cystectomy: a statistical model. BJU Int 2014;113:726–32.

44. Modh RA, Mulhall JP, Gilbert SM. Sexual dysfunction after cystectomy and urinary diversion. Nat Rev Urol 2014;11:445–53.

45. Matsuda T, Aptel I, Exbrayat C, et al. Determinants of quality of life of bladder cancer survivors five years after treatment in France. Int J Urol 2003;10:423–9.

46. Resnick MJ, Koyama T, Fan KH, et al. Long-term functional outcomes after treatment for localized prostate cancer. N Engl J Med 2013;368:436–45.

47. Gilbert SM, Wood DP, Dunn RL, et al. Measuring health-related quality of life outcomes in bladder cancer patients using the Bladder Cancer Index (BCI). Cancer 2007;109:1756–62.

48. Månsson Å, Al Amin M, Malmström PU, et al. Patient-assessed outcomes in Swedish and Egyptian men undergoing radical cystectomy and orthotopic bladder substitution-a prospective comparative study. Urology 2007;70:1086–90.

49. Kikuchi E, Horiguchi Y, Nakashima J, et al. Assessment of long-term quality of life using the FACT-BL questionnaire in patients with an ileal conduit, continent reservoir, or orthotopic neobladder. Jpn J Clin Oncol 2006;36:712–6.

50. Goossens-Laan CA, Kil PJ, Bosch JL, et al. Patient-reported outcomes for patients undergoing radical cystectomy: a prospective case-control study. Support Care Cancer 2014;22:189–200.

51. Hedgepeth RC, Gilbert SM, He C, et al. Body image and bladder cancer specific quality of life in patients with ileal conduit and neobladder urinary diversions. Urology 2010;76:671–5.

52. Vakalopoulos I, Dimitriadis G, Anastasiadis A, et al. Does intubated uretero-ureterocutaneostomy provide better health-related quality of life than orthotopic neobladder in patients after radical cystectomy for invasive bladder cancer? Int Urol Nephrol 2011;43:743–8.

53. Hekal IA, El-Bahnasawy MS, Mosbah A, et al. Recoverability of erectile function in post-radical cystectomy patients: subjective and objective evaluations. Eur Urol 2009;55:275–83.

54. Zippe CD, Raina R, Massanyi EZ, et al. Sexual function after male radical cystectomy in a sexually active population. Urology 2004;64:682–5.

55. Schoenberg MP, Walsh PC, Breazeale DR, et al. Local recurrence and survival following nerve sparing radical cystoprostatectomy for bladder cancer: 10-year followup. J Urol 1996;155:490–4.

56. Bhatt A, Nandipati K, Dhar N, et al. Neurovascular preservation in orthotopic cystectomy: impact on female sexual function. Urology 2006;67:742–5.

57. Berman L, Berman J, Felder S, et al. Seeking help for sexual function complaints: what gynecologists

need to know about the female patient's experience. Fertil Steril 2003;79:572–6.

58. Stenzl A, Colleselli K, Poisel S, et al. Rationale and technique of nerve sparing radical cystectomy before an orthotopic neobladder procedure in women. J Urol 1995;154:2044–9.

59. Schoenberg M, Hortopan S, Schlossberg L, et al. Anatomical anterior exenteration with urethral and vaginal preservation: illustrated surgical method. J Urol 1999;161:569–72.

60. Zippe CD, Raina R, Shah AD, et al. Female sexual dysfunction after radical cystectomy: a new outcome measure. Urology 2004;63:1153–7.

61. Horenblas S, Meinhardt W, Ijzerman W, et al. Sexuality preserving cystectomy and neobladder: initial results. J Urol 2001;166:837–40.

Adjuvant Therapy in Muscle-Invasive Bladder Cancer and Upper Tract Urothelial Carcinoma

Tala Achkar, MD[a], Rahul A. Parikh, MD, PhD[b],*

KEYWORDS

- Muscle-invasive bladder cancer (MIBC) • Adjuvant chemotherapy • Neoadjuvant chemotherapy
- Urothelial cancer • Micrometastases

KEY POINTS

- The definitive therapy for muscle-invasive bladder cancer (MIBC) is radical cystectomy or radiation to the bladder.
- There is a benefit of 5% to 10% absolute improvement in 5-year overall survival (OS) for the use of neoadjuvant cisplatin-based chemotherapy based on prospective clinical studies; however, this is lacking for adjuvant cisplatin-based therapy.
- Patients with MIBC are frequently upstaged at the time of definitive surgery, adjuvant chemotherapy provides the opportunity to treat patients based on their actual pathologic stage.
- Randomized trials with adjuvant cisplatin-based chemotherapy in MIBC have failed to accrue enough patients, and thus, failed to demonstrate a statistically significant improvement in 5-year OS compared with cystectomy alone.
- Patients who did not receive neoadjuvant chemotherapy but have high-risk disease (defined as T3, T4 disease, or presence of nodal metastases) after radical cystectomy should be considered for adjuvant cisplatin-based chemotherapy.

INTRODUCTION
Neoadjuvant Versus Adjuvant Therapy

Adjuvant therapy is the use of chemotherapy, immunotherapy, or radiation for bladder cancer after definitive surgery in the absence of detectable disease. The goal of adjuvant therapy is to reduce the risk of relapse from micrometastatic disease. Neoadjuvant therapy is the use of chemotherapy, immunotherapy, or radiation before definitive surgery. The goal of neoadjuvant therapy is to shrink the tumor and reduce the risk of relapse from micrometastatic disease. Neoadjuvant chemotherapy may be better tolerated because it is administered before surgery.

The key differences between adjuvant and neoadjuvant therapies are summarized in **Table 1**.

For muscle-invasive bladder cancer (MIBC), neoadjuvant chemotherapy using a cisplatin-based regimen is considered the standard of care based on statistically significant improvement in median overall survival (OS) and 5-year OS in prospective clinical trials and meta-analyses.

Conflicts of Interest: The authors have nothing to disclose.
[a] Department of Medicine, Division of Hematology-Oncology, University of Pittsburgh Medical Center, 5150 Centre Avenue, Pittsburgh, PA 15232, USA; [b] Department of Medicine, Division of Medical Oncology, University of Kansas Medical Center, 2330 Shawnee Mission Parkway, Suite 210, MS 5003, Westwood, KS 66205, USA
* Corresponding author.
E-mail address: rparikh2@kumc.edu

urologic.theclinics.com

Table 1
Key differences between adjuvant and neoadjuvant therapies

Neoadjuvant Therapy	Adjuvant Therapy
Given before definitive surgery or radiation	Given after definitive surgery or radiation
May shrink the tumor before surgery	May be difficult to administer following morbidity from surgery
Treats micrometastatic disease present at the time of diagnosis	Treats micrometastatic disease after surgery
Allows evaluation of the primary tumor for response, better prognostication and tissue correlatives in response to chemotherapy	Allows selection of appropriate high-risk patients after complete pathologic evaluation
May result in a delay in surgical management	Avoids any delay in surgical management, but can result in a delay in receiving chemotherapy

This article focuses on the prior studies with adjuvant chemotherapy in bladder cancer. The authors summarize these studies and present their recommendations for the use of adjuvant chemotherapy in these patients.

Patient Case

Mr Bond is a 57-year-old man who presented with hematuria. On cystoscopy, he was noted to have a mass in the bladder, staged as T2 disease on transurethral resection of his bladder tumor (TURBT). He has normal renal function and hearing. He was counseled on the use of cisplatin-based neoadjuvant chemotherapy. He refused chemotherapy given concerns regarding the side effects of hearing loss and renal dysfunction with cisplatin. He proceeded to radical cystectomy and was noted to have T4N1 disease on final pathology. Using a Bladder Cancer Recurrence Normogram (https://www.mskcc.org/nomograms/bladder/post_op), you inform the patient that his risk of recurrence in the next 5 years is 92%. What is the next step in the management of this patient?

Muscle-Invasive Bladder Cancer

MIBC is defined as clinical stage T2-T4a and accounts for approximately one-third of bladder

cancer presentations.[1] Approximately 50% of patients with MIBC develop metastatic disease, thought to be due to the presence of occult metastatic disease present at the time of initial diagnosis.[1] Patients with T2 bladder cancer achieve high cure rates of approximately 80% with radical cystectomy alone. However, in patients with T3 disease, this cure rate reduces to approximately 60%, and in T4 disease, to approximately 45%. In patients with lymph node involvement, cure rates decrease to approximately 35%.[2] Thus, the patients with the highest recurrence rates are those with T3 or T4 disease and positive lymph node involvement (**Table 2**).

Despite potentially curative surgery, approximately 50% of patients with stage T2b-4 MIBC develop metastatic disease within 2 years.[3] The median time to recurrence in patients with node-positive disease is approximately 12 months, and these patients usually present with distant recurrences.[2] A study showed that overall 2- or 3-year disease-free survival (DFS) correlates with OS and can be a surrogate for 5-year OS in patients with bladder cancer treated with radical cystectomy.[4]

According to the National Comprehensive Cancer Network (NCCN) guidelines, treatment is primarily surgical in patients with no evidence of nodal disease, with consideration of neoadjuvant chemotherapy, particularly in the case of T2-4 disease. Adjuvant chemotherapy is considered based on pathologic risk as well as positive lymph nodes, and T3 or T4 lesions.[5] Therefore, in patients who did not receive neoadjuvant chemotherapy, and who have a higher risk of recurrence, the benefits and adverse effects of cisplatin-based adjuvant chemotherapy should be discussed with the patient.

The Second International Consultation on Bladder Cancer recommends adjuvant cisplatin-based chemotherapy in patients with T3/T4 and/or lymph node–positive bladder cancer following cystectomy, if they have not received prior cisplatin-based neoadjuvant chemotherapy and are medically fit (grade B).[3] They also recommend against the use of non-cisplatin-based combination chemotherapy in the adjuvant setting (grade A).[3]

Table 2
Recurrence risk based on extent of muscle and nodal invasion from bladder cancer

	T2	T3	T4	Lymph Nodes Involved
Recurrence risk, %	20	40	55	65

Cisplatin-based neoadjuvant chemotherapy has demonstrated a clear 5-year OS benefit in MIBC.[6] It also provides an ability to treat potential micrometastatic disease early in the treatment course, particularly before the possible morbidity associated with surgery while the patients are still fit. In addition, neoadjuvant chemotherapy uniquely allows the evaluation of a tumor's response to the treatment regimen and further tumor tissue analysis. In the adjuvant setting, chemotherapy can be given based on complete pathologic staging, as opposed to in the neoadjuvant setting when it is based on clinical staging, therefore selecting out the high risk patients who will most likely benefit from adjuvant treatment.[7] In fact, approximately 42% of patients with T2 disease on TURBT are upstaged at the time of radical cystectomy.[8] Also, the use of adjuvant chemotherapy does not delay upfront definitive surgery.[8]

Overall, the studies that have been conducted in order to evaluate the efficacy of adjuvant chemotherapy have been lacking in quality overall, as is described in later discussion. The lack of quality is partly due to issues with poor patient accrual in the studies, and difficulty in selecting appropriate candidates due to the absence of useful biomarkers in this disease.[7]

Adjuvant Studies

Retrospective studies

A large retrospective study of 3947 patients with bladder cancer treated with radical cystectomy and lymphadenectomy analyzed the benefit of adjuvant chemotherapy in patients divided into quintiles based on disease risk.[9] The higher the quintile, the higher risk the disease, and the lower the patient's predicted survival. In the lower 2 quintiles, adjuvant chemotherapy was associated with decreased survival (hazard ratio [HR] 6.21 and 2.20, respectively); however, the fifth (and highest) quintile patients experienced significant benefit from adjuvant chemotherapy (HR 0.75, $P = .002$), with an improvement in survival by approximately 5.8 weeks.[9]

Another retrospective study reviewed 424 patients who underwent radical cystectomy and lymph node dissection and selected 101 patients who had T3 bladder cancer.[10] They found that adjuvant chemotherapy was significantly associated with an improved OS (HR 0.35, $P = .004$) and disease-specific survival (DSS; HR 0.33, $P = .022$) but only in the T3b subgroup (macroscopic invasion of the perivesical fat).

Randomized clinical trials

A published phase I/II study compared 2 adjuvant chemotherapy arms to control patients (observation after radical cystectomy), one with gemcitabine and doxorubicin followed by paclitaxel and cisplatin given to patients with normal renal function and the other with gemcitabine and doxorubicin followed by paclitaxel and carboplatin given to patients with impaired renal function.[11] There were a total of 50 patients in both chemotherapy arms. OS was higher for protocol patients compared with controls, 4.6 years in those with good renal function versus 2.5 years ($P = .03$), and 3.4 years in those with poor renal function versus 2 years ($P = .04$). There was no statistically significant difference in DSS, thought to be secondary to missing data in the control data set.

A randomized clinical trial to investigate the efficacy of adjuvant chemotherapy in bladder cancer was reported in 1989.[12] There were a total of 125 patients, and 32 patients had lymph node–positive disease and were treated with 4 cycles of cisplatin followed by methotrexate. Ninety-two patients had no lymph node involvement and were randomized to chemotherapy versus observation. They did not find a statistically significant difference in OS or DFS, which may have been secondary to their small patient numbers and small sample size. Similarly, in another trial, 77 patients were assigned to observation or adjuvant cisplatin monotherapy and did not show a difference in OS between the 2 groups, even when stratified by lymph node status.[13]

In another small randomized trial, 49 patients were randomized to either chemotherapy (26 patients) or observation after cystectomy (23 patients).[14,15] Chemotherapy was 3 cycles of either methotrexate, vinblastine, adriamycin, and cisplatin (MVAC) or MVEC with adriamycin substituted by epirubicin. Progression-free survival (PFS) was 66.9 months in the chemotherapy arm, and 11.6 months in the control arm. Median OS was 35.1 months and 20.4 months in the chemotherapy and control arms, respectively, which were statistically significant.

In a small randomized trial, 91 patients were randomized to either chemotherapy or observation following cystectomy.[16] Most patients were given a combination of cisplatin, doxorubicin, and cyclophosphamide. At 3 years, 30% of the patients in the chemotherapy group recurred compared with 54% in the observation group ($P = .011$). The probability of disease-specific death at 3 years was 0.29 in the chemotherapy group compared with 0.50 in the observation group ($P = .099$). The median time to progression in the entire cohort was 1.92 years in the observation arm compared with 6.58 years in the chemotherapy arm. The median OS was 2.41 years in the observation arm compared with 4.25 years in the chemotherapy arm. This study provided encouragement for developing larger phase 3 studies evaluating cisplatin-based combination therapy in the adjuvant setting.

In a prospective randomized clinical trial of adjuvant chemotherapy, patients with T3b or T4 bladder cancer with or without lymph node involvement were randomized to adjuvant chemotherapy with 4 cycles of cisplatin, methotrexate, and vinblastine (CMV) versus observation after radical cystectomy.[17] There were 25 patients in the chemotherapy arm, and 25 patients in the observation arm. Median time to progression was 26 months in the adjuvant arm compared with 12 months in the observation arm ($P = .01$). Median OS was 63 months in the adjuvant arm compared with 36 months in the observation arm; however, this was not statistically significant ($P = .32$), potentially because those patients in the observation arm who recurred then received chemotherapy with CMV, and also because of the very small size of the study.

A phase III Italian multicenter clinical trial randomized patients within 10 weeks of radical cystectomy to adjuvant chemotherapy with gemcitabine and cisplatin versus observation with treatment at relapse.[18] The trial was prematurely closed because of low accrual rates, with a total of 194 patients. Five-year OS was 53.7% in the control group and 43.4% in the adjuvant treatment group, which was not statistically significant ($P = .24$). In patients with lymph node–negative disease, 5-year OS was 73.2% in the control arm versus 64.5% in the chemotherapy arm ($P = .65$), and in patients with lymph node involvement, it was 27.6% in the control arm versus 25.8% in the chemotherapy arm ($P = .71$). There was also no statistically significant difference in DFS.

In a recent randomized phase III trial conducted by the European Organization for Research and Treatment of Cancer (EORTC 30994), 284 patients were randomly assigned to adjuvant chemotherapy (4 cycles of gemcitabine, cisplatin, or high-dose MVAC, or MVAC) or chemotherapy at relapse after cystectomy.[19] One hundred forty-one patients were assigned to the immediate therapy group, and 143 were assigned to the deferred treatment group. There was no significant difference in OS in the immediate treatment group as compared with the deferred treatment group (HR 0.78, $P = .13$). However, there was a significant difference in PFS with an HR of 0.54 ($P<.0001$) in the immediate treatment group compared with the deferred treatment group. Unfortunately, this trial had a planned enrollment of 1344 patients

and accrued only a fraction of these patients (~21%) before closure.

Lehmann and colleagues[20] conducted a phase III trial of adjuvant gemcitabine monotherapy administered after surgery versus at the time of progression in cisplatin-ineligible patients. They recruited 120 of 178 planned patients with locally advanced bladder cancer. The patients were randomized to 6 cycles of adjuvant gemcitabine monotherapy within 12 weeks of surgery or treatment at relapse. The trial was closed due to slow accrual. They were unable to meet their prespecified difference in PFS ($P = .335$), DSS ($P = .622$), or OS ($P = .426$). There was a trend for OS in favor of immediate adjuvant chemotherapy; however, as noted, this was not statistically significant. Paz-Ares and colleagues[21] conducted a trial comparing adjuvant paclitaxel, gemcitabine, and cisplatin (PGC) with observation after cystectomy. They recruited 142 patients, 74 of whom were randomized to observation and 68 of whom were randomized to treatment with PGC. This study also closed early due to poor recruitment. However, both OS ($P<.0009$) and DFS ($P<.0001$) were significantly prolonged in the PGC arm compared with observation. At 30 months of follow-up, 45 patients died in the control arm compared with only 24 patients in the PGC arm.

A phase III trial compared perioperative chemotherapy with MVAC versus adjuvant chemotherapy, where perioperative chemotherapy was given as 2 cycles in the neoadjuvant setting and 3 cycles in the adjuvant setting. There were a total of 140 patients, and the study showed no difference in outcome in the 2 groups.[22]

Systematic reviews and meta-analyses

Randomized clinical trials have been unable to answer the question of whether adjuvant chemotherapy in bladder cancer provides statistically significant improvement in OS. Most of these prospective clinical studies have faced the problem of poor accrual and thus have been underpowered to answer this question. Subsequently, several meta-analyses and/or observational studies were performed to bridge this gap.

Galsky and colleagues[23] conducted a meta-analysis using the National Cancer Data Base (NCDB), which is representative of nearly 70% of all newly diagnosed cancers in the United States. A total of 5653 patients with T3-4 and/or N+ bladder cancer were included in the study, and 23% of them received adjuvant chemotherapy after radical cystectomy. There was an improvement in OS with adjuvant chemotherapy (HR 0.70; confidence interval [CI] 0.64–0.76), and this association with improved survival was seen in subgroup analyses as well, taking into consideration the patient performance status.[23] This retrospective study however failed to account for the number of patients who received cisplatin-based versus a non-cisplatin-based regimen. Also, they could not explain the chronology and type of treatment received after disease recurrence, which may have affected their outcome.

Leow and colleagues[24] performed a systematic review and meta-analysis of studies of adjuvant chemotherapy in upper tract urothelial carcinoma (UTUC). This review included 9 retrospective studies and 1 prospective study with a total of 482 patients. The pooled HR for OS was 0.43 ($P = .023$) in the cisplatin-based studies compared with surgery alone. This benefit was not seen in non-cisplatin-based regimens. Given most of these studies were retrospective, with a small sample size, there is not enough strength of evidence to make recommendations on adjuvant chemotherapy based on this meta-analysis alone.

Ruggeri and colleagues[25] pooled 5 randomized phase III trials with a total of 350 patients in order to examine whether adjuvant chemotherapy increases the DFS and OS of patients with MIBC after radical cystectomy. There was a significant benefit in OS (relative risk [RR] 0.74, $P = .001$) and DFS (RR 0.65, $P<.0001$) in patients who received adjuvant chemotherapy compared with those who did not.

A Cochrane meta-analysis compiled individual patient data from 6 randomized controlled trials with a total of 491 patients.[26] All the trials used cisplatin in adjuvant treatment in combination with other chemotherapeutic agents with the exception of one trial, which used cisplatin monotherapy. The overall HR for risk of death was 0.75 (95% CI 0.60–0.96) in the adjuvant chemotherapy arm. There was also a 32% decrease in the risk of recurrence or death in the chemotherapy arm compared with control ($P = .004$) (**Table 3**).

Adjuvant Therapy for Cisplatin-Ineligible Urothelial Carcinomas

Gemcitabine was evaluated in cisplatin-ineligible patients, 6 cycles as adjuvant therapy within 12 weeks of definitive surgery or at disease progression. One hundred fourteen patients were eligible for analysis; the PFS at 3 years was 50% and OS at 3 years was 49% with adjuvant gemcitabine compared with PFS of 40% and OS of 48% with deferred gemcitabine. Thus, their primary endpoint of a 15% improvement in PFS at 3 years with adjuvant gemcitabine compared with deferred treatment did not meet statistical significance.[20] In a nonrandomized study, 50 patients

with high-risk urothelial carcinoma were treated with sequential chemotherapy. This treatment consisted of doxorubicin and gemcitabine followed by paclitaxel and cisplatin in cisplatin-eligible patients and doxorubicin with gemcitabine followed by paclitaxel and carboplatin in cisplatin-ineligible subjects. In this small study, adjuvant sequential chemotherapy did not improve DSS, the primary endpoint compared with surgery alone.[11] Thus, because of poor efficacy and lack of both prospective and retrospective data, there is no evidence to support the use of non-cisplatin-based regimens in the adjuvant setting. There are several studies ongoing with checkpoint inhibitors in the adjuvant setting for patients with cisplatin-ineligible disease.

Adjuvant Therapy for Upper Tract Urothelial Carcinomas

UTUCs constitute a small proportion (~5%–8%) of all urothelial malignancies. The definitive management for these patients is radical nephroureterectomy. There is very limited prospective evidence to support the use of adjuvant cisplatin-based chemotherapy in UTUC. A recent retrospective study, using the NCDB, studied 3253 patients who received adjuvant chemotherapy or observation after radical nephroureterectomy for T3/T4 or node-positive UTUC. Adjuvant chemotherapy was associated with a statistically significant improvement in OS benefit (HR 0.77, CI 0.68–0.88). This treatment effect was consistent across subgroups irrespective of age, Charlson comorbidity index, pathologic stage, and surgical margin status. Just like the bladder cancer study, this study is limited because there is no information on the type of chemotherapy regimen or subsequent therapy at disease recurrence.[24] Also, because several of these patients may have compromised renal function because of age and the presence of a solitary kidney, it is unclear what effects cisplatin-based chemotherapy had on their renal function.

Ongoing Clinical Studies

There are multiple ongoing clinical trials evaluating adjuvant therapies for locally advanced bladder cancer, including a phase II trial of adjuvant sunitinib in patients who have already received neoadjuvant chemotherapy followed by cystectomy for high-risk urothelial carcinoma (NCT01042795). For patients with stage II and/or stage III (T2-T4a, NX, or N0) bladder cancer, there are 2 combined modality studies, which involve the use of upfront chemoradiation followed by adjuvant chemotherapy if the tumor persists after surgery. The first

Table 3
A summary of adjuvant studies performed for locally advanced muscle-invasive bladder cancer

Reference	Type of Study	Design	Findings
Svatek et al,[9] 2010	Retrospective	3947 patients with bladder cancer who received radical cystectomies and did not receive neoadjuvant chemotherapy; 23.6% received adjuvant chemotherapy	Adjuvant chemotherapy was associated with improved survival (HR 0.83, P = .017). Increasing benefit over higher-risk groups
Kim et al,[10] 2015	Retrospective	424 patients with bladder cancer who received radical cystectomies and did not receive neoadjuvant chemotherapy	Adjuvant chemotherapy was associated with improved survival (P = .018) but not DSS. However, both DSS and OS were improved in stage T3b
Gallagher et al,[11] 2009	Phase 2 trial	50 patients were treated with 2 different adjuvant protocols. Protocol A was with doxorubicin and gemcitabine followed by paclitaxel and cisplatin. Protocol B (renally impaired patients) was doxorubicin and gemcitabine followed. by paclitaxel and carboplatin	OS was improved in patients in both protocol groups as compared with controls. DSS was not improved in either protocol group compared with controls
Bono et al,[12] 1989	Randomized trial	125 patients with locally advanced bladder cancer. 32 patients with node-positive disease were treated with sequential cisplatin and methotrexate. 92 node-negative patients were randomized to the same chemotherapy regimen vs observation	No statistically significant difference in OS or PFS
Studer et al,[13] 1994	Randomized trial	77 patients with locally advanced bladder cancer stratified by nodal status and then randomly assigned to either observation or 3 adjuvant cycles of cisplatin	There was no statistically significant difference in OS between the groups in either the node-positive or node-negative groups compared with controls
Lehmann et al,[14] 2006; Stockle et al,[15] 1992	Randomized trial	49 patients with locally advanced bladder cancer randomized to either observation or adjuvant chemotherapy with 3 cycles of MVAC/MVEC	There was an improvement in PFS (HR 2.84, P = .002), OS (HR 1.75, P = .069), and DSS (HR 2.52, P = .007) in the adjuvant chemotherapy group compared with controls
Skinner et al,[16] 1991	Randomized trial	91 patients with locally invasive bladder cancer were randomized to either 4 cycles of adjuvant cisplatin, doxorubicin, and cyclophosphamide or observation	Median OS was 4.3 y in the chemotherapy group vs 2.4 y in the observation group (P = .0062)

Study	Type	Description	Results
Freiha et al,[17] 1996	Randomized trial	50 patients were randomized to either 4 adjuvant cycles of CMV or observation. Those in the observation group who relapsed were treated with CMV	PFS was 37 mo in the chemotherapy group vs 12 mo in the observation group ($P = .01$). Median OS was 63 mo in the chemotherapy group vs 36 mo in the observation group, but this was not statistically significant ($P = .32$)
Cognetti et al,[18] 2012	Randomized trial	194 patients were randomly assigned to observation vs adjuvant chemotherapy. There were 2 chemotherapy arms, both with cisplatin and gemcitabine on different schedules	There was no difference in OS and PFS between the arms
Sternberg et al,[19] 2015	Randomized trial	284 patients were randomly assigned to immediate treatment with 4 cycles of gemcitabine plus cisplatin, high-dose MVAC, or MVAC or chemotherapy at relapse with 6 cycles of MVAC	There was no significant difference in OS. There was a statistically significant difference in PFS (HR 0.54, $P<.0001$)
Lehmann et al,[20] 2013	Randomized trial	120 patients with locally advanced bladder cancer were randomized to single-agent adjuvant gemcitabine	Trial was closed early due to slow accrual. There was no statistically significant difference in PFS, DSS, or OS
Paz-Ares et al,[21] 2010	Randomized trial	142 patients randomized to observation or adjuvant treatment with PGC	Trial closed due to poor recruitment. OS was significantly prolonged in the chemotherapy arm ($P<.0002$), as was PFS ($P<.0001$) and DSS ($P<.0002$)
Millikan et al,[22] 2001	Randomized trial	140 patients with locally advanced bladder cancer were randomized to 5 cycles of adjuvant MVAC or perioperative MVAC (2 neoadjuvant cycles, and 3 adjuvant cycles)	There was no difference in OS based on the sequence of chemotherapy
Galsky et al,[23] 2016	Retrospective study	5653 patients with locally advanced bladder cancer. 23% received adjuvant chemotherapy	There was an improvement in OS with adjuvant chemotherapy (HR 0.70)

of these studies is investigating the effectiveness of radiation therapy with cisplatin and paclitaxel followed by surgery and adjuvant cisplatin with gemcitabine for any residual disease noted after chemoradiation (NCT00003930). The study has been completed but not yet published. A second phase II trial evaluates transurethral surgery and radiation with cisplatin and paclitaxel or cisplatin and 5-fluorouracil followed by selective bladder preservation and gemcitabine with paclitaxel and cisplatin as adjuvant chemotherapy (NCT00055601). NCT00006105 is a phase II trial that has completed accrual investigating adjuvant gemcitabine, cisplatin, and amifostine as a chemoprotectant. There is a phase III trial to compare adjuvant cisplatin and gemcitabine with sequential doxorubicin, gemcitabine, ifosfamide, paclitaxel, and cisplatin (NCT00014534). This study has completed; however, it has not yet published its data. A phase III trial of adjuvant chemotherapy versus deferred chemotherapy after radical cystectomy with MVAC has also completed accrual (NCT00028756). Immunotherapy is also being investigated in the adjuvant setting.

Role of Molecular Analyses on Adjuvant Therapy

In the era of whole- and targeted exome sequencing, it is important to evaluate patients for both prognostic and predictive biomarkers. Several predictive biomarkers are currently being evaluated in bladder cancer and are discussed later.

High-grade MIBCs are characterized by alterations in p53, a tumor suppressor protein, and it is reported to be mutated in 50% of invasive bladder cancers.[27] A phase III clinical trial will determine whether TP53 alteration is prognostic in urothelial cancer and predictive for benefit from MVAC adjuvant chemotherapy given prior published retrospective studies.[28] They selected patients with T1/T2N0 disease with TP53 alterations because despite the lower-risk stage, they have a higher risk of recurrence based on TP53 status. A total of 114 patients with p53 alterations were randomly assigned to adjuvant chemotherapy or observation. Accrual was halted based on futility, and no difference in PFS in either group was found.[28]

Activating mutations of FGFR3 are found in a large proportion of non-MIBCs, but are also present in 10% to 20% of MIBC.[27] This finding with FGFR alterations in bladder cancer has led to the development of targeted drugs to FGFR3, including dovitinib, which is an FGFR inhibitor with preclinical activity in FGFR3-mutant and overexpression bladder cancer cell lines. In a phase II study, 44 patients with urothelial carcinoma with either mutant or wild-type FGFR3 were treated with dovitinib. The study was terminated because dovitinib was not active in patients with urothelial carcinoma regardless of FGFR3 mutation status.[29] Another phase II study of JNJ-42756493, a pan-FGFR inhibitor in patients with advanced urothelial carcinoma in patients with FGFR alterations, is currently underway.[30] Another phase II trial using BGJ398, an FGFR inhibitor in patients with metastatic urothelial carcinoma with activating FGFR3 mutations, showed a notable 36% overall response rate in this pretreated population. Plimack and colleagues[31] sought to determine whether there were genomic alterations that would predict response to DNA-damaging chemotherapy in MIBC given that approximately 30% of patients achieve a response to neoadjuvant chemotherapy. ATM, RB1, and FANCC are mutated in 11%, 14%, and 2% of urothelial carcinomas, respectively, and each plays a role in DNA repair. They found that, as predicted, alterations in these genes led to increased sensitivity to chemotherapy and thus correlated with pathologic response ($P<.001$), PFS ($P = .0085$), and OS ($P = .007$). To test a similar concept, Van Allen and colleagues[32] studied ERCC2, which is mutated in 7% to 12% of urothelial carcinomas. ERCC2 is part of the nucleotide excision repair pathway and loss of function correlates with cisplatin sensitivity, whereas overexpression correlates with cisplatin resistance. They performed whole-exome sequencing of tumors from patients before being treated with neoadjuvant cisplatin-based chemotherapy. Among 3277 genes, ERCC2 was the only one that was enriched in the cisplatin responders, with somatic mutations occurring in this cohort ($P<.001$).[32] Once validated for metastatic disease, it may be reasonable to consider clinical studies with these molecular markers and targeted agents in the perioperative setting.

SUMMARY/DISCUSSION

To return to the case of Mr Bond, he had lymph node involvement at the time of surgery, with a high risk of disease recurrence (92% over 5 years). He also did not receive neoadjuvant chemotherapy. Given this, and the data summarized above, the authors recommend that he undergo adjuvant chemotherapy with a cisplatin-based regimen.

Given that nearly half of all patients with MIBC will develop metastatic disease thought to be secondary to micrometastatic disease at the time of diagnosis, there is a pressing need to improve perioperative therapy for these patients.[1] Unfortunately, there have been mixed results from the randomized trials that have investigated the role of adjuvant cisplatin-based chemotherapy in MIBC. Overall, these prospective trials have been underpowered because of issues with patient accrual, with several of them closing early as a result of this. It is also difficult to compare the results from these studies given that there is no standard adjuvant chemotherapy regimen. Many patients in the studies did not receive the same number of adjuvant chemotherapy cycles because of various reasons, including toxicities and patient refusal. In addition, some studies stratified patients by lymph node status, whereas others did not. In an attempt to answer the question, meta-analyses have been conducted and have shown an OS benefit for adjuvant chemotherapy in MIBC. Although not ideal, these retrospective studies provide some valuable information on the role of adjuvant cisplatin-based chemotherapy, especially in patients with high-risk disease like the patient in the clinical scenario.

Although neoadjuvant chemotherapy remains the standard of care, the NCCN guidelines as well as the recently released American Urological Association guidelines for MIBC recommend the consideration of adjuvant chemotherapy in patients with high-risk disease (T3 or T4 or node-positive) who have not received neoadjuvant chemotherapy.

There are several clinical trials that are currently underway, some of which have been completed but not yet published. Until the time that we have prospective data, we will need to counsel patients and use our best clinical judgment to determine whether patients are good candidates for adjuvant cisplatin-based chemotherapy. The authors recommend that adjuvant chemotherapy should be considered for patients with high-risk disease, who did not receive neoadjuvant cisplatin-based chemotherapy. The authors do not recommend the use of non-cisplatin-based regimens for adjuvant chemotherapy because of a lack of prospective and retrospective evidence. The data from DNA-sequencing and adjuvant clinical trials with immunotherapy may provide an answer to the use of targeted agents or immunotherapy as adjuvant therapy for locally advanced bladder cancer.

REFERENCES

1. Calabro F, Sternberg CN. Neoadjuvant and adjuvant chemotherapy in muscle-invasive bladder cancer. Eur Urol 2009;55(2):348–58.
2. Stein JP, Lieskovsky G, Cote R, et al. Radical cystectomy in the treatment of invasive bladder cancer: long-term results in 1,054 patients. J Clin Oncol 2001;19(3):666–75.
3. Sternberg CN, Bellmunt J, Sonpavde G, et al. ICUD-EAU International Consultation on Bladder Cancer 2012: chemotherapy for urothelial carcinoma-neoadjuvant and adjuvant settings. Eur Urol 2013; 63(1):58–66.
4. Sonpavde G, Khan MM, Lerner SP, et al. Disease-free survival at 2 or 3 years correlates with 5-year overall survival of patients undergoing radical cystectomy for muscle invasive bladder cancer. J Urol 2011;185(2):456–61.
5. Network NCC. Bladder cancer (version 5.2017). Available at: https://www.nccn.org/professionals/physician_gls/pdf/bladder_blocks.pdf. Accessed October 30, 2017.
6. Yin M, Joshi M, Meijer RP, et al. Neoadjuvant chemotherapy for muscle-invasive bladder cancer: a systematic review and two-step meta-analysis. Oncologist 2016;21(6):708–15.
7. Lu K. Adjuvant chemotherapy in locally advanced bladder cancer. Lancet Oncol 2015;16(3):e103–4.
8. Meeks JJ, Bellmunt J, Bochner BH, et al. A systematic review of neoadjuvant and adjuvant chemotherapy for muscle-invasive bladder cancer. Eur Urol 2012;62(3):523–33.
9. Svatek RS, Shariat SF, Lasky RE, et al. The effectiveness of off-protocol adjuvant chemotherapy for patients with urothelial carcinoma of the urinary bladder. Clin Cancer Res 2010;16(17): 4461–7.
10. Kim HS, Piao S, Moon KC, et al. Adjuvant chemotherapy correlates with improved survival after radical cystectomy in patients with pT3b (macroscopic perivesical tissue invasion) bladder cancer. J Cancer 2015;6(8):750–8.
11. Gallagher DJ, Milowsky MI, Iasonos A, et al. Sequential adjuvant chemotherapy after surgical resection of high-risk urothelial carcinoma. Cancer 2009;115(22):5193–201.
12. Bono AV, Benvenuti C, Reali L, et al. Adjuvant chemotherapy in advanced bladder cancer. Italian Uro-Oncologic Cooperative Group. Prog Clin Biol Res 1989;303:533–40.
13. Studer UE, Bacchi M, Biedermann C, et al. Adjuvant cisplatin chemotherapy following cystectomy for bladder cancer: results of a prospective randomized trial. J Urol 1994;152(1):81–4.
14. Lehmann J, Franzaring L, Thuroff J, et al. Complete long-term survival data from a trial of adjuvant chemotherapy vs control after radical cystectomy for locally advanced bladder cancer. BJU Int 2006; 97(1):42–7.
15. Stockle M, Meyenburg W, Wellek S, et al. Advanced bladder cancer (stages pT3b, pT4a, pN1 and pN2): improved survival after radical cystectomy and 3 adjuvant cycles of chemotherapy. Results of a

controlled prospective study. J Urol 1992;148(2 Pt 1):302–6 [discussion: 306–7].

16. Skinner DG, Daniels JR, Russell CA, et al. The role of adjuvant chemotherapy following cystectomy for invasive bladder cancer: a prospective comparative trial. J Urol 1991;145(3):459–64 [discussion: 464–7].

17. Freiha F, Reese J, Torti FM. A randomized trial of radical cystectomy versus radical cystectomy plus cisplatin, vinblastine and methotrexate chemotherapy for muscle invasive bladder cancer. J Urol 1996;155(2):495–9 [discussion: 499–500].

18. Cognetti F, Ruggeri EM, Felici A, et al. Adjuvant chemotherapy with cisplatin and gemcitabine versus chemotherapy at relapse in patients with muscle-invasive bladder cancer submitted to radical cystectomy: an Italian, multicenter, randomized phase III trial. Ann Oncol 2012;23(3):695–700.

19. Sternberg CN, Skoneczna I, Kerst JM, et al. Immediate versus deferred chemotherapy after radical cystectomy in patients with pT3-pT4 or N+ M0 urothelial carcinoma of the bladder (EORTC 30994): an intergroup, open-label, randomised phase 3 trial. Lancet Oncol 2015;16(1):76–86.

20. Lehmann J, Kuehn M, Fischer C, et al. Randomized phase III study of adjuvant versus progression-triggered treatment with gemcitabine (G) after radical cystectomy (RC) for locally advanced bladder cancer (LABC) in patients not suitable for cisplatin-based chemotherapy (CBC) (AUO-trial AB22/00). J Clin Oncol 2013;31(6_suppl):250.

21. Paz-Ares LG, Solsona E, Esteban E, et al. Randomized phase III trial comparing adjuvant paclitaxel/gemcitabine/cisplatin (PGC) to observation in patients with resected invasive bladder cancer: results of the Spanish Oncology Genitourinary Group (SOGUG) 99/01 study. J Clin Oncol 2010;28(18_suppl):LBA4518.

22. Millikan R, Dinney C, Swanson D, et al. Integrated therapy for locally advanced bladder cancer: final report of a randomized trial of cystectomy plus adjuvant M-VAC versus cystectomy with both preoperative and postoperative M-VAC. J Clin Oncol 2001;19(20):4005–13.

23. Galsky MD, Stensland KD, Moshier E, et al. Effectiveness of adjuvant chemotherapy for locally advanced bladder cancer. J Clin Oncol 2016;34(8):825–32.

24. Leow JJ, Martin-Doyle W, Fay AP, et al. A systematic review and meta-analysis of adjuvant and neoadjuvant chemotherapy for upper tract urothelial carcinoma. Eur Urol 2014;66(3):529–41.

25. Ruggeri EM, Giannarelli D, Bria E, et al. Adjuvant chemotherapy in muscle-invasive bladder carcinoma: a pooled analysis from phase III studies. Cancer 2006;106(4):783–8.

26. Advanced Bladder Cancer (ABC) Meta-analysis Collaboration. Adjuvant chemotherapy for invasive bladder cancer (individual patient data). Cochrane Database Syst Rev 2006;(2):CD006018.

27. Ye F, Wang L, Castillo-Martin M, et al. Biomarkers for bladder cancer management: present and future. Am J Clin Exp Urol 2014;2(1):1–14.

28. Stadler WM, Lerner SP, Groshen S, et al. Phase III study of molecularly targeted adjuvant therapy in locally advanced urothelial cancer of the bladder based on p53 status. J Clin Oncol 2011;29(25):3443–9.

29. Milowsky MI, Dittrich C, Duran I, et al. Phase 2 trial of dovitinib in patients with progressive FGFR3-mutated or FGFR3 wild-type advanced urothelial carcinoma. Eur J Cancer 2014;50(18):3145–52.

30. Siefker-Radtke AO, Mellado B, Decaestecker K, et al. A phase 2 study of JNJ-42756493, a pan-FGFR tyrosine kinase inhibitor, in patients (pts) with metastatic or unresectable urothelial cancer (UC) harboring FGFR gene alterations. J Clin Oncol 2016;34(15_suppl):TPS4575.

31. Plimack ER, Dunbrack RL, Brennan TA, et al. Defects in DNA repair genes predict response to neoadjuvant cisplatin-based chemotherapy in muscle-invasive bladder cancer. Eur Urol 2015;68(6):959–67.

32. Van Allen EM, Mouw KW, Kim P, et al. Somatic ERCC2 mutations correlate with cisplatin sensitivity in muscle-invasive urothelial carcinoma. Cancer Discov 2014;4(10):1140–53.

Endoscopic Approaches to Upper Tract Urothelial Carcinoma

Firas G. Petros, MD, Roger Li, MD, Surena F. Matin, MD*

KEYWORDS

- Endoscopy • Ureteroscopy • Ureteral cancer • Laser • Upper-tract urothelial carcinoma

KEY POINTS

- All data supporting endoscopic management of upper-tract urothelial carcinoma are based on level 3 evidence, with no prospective studies available.
- Endoscopic management can be performed retrograde by ureteroscopy, or antegrade by percutaneous ureteropyeloscopy, as indicated.
- A variety of tools are available for tumor sampling and resection; although most of these were developed for treatment of stone disease, they can be improvised by urologists to adequately biopsy and treat tumors.
- Topical therapy may help reduce recurrences, but newer paradigms that are being prospectively tested may hold greater promise for efficacious treatment.
- Surveillance of the upper tract and bladder is mandatory after endoscopic management.

▶ **Video content accompanies this article at http://www.urologic.theclinics.com.**

INTRODUCTION

Upper urinary tract urothelial carcinoma (UTUC) is uncommon and accounts for only 5% to 10% of all urothelial carcinomas.[1] Traditionally, radical nephroureterectomy (RNU) was considered the standard of care for UTUC. With increasing experience and enhanced technology, endoscopy for UTUC has increasingly been used.[2] This article summarizes the evidence for endoscopic management of UTUC in conjunction with our experience, highlighting the indications for its use and pitfalls.

DIAGNOSIS OF UPPER-TRACT UROTHELIAL CARCINOMA

Endoscopic evaluation is critical for the initial diagnosis and risk stratification of UTUC. Data gathered during endoscopy are not only useful for diagnosis of UTUC but also for prognosis and treatment planning, providing assessment for multilocality, multifocality, tumor architecture, and tumor biopsy, all highly relevant factors when determining an optimal treatment plan.

Urine-Based Studies

Positive cytology after a negative cystoscopic examination may be the first sign of UTUC.[2] However, cytologic examination of voided urine has poor sensitivity in detecting the rare malignant exfoliated cells from UTUC. Furthermore, false-positive rates caused by instrumentation effects and/or incidental inflammatory processes may be as high as 50%.[3] Site-directed collection via

Disclosure: F.G. Petros and R. Li have nothing to disclose. S.F. Matin serves as consultant for Taris Biomedical, Urogen Corp., CSATS, and Peloton Therapeutics. Research grant support from the AT&T Foundation and Specialized Programs in Oncology Research (SPORE PAR-14-353).
Department of Urology, UT MD Anderson Cancer Center, 1515 Holcombe Boulevard, Houston, TX 77030, USA
* Corresponding author. Department of Urology Unit 1373, UT MD Anderson Cancer Center, 1515 Holcombe Boulevard, Houston, TX 77030.
E-mail address: surmatin@mdanderson.org

Urol Clin N Am 45 (2018) 267–286
https://doi.org/10.1016/j.ucl.2017.12.009
0094-0143/18/© 2018 Elsevier Inc. All rights reserved.

urologic.theclinics.com

endoscopic measures (selective washings) have been shown to increase sensitivity for the detection of both high-grade (69% sensitivity, 85% positive predictive value [PPV]) and muscle-invasive UTUC (76% sensitivity, 89% PPV). Nevertheless, cytology alone may not be sufficient to predict pathologic findings of high-grade or muscle-invasive UTUC.[4]

In contrast, cytology can compensate for nondiagnostic or ambiguous endoscopic biopsy results. Kleinmann and colleagues[5] showed that diagnosis can be made by cytologic evaluation in almost all (91%) patients with nondiagnostic endoscopic biopsies. Furthermore, in patients with grade 2 tumors found on endoscopic biopsy, concomitant positive cytology increased the risk of upgrading[6] and upstaging to muscle-invasive UTUC[7] on RNU pathology. In patients managed with ureteroscopic laser ablation, abnormal cytology pretreatment also portended increased risk of recurrence (94.1% vs 47.1%; $P = .0026$).[8] Cytology from selective washings may also be the only indication for upper-tract carcinoma in situ (UTCIS), if no tumors are seen on a high-quality ureteroscopic evaluation.

Fluorescent in situ hybridization (FISH), a urine-based cytogenetic analysis, has also been used to diagnose UTUC. Compared with cytology, FISH consistently showed superior sensitivity (77%–100%) while maintaining comparable specificity in detecting UTUC on both voided[9] and selective washings.[10] In a multicenter study using selective washings, a group from Italy was able to achieve 100% sensitivity in detecting UTUC in 21 patients.[10] However, for UTUC, a high sensitivity would translate to a significant number of potentially negative ureteroscopic evaluations, which are more invasive than cystoscopy. Whether FISH can be used to reliably rule out UTUC requires validation in larger studies.

Ureteroscopy and Biopsy

Owing to difficult access and limited tissue samples, ureteroscopy (URS) biopsy of UTUC can be extremely challenging. In an attempt to obviate biopsy, many studies have assessed the adequacy of morphologic evaluation by URS inspection in predicting pathologic grading. The available evidence suggests gross underestimation of the tumor grading by endoscopic inspection, underscoring the importance of histology.[11,12] However, the visual architecture of tumors has been found to have strong predictive ability. Sessile-appearing tumors are consistently found to be associated with high-stage disease.[7,11]

In addition to increasing diagnostic accuracy, diagnostic URS with biopsy was found to shift management of UTUC toward less morbid options. Use of RNU was reduced by 20%, with only 5 URS needed to downgrade 1 patient from planned RNU to organ-sparing management. The investigators were careful to point out several scenarios in which URS evaluation may be avoided: (1) nonfunctioning kidney; (2) history of ipsilateral UTUC; (3) positive cytology with multifocal lesions on imaging. In each of these cases the investigators suggest avoiding URS and proceeding with RNU. A fourth scenario, a positive biopsy of a regional lymph node, would indicate the need for chemotherapy as initial primary therapy.

A few concerns regarding the routine use of URS biopsy have been allayed. Kulp and Bagley[13] addressed the fear of metastatic spread via pyelovenous and pyelolymphatic backflow by examining the surgical specimens from RNU. On histologic examination, no free-floating tumor cells were found in the vascular or lymphatic spaces of the submucosa or renal parenchyma surrounding the tumor. In a subsequent clinical study, Hendin and colleagues[14] showed the lack of difference in metastasis rates after RNU in patients receiving preoperative URS with a variety of irrigation systems versus those who did not. A second concern is possible bladder implantation by sloughed UTUC cells during URS leading to increased intravesical recurrences. Although Ishikawa and colleagues[15] found similar rates of intravesical recurrence in patients with or without preoperative URS (60% vs 59%; $P = .9$), others described a higher incidence of intravesical recurrence in patients having undergone URS (hazard ratio, 1.44–2.58).[16] The use of perioperative intravesical chemotherapy has been adopted after RNU to reduce intravesical recurrence, but the utility in the setting of diagnostic URS has not been investigated. A third concern pertains to the delay in definitive treatment, which has previously been linked to numerous adverse pathologic features such as advanced stage, grade, and lymphovascular invasion (LVI), as well as increased disease recurrence and cancer-specific mortality.[17] However, the interval from diagnosis on imaging to RNU caused by diagnostic URS has not been found to impair cancer-specific survival, recurrence-free survival, or metastasis-free survival.[18]

Drawing from their extensive experience, Tawfiek and colleagues[19] first described detailed methods of ureteroscopic inspection and biopsy. Emphasis was placed on obtaining multiple urine and washing samples before and after biopsy. Subsequently, Guarnizo and colleagues[20] also proposed multiple, quality biopsies to ensure sufficient tissue for diagnosis. The choice of biopsy instrument depends on the morphology of the tumor. Ureteroscopic forceps (eg, Piranha forceps [Boston Scientific, Marlborough, MA], BIGopsy forceps [Cook Medical, Bloomington, IN]) are best suited for sessile tumors. Although the BIGopsy forceps is capable of larger biopsy specimens with less architectural distortion, its large size also requires cumbersome backloading through the ureteroscope, and impairs instrument deflection and visualization.[21] For papillary tumors, stainless steel wire or nitinol baskets are capable of excising tumor and can be effectively used to debulk large-volume papillary tumors.[22]

Because of the limited biopsy tissue, special processing and evaluation techniques may also enhance diagnostic yield.[19] Fresh specimen should be promptly delivered to the cytopathology laboratory. By using the cytospin technique and creating cell blocks to visualize tissue architecture, the ability to grade biopsied tumors was increased from 43% to 97%.[19] Whenever possible, analysis of the specimen should be performed at high-volume centers and/or pathologic units with sufficient experience with UTUC.

Overall, there is adequate concordance (69%–91%) between the grades on endoscopic biopsy and on RNU specimen.[23] One caveat is that low-grade tumors on URS biopsy may have a high tendency to be upgraded on the final specimen. In a Mayo Clinic study, 96% of the clinical grade 1 tumors were found to be upgraded on final pathologic evaluation.[24] Biopsy technique details are critically important when assessing the risk for upgrading, as discussed further later. The discordance between the endoscopic and final pathologic grading on these clinically low-risk tumors needs to be considered, as does biopsy technique and sampling, when organ-sparing treatment is pursued.

In contrast, URS staging is often suboptimal because of insufficient tissue on the biopsy specimen.[7] For instance, up to 45% of cTa tumors on endoscopic biopsy may be understaged.[20] However, tumor stage classification in these cases is to be questioned, because a cTa can only be classified as such if lamina propria is present. If it is not, then invasion cannot be assessed and the tumor is more correctly classified as a cTx. Obtaining muscle is even more uncommon, and thus a cT2 is not a typical classification that can be assigned. Thus, from a URS staging perspective, the most appropriate classifications are cTx, cTa, cTis, cT1, and, rarely, cT2 disease. Imaging studies showing parenchymal or periureteral invasion allow classification of cT3-4 disease. As a result, biopsy grade has been relied on as a surrogate predictor for final pathologic stage, with 68% to 100% of grade 1 biopsies correctly predicting noninvasive stage (≤pT1) and 62% to 100% of grade 3 biopsies predicting invasive disease (≥pT2).[23,25–27] Even so, many groups continue to report suboptimal diagnostic yield secondary to inadequate biopsy tissue compounded by crush artifacts on the specimen.[28,29] Altogether, 20% or more of the specimen may be nondiagnostic, with grading and staging discrepant in many more cases on the endoscopic and surgical specimens.[29] Technical factors play a significant role in these findings, such as the number and amount of biopsies obtained, the size of the tumor (directly relating to adequate tumor sampling), and use of access sheaths, which greatly facilitate sampling. To improve diagnostic accuracy, nomograms incorporating biopsy information with other preoperative parameters have been developed. Brien and colleagues[26] found that the combined findings of hydronephrosis on cross-sectional imaging, positive urine cytology, and high-grade UTUC on biopsy had 89% positive predictive value for greater than pT1 disease, and 75% PPV for non–organ-confined disease (>pT2). Margulis and colleagues[30] used a backward step-down selection process and achieved the most informative and parsimonious model incorporating biopsy grade, tumor architecture (sessile vs papillary), and location on URS (ureter vs renal pelvis) to predict for non–organ-confined disease at RNU with 76.6% accuracy. The European Association of Urology guidelines suggest that low-risk tumors can be classified based on finding of unifocal noninvasive disease on computed tomography (CT) urogram with tumor size less than 2 cm of low grade both on cytology and URS biopsy.[2] These tumors are their suggested ideal candidates for endoscopic management based on consensus opinion and level 3 data.

New Technologies Being Developed

With the advent of new miniaturized imaging technologies, several have been tailored for ureteroscopic use. Matin and colleagues[31] assessed the use of endoluminal ultrasonography and found 67% PPV and 100% negative predictive value in staging UTUC. A follow-up study of this technology with larger patient numbers shows that endoluminal ultrasonography has poor predictive ability for advanced stage, although it is largely accurate to confirm noninvasive disease (Fig. 1). Technologies that have been established in the imaging of bladder cancer have also been adopted for the diagnosis of UTUC: narrow band imaging and

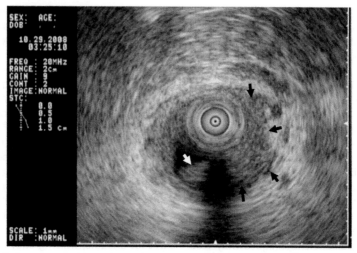

Fig. 1. Endoluminal ultrasonography in the midureter showing a small papillary tumor (*white arrowhead*), in addition to a sessile invasive tumor (*black arrows*). (*Courtesy of* S.F. Matin, MD, Houston, TX, 2017.)

blue light photodynamic diagnosis have subjectively improved endoscopic visualization of UTUC, but they do not assist with staging.[32,33] Optical coherence tomography (OCT) is a technology analogous to ultrasonography in regard to assessment of tumor invasion, using backscattered light to produce cross-sectional images with micrometer scale resolution. Staging using OCT was found to be accurate on the final RNU specimen in 7 of 8 patients with UTUC.[34] In addition, confocal laser endomicroscopy is a promising technology to provide real-time histologic characterization, delivering in-vivo high-resolution images of tissue architecture and morphology using a low-energy laser light source and photosensitizer during URS.[35] This technology holds the promise of improving tumor sampling for grading but does not provide staging information directly. The diagnostic information captured by these newer technologies may further help direct treatment decisions for successful oncologic outcomes, but more research with larger patient numbers is still needed.

IMPERATIVE AND ELECTIVE INDICATIONS FOR KIDNEY-SPARING SURGERY AND ENDOSCOPIC TREATMENT OF UPPER-TRACT UROTHELIAL CARCINOMA

Imperative indications for kidney-sparing surgery and endoscopic management (retrograde or antegrade approach) for UTUC include those patients with contraindications to radical resection, such as solitary functioning kidney caused by absent or nonfunctioning contralateral kidney, bilateral UTUC tumors, baseline renal insufficiency, poor

candidates for hemodialysis or renal transplant, or patients with significant medical comorbidities.[36] In selected subsets, these patients may be at considerable competing risk of death because of underlying comorbidities precluding definitive surgery, or may be at high risk for reduced survival from end-stage renal disease if their kidneys were removed.[36] Furthermore, radical nephrectomy in patients with renal cortical tumors has been found to be a significant risk factor for development of chronic kidney disease.[36] Therefore, while preserving renal function, endoscopic management offers extended indications for cancer and symptom control in this cohort of patients to prevent local recurrence and disease progression. **Fig. 2** shows a suggested algorithm for endoscopic management of suspicious upper-tract lesions.

In contrast, kidney-sparing procedures, including partial nephrectomy, segmental ureterectomy, and endoscopic management via URS or percutaneous approach, are traditionally reserved for patients with low-risk non–muscle-invasive UTUC defined as (pT0-1) low-grade tumors, which were described in up to 56% of UTUC following RNU.[37] Hence, for this purpose, elective indications of endoscopic ablation takes into consideration patient and tumor factors, including clinical, radiographic, endoscopic, and pathologic characteristics focusing on compliant patients with low-grade, low-volume solitary lesions[36] consistent with the 2017 update consensus criteria for risk stratification of UTUC described by the European Association of Urology.[2] **Table 1** details our ideal conditions for endoscopic management of low-grade UTUC.

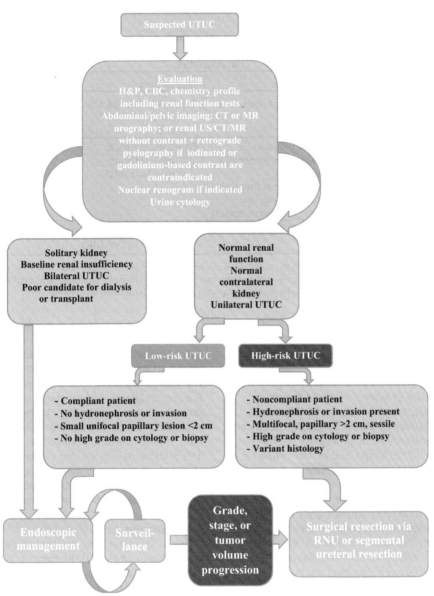

Fig. 2. Suggested algorithm for kidney-sparing endoscopic treatment of patients with UTUC. CBC, complete blood count; H&P, history and physical examination; MR, magnetic resonance; US, ultrasonography. (*Courtesy of* S.F. Matin, MD, Houston, TX, 2017.)

Retrograde Endoscopic Management

The principal advantage of URS in the management of UTUC is that it can offer both diagnostic and potentially therapeutic treatment options with the ability to have the procedure performed as an outpatient. Furthermore, URS helps maintain urothelial integrity of the upper urinary tract with the benefit of low morbidity.[36] The technical evolution in endoscopy as well as the innovations in optics and digital and laser technologies has allowed better visualization and effective treatment. Similarly, refinement in instruments used

for endoscopic biopsies permitted larger tumor specimens to be biopsied and thus improved pathologic staging. However, this instrumentation remains limited because of size constraints. Semi-rigid URS is often used to access distal and mid-ureteral tumors, whereas higher lesions located at the proximal ureter, renal pelvis, and calyces require flexible URS. When feasible, the use of ureteral access sheaths allows for atraumatic and facile reinsertion of the flexible URS, and continuous flow irrigation achieves an optimized intraoperative visualization while intrarenal low

Table 1
Ideal low-risk indications for endoscopic treatment of upper-tract urothelial carcinoma

Characteristics			
Clinical	Radiographic	Endoscopic	Pathologic
No untreated urothelial carcinoma of bladder	No hydronephrosis	Tumor endoscopically controlled in 1–2 sessions	Confirmed low grade on biopsy
Compliance with surveillance imaging and ureteroscopy	No local invasion or infiltration (urothelial thickening, parenchymal invasion, fat stranding, or enlarged lymph nodes)	Papillary, unifocal tumor without sessile features[a]	Negative selective upper-tract cytology for high-grade cancer[a]
—	—	Thorough evaluation of entire upper tract	—

[a] If no tumors are visible after thorough evaluation of the entire upper tract and selective washings show high-grade urothelial cancer, this is suggestive of carcinoma in situ, which can be considered for primary treatment with topical bacillus Calmette-Guérin (BCG) via nephrostomy tube or cystoscopically placed ureteral catheter (see **Fig. 8**).

pressure is maintained.[36] The authors find that access sheaths make a critical difference in the ability to obtain adequate tumor sampling by facilitating multiple passes and allowing for complete resection or laser ablation of tumors.

In contrast, the drawbacks of URS include the potential inability to obtain adequate tissue samples for assessment of prognostic factors such as primary tumor stage and/or the presence of LVI.[38] In addition, the limited size of the working channel of the URS coupled with the use of larger endoscopic tools in an attempt to obtain larger specimens of lesions cause significant decrease in flow of irrigation and consequently poor visualization if any hematuria is present, with theoretic potential of risking tumor cells seeding with the generated pressure resulting in pyelolymphatic backflow.[39]

Cystoscopy of the urinary bladder usually precedes upper-tract URS. A thorough examination of the bladder is essential to confirm the presence or absence of associated bladder lesions. Selective urinary cytology is often obtained before instrumentation or instillation of contrast agent to reduce the degenerative effects on cell viability and architectural organization.[40] Upper-tract wash (barbotage) cytology is usually acquired; the authors usually obtain at least 20 to 30 mL of saline barbotage in order to maximize diagnostic yield. We find that this is more easily done using a multi–side-hole ureteral catheter (Royal Flush or Beacon Tip catheter, Cook Medical, Bloomington, IN) or through an access sheath already in place with its obturator, and placing these in the upper ureter or renal pelvis, rather than the traditional method of placing a catheter at the intramural ureter, in order to avoid contamination from the bladder. Given the 4% to 6% risk of synchronous bilateral UTUC, it is prudent to assess the contralateral upper tract via either axial cross-sectional urography before endoscopic evaluation or by retrograde pyelogram at the time of the present endoscopic assessment.[41] The authors usually do not perform contralateral URS unless there is a cause, suspicion, or other reason to investigate an abnormality, so as not to risk any strictures on the normal side.

Laser ablation
Depending on the size, morphologic architecture, and location of the UTUC tumors, biopsies can be obtained using biopsy forceps, stone basket, graspers, as well as brushes. **Fig. 3** shows our most commonly used tools. We find the most useful instruments to be the 3-F cup biopsy forceps (Piranha forceps, Boston Scientific, Marlborough, MA); a 1.7-F nitinol basket (NGage Nitinol Stone Extractor, Cook Medical, Bloomington, IN); and occasionally a steel wire basket (Atlas Wire Stone Extractor, Cook Medical, Bloomington, IN). There are advantages and disadvantages of these instruments, detailed in **Table 2**. It is important to obtain multiple specimens to avoid inconclusive results, which can reach up to 25%.[29] The technique of biopsy is critical to obtain an adequate sample, such as by pushing the biopsy forceps, not pulling (**Fig. 4** and Video 1).

Following biopsy, the laser can either be used to achieve hemostasis or used for tumor resection and fulguration of the tumor bed.[42] Two types of

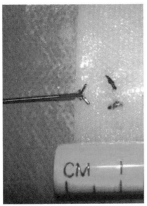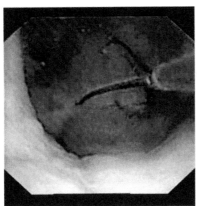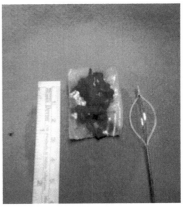

Fig. 3. A variety of tools used to biopsy or resect ureteral and renal pelvis tumors. Our go-to tools are the 3-F cup biopsy forceps (*left*) using the push technique, and the 1.7-F nitinol basket (*middle*), primarily in the renal pelvis/calyces/lower pole and whenever there is hematuria and flow needs to be maintained. The 3-F steel wire basket (*right*) is ideal for larger tumors in the ureter and if no hematuria is present. (*Courtesy of* S.F. Matin, MD, Houston, TX, 2017.)

lasers are most commonly used for ablation. The holmium:yttrium-aluminum-garnet (YAG) laser, which is a pulsed laser with a wavelength of 2.1 μm and a depth of penetration of less than 0.5 mm. At a lower energy and higher pulse duration, it causes tissue coagulation and ablation.[42] The holmium energy is strongly absorbed by water, resulting in minimal thermal injury to the surrounding tissue. However, direct contact of the laser fiber with the tissue during treatment is necessary, and for larger tumors the effect is not substantial, requiring a long time to perform ablation.[43] A 120 W version may allow more efficient ablation. Alternatively, the neodymium-doped (Nd):YAG laser, at a wavelength of 1.064 μm and penetration depth of 5 to 6 mm in tissue or water, can be used to destroy tissue with coagulation without needing direct contact of the laser fiber with target tissue.[44] Ideally, the type of laser used for ablation is dictated by the size and location of the UTUC lesion, but in reality many centers may have only one or the other available. For small

Table 2
Specifications of most commonly used ureteroscopic forceps and baskets for biopsy of upper-tract urothelial lesions

Instrument	Size	Advantage	Disadvantage
Piranha cup biopsy forceps	3-F	Can biopsy sessile tumors, flat tumors, or areas suspicious for carcinoma in situ	Size reduces irrigant flow and limits URS deflection
BIGopsy forceps	2.4-F	Large jaw allows better tumor sampling	Must use access sheath and back-load jaw; limited visualization and deflection
NGage nitinol basket	1.7-F or larger	Small size allows irrigant flow and better visualization if hematuria is present; URS deflection minimally affected; tipless configuration ideal for calyceal tumors	May not provide as good a bite as steel wire basket. May not work on sessile tumors
Atlas steel wire basket	3-F	Ideal for larger ureteral tumors; can shear off large biopsy specimens	Significantly limits irrigant flow with poor visualization if hematuria is present; limited URS deflection; tipped design not ideal for calyceal or some renal pelvis tumors

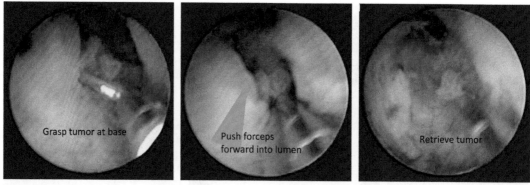

Fig. 4. Video stills showing the push technique using 3-F cup biopsy forceps for optimal tissue retrieval. The most frequent error is to grasp the tumor and pull back. These small instruments do not have the jaw strength to tear off tumor, thus most of the tissue slides out, resulting in minute specimens 1 to 2 mm³ in size; in contradistinction, if the biopsy forceps is pushed after grasping the tumor, larger specimens are obtained. The tumor is grasped at its base (*left*), the forceps is then pushed forward, into the lumen of the ureter to avoid perforation, shearing off the entire grasped tissue (*middle*). Resected tumor is then retrieved (*right*). This technique can be repeated multiple times, with the lowermost edge of tumor grasped, pushed, let go, regrasped, and pushed again, until it is detached at its base once a significant portion is separated from the wall. (*Courtesy of* S.F. Matin, MD, Houston, TX, 2017.)

superficial tumors, holmium laser ablation is preferred to protect the ureteral wall, with a thermal injury zone of 0.5 to 1.0 mm.[45] For larger tumors, Nd:YAG laser can be used because it has deeper penetration energy.[36,42] Again, technique is critical to the successful use of these instruments, for ablation and even for resection. The holmium laser can be used as an incising or resection tool; for example, to carve out a sessile or papillary tumor, which can then be removed with a forceps or basket as shown in **Fig. 5** and Video 1. If ablating a larger tumor, ideally ablation

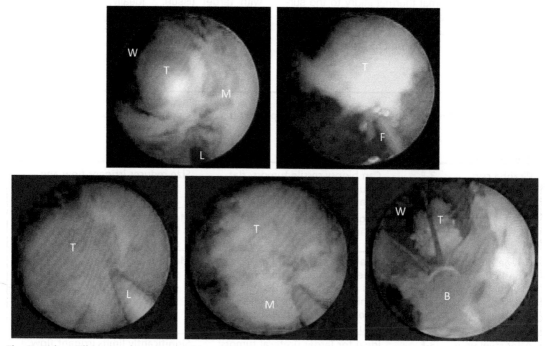

Fig. 5. Video still images from 2 case videos showing laser resection using 200-μm Holmium laser fiber (L). The laser fiber is first used to circumscribe the tumor (T); the tumor can be elevated at its base using the tip of the laser fiber, detaching it from the underlying lamina or muscularis (M). Once the specimen is largely detached, a biopsy forceps (F) or basket (B) can be used to detach and retrieve the specimen. Top panels show resection of a sessile tumor, whereas the lower panels show resection of a papillary tumor with a broad base. W, safety wire. (*Courtesy of* S.F. Matin, MD, Houston, TX, 2017.)

can be performed at or near the vascular pedicle first to cause a vascular amputation of tumor and minimize problematic hematuria, which can slow down the procedure significantly.

The primary complications associated with retrograde endoscopic management can be divided into intraoperative complications, including low-grade ureteral injuries, such as mucosal contusion, superficial mucosal erosion, or false passage, versus high-grade ureteral injuries in the form of ureteral perforation, intussusception, and avulsion. Postoperative complications of retrograde URS include development of ureteral strictures. In general, low-grade ureteral complications are very common and are even to be expected in some cases of URS management and have been reported to occur in approximately 87%.[46] These complications are often caused by wire deployment, URS manipulation, advancement of ureteral access sheath or endoscopic instruments, and misfired energy. When recognized intraoperatively, completion of the procedure is possible, with extreme care taken to avoid crossing the area of injury to prevent more significant ureteral perforation. However, false passage, perforation, and the other high-grade complications are much more problematic and should be avoided at all cost. When concerns for higher grade injuries exist, it is reasonable to abort the procedure and place a ureteral stent.

High-grade ureteral complications are remarkably rare in contemporary practice. Historically, ureteral perforation was reported to occur in approximately 10%.[47] However, a recently reported URS global study of 11,885 patients described a 1% rate of ureteral perforation and exceedingly lower rate of ureteral avulsion of 0.1%.[48] Similarly, ureteral intussusception is a rare complication of retrograde URS of unknown incidence rate. These complications are caused by similar mechanisms to low-grade injuries with entrapment of ureteral wall in the basket used to remove large stones or tissue specimens, for example, resulting in either intussusception or avulsion injuries. Once a ureteral perforation is identified intraoperatively, the procedure should be aborted and placement of a ureteral stent or percutaneous nephrostomy should be performed.[36] The best treatment of intussusception or avulsion injuries is prevention and avoiding blind basketing or application of excessive force to remove these baskets. Often, these types of injury require nephrostomy tube placement followed by nephroureterectomy. In contrast, postoperative complications in the form of ureteral strictures following retrograde URS have been reported to occur in up to 14% of patients.[36] Endoscopic management with balloon dilation, laser incision, and stenting is often reserved for nonmalignant, nonischemic, non–radiation-induced, nonrecurrent strictures of less than 1.5 cm in length, without significant hydronephrosis of the affected kidney and with good renal function.[49] In our practice, whenever possible we perform prestenting to allow for passive dilation for 1 to 2 weeks before URS, especially if we anticipate a narrow distal or intramural ureter.

Electrocautery resection and fulguration

A 10.5 to 13 F rigid ureteral resectoscope (Karl Storz Endoscopy, Tuttlingen, Germany) has been used to resect or ablate distal, midureteral, and proximal ureteral tumors using a electrocautery loop similar to transurethral resection of bladder tumor.[50] However, this instrument is not readily available in current practice and is infrequently used. As previously discussed, biopsy and debulking excision of a large tumor can be performed using grasping forceps or tipless nitinol or flat wire steel baskets with fulguration of the base achieved. Caution must be exercised to not fulgurate larger areas of the ureteral wall, particularly in circumferential fashion, because this may result in development of ureteral strictures. A ureteroscopic Bugbee electrode can also be used to perform tumor ablation; this is particularly useful for lower pole tumors when the laser fiber does not allow full deflection of the URS. The energy level should be decreased significantly (compared with use in the bladder), because perforation can easily occur. Also, electrocautery causes gas bubble formation, which can impede the view.

Oncologic outcomes

With the absence of level I evidence for oncologic outcomes following URS management, most of the data are driven from small retrospective cohort series providing, at best, level III evidence (**Table 3**). With a minimum of 2 years of follow-up, in most of these studies selection bias is evident by selecting those with highly favorable tumor features (low-volume and low-grade tumors on biopsy) as well as lower overall survival compared with cancer-specific survival rates resulting from underlying patient comorbidity, which drove the selection to less invasive measures. Overall, these studies report 65% and 44% rates of UTUC and intravesical recurrences after endoscopic treatment, respectively, with 33% progressing toward RNU or ureterectomy. These rates are consistent with a recent systematic review showing 52% and 34% recurrences of UTUC and bladder, respectively, after endoscopic management.[23]

Table 3
Oncologic outcomes of retrograde endoscopic management for upper-tract urothelial carcinoma[a] with a minimum of 2 years of follow-up

Study	N	URS Bx (LG/HG)	Follow-up (mo)	Upper-Tract/ Bladder Recurrence (%)	Progression to Surgical Resection (%)	OS (%)	CSS (%)
Grasso et al,[81] 2012	82	66/16	38	81/57	19	74	87
Thompson et al,[12] 2008	76	14/18/8[b]	55	55/45	33	NR	85
Cutress et al,[82] 2012	73	34/19/6[b]	54[e]	69/43	19	70	89
Pak et al,[83] 2009	57	NR	53	90/NR	19	93	95
Lucas et al,[84] 2008	39	27/12	33	44/NR	28	62	82
Krambeck et al,[85] 2007	37	2/13/7[b]	32	62/35	30	35	70
Cornu et al,[86] 2010	35	16/6	24	60/40	11	100	100
Johnson et al,[87] 2005	35	35/6/14[b]	32	68/60	3	NR	100
Gadzinski et al,[88] 2010	34	NR	58	84/NR	32	75	100
Daneshmand et al,[89] 2003	30	7/6/14[b]	31	90/23	13	77	97
Matsuoka et al,[90] 2003	27	10/2/0[b]	33	33/19	NR	NR	89
Roupret et al,[91] 2006	27	19/8	52	15/22	26	77	81
Hoffman et al,[80] 2014	25	21	26	36/44	0	NR	100
Reisiger et al,[92] 2007	10	10/0/0[b]	73	50/70	10	100	100
Engelmyer and Belis[93] 1996	10	10/0	43	70/NR	0	90	100
Overall	597		24–58	65[c]/44[d]	0–33	35–100	70–100

Abbreviations: Bx, biopsy; CSS, cancer-specific survival; HG, high grade; LG, low grade; NR, not reported; OS, overall survival.
[a] Patients with low-grade and high-grade findings on biopsy were included.
[b] Grade reported by older grading system (G1/G2/G3).
[c] Local recurrence reported in 15 studies (386 out of 597 patients).
[d] Bladder recurrence reported in 11 studies (199 out of 457 patient).
[e] Median follow-up provided.

Predictors of UTUC recurrence are largely related to tumor characteristics such as tumor size, tumor grade, multifocality, and history of bladder cancer.[51]

Percutaneous Endoscopic Management

The antegrade percutaneous endoscopic approach is usually reserved for patients with low-grade, large-volume UTUC that could be either anatomically or technically challenging to treat via retrograde URS, including those in the lower pole. It is considered the standard approach for patients with urinary diversions. After gaining percutaneous access, the cup biopsy forceps, resectoscope, or laser can be used. Furthermore, percutaneous management provides access for antegrade instillation of adjuvant topical therapy.[52,53]

The main advantage of percutaneous management is the ability to use larger caliber tools such as the rigid nephroscope; flexible pyeloscope/cystoscope to allow inspection of the renal pelvis and calyces; antegrade flexible URS to evaluate the ureter for multifocal tumor; and the resectoscope with loop cautery, which can be used for efficient debulking and resections of larger tumors. The availability of a bipolar resectoscope allows resection of large tumors using saline irrigation, thereby decreasing risks of electrolyte disturbances associated with hypotonic irrigation.[54] Some studies have reported lower rates of local upper-tract and bladder recurrences with the percutaneous approach compared with retrograde endoscopic approach used in the treatment of UTUC.[23]

The principal disadvantages of the antegrade approach have been related to the invasive nature compared with retrograde endoscopy. As such, the integrity of the urothelium of upper urinary tract is interrupted, which could theoretically increase the risk of tumor seeding in the percutaneous tract.[55] The primary complications associated with percutaneous endoscopic management are bleeding requiring blood transfusion in 17% to 37%, kidney failure necessitating dialysis in 2%, and need for emergent nephrectomy or angioembolization in 1% for acute hemorrhage.[23] Other complications, including pleural injury causing development of pneumothorax or hydrothorax (this can largely be prevented by accessing lower pole posterior calyx), colonic injury, infection, and intrarenal strictures and perforations, can occur with the antegrade approach.[56,57]

Oncologic outcomes

Data for the oncologic outcome of the percutaneous management of UTUC with a minimum of 2 years of follow-up are summarized in **Table 4**, showing a total of 361 patients from 8 retrospective studies with median follow-up of up to 66 months. UTUC and intravesical recurrences occurred in 40% and 24%, respectively. A common observation among these studies is that disease recurrence, progression, and cancer-specific survival is associated with tumor grade.[56] Overall, disease progression requiring RNU or ureterectomy occurred in 6% to 50%, likely because of inclusion of more patients with high-grade UTUC for percutaneous management compared with retrograde endoscopic approach (60% vs 35%, respectively).

Upper-Tract Urothelial Carcinoma After Cystectomy

The prevalence of UTUC in patients with a history of bladder cancer treated with radical cystectomy is 0.75% to 6.4% in long-term follow-up studies.[58] Most UTUC cases (71%) develop within 5 years following bladder cancer diagnosis and treatment, whereas only 6% of UTUCs develop 10 years after bladder cancer diagnosis.[59] In contrast, patients with UTUC have a 15% to 50% risk of developing bladder cancer following RNU.[60] Patients with high-grade invasive bladder cancer, bladder carcinoma in situ, multifocal disease, multiple recurrences, positive ureteral and/or urethral margins at the time of cystectomy, and history of UTUC are more likely to develop UTUC after cystectomy.[58] When UTUC develops in patients with a urinary diversion, access to the upper tract can be challenging. Percutaneous access to the upper tract is often required (discussed earlier), although retrograde access via the urinary diversion can sometimes be performed.[61,62]

Our high-volume cystectomy practice results in a large number of patients referred for workup of upper-tract lesions after diversion. The practice pattern that we have developed in these cases is the following: (1) perform an in-office loopogram/pouchogram and flexible cystoscopy to evaluate accessibility of the upper tract. (2) If it is accessible, washings for cytology, a retrograde pyelogram, and stent placement are done. A formal URS evaluation under anesthesia is then scheduled. (3) If the upper tract is not accessible, and often it is not because of tortuosity of the ileal conduit or complex angulation of the pouch chimney (**Figs. 6** and **7**), we then schedule antegrade evaluation through a nephrostomy access.

Table 4
Oncologic outcomes of antegrade percutaneous management for upper-tract urothelial carcinoma[a] with a minimum of 2 years of follow-up

Study	N	Biopsy (LG/HG)	Follow-up (mo)	Upper-Tract/ Bladder Recurrence (%)	Progression to Surgical Resection (%)	OS (%)	CSS (%)
Motamedinia et al,[94] 2016	141	73/64	66[e]	37 LG, 63 HG/NR	13	40	NR
Rastinehad et al,[95] 2009	89	50/39	61	33/NR	13	68	NR
Palou et al,[96] 2004	34	7/21/5[b]	51	41/NR	26	74	94
Patel et al,[97]	26	11/11/1[b]	45	35/42	6	75	91
Roupret et al,[79] 2007	24	17/7	62[e]	13/17	21	79	83
Goel et al,[98] 2003	20	15/5	64	65/15	50	NR	75
Clark et al,[99] 1999	17	6/7/4[b]	24	33/NR	12	75	82
Plancke et al,[100] 1995	10	6/3/1[b]	28	10/10	10	90	100
Overall	361		24–66	40[c]/24[d]	6–50	40–90	75–100

[a] Patients with low-grade and high-grade findings on biopsy were included.
[b] Grade reported by older grading system (G1/G2/G3).
[c] Local recurrence reported in 8 studies (144 out of 361 patients).
[d] Bladder recurrence reported in 4 studies (19 out of 80 patients).
[e] Median follow-up provided.

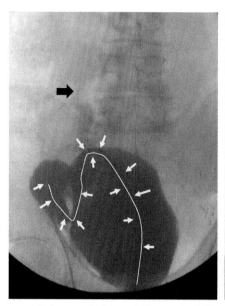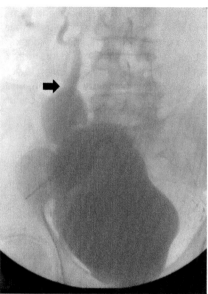

Fig. 6. Fluoroscopic images during pouchoscopy while attempting to access the right ureter for work-up of a filling defect seen on imaging. The flexible cystoscope is seen with an S-shaped curve (*left; white line* and *arrows*), limiting the ability to further manipulate or advance the scope. The location of the right ureteral orifice, seen in subsequent fluoroscopy image, is shown by the black arrow. When the wire is introduced to attempt to cannulate the ureter, the flexible cystoscope loses its deflection (*right*). (*Courtesy of* S.F. Matin, MD, Houston, TX, 2017.)

TOPICAL THERAPY FOR UPPER-TRACT UROTHELIAL CARCINOMA

Because 30% to 70% of patients with UTUC experience local recurrence within the upper tract following endoscopic management,[63] the goal of adjuvant topical therapy is to decrease the risk of local recurrence after complete endoscopic ablation, similar to our expectations for bladder cancer.[52] The role of intravesical treatment at or following RNU is well established based on 2 randomized controlled trials showing diminished risk of intravesical recurrence down to 16% following RNU with single intravesical instillation of chemotherapy.[64,65] Patients with UTUC having disease managed with kidney-sparing approaches may have greater risk for intravesical recurrence. Although there are no direct data, the experience in bladder cancer as well as the postnephroureterectomy data suggest that post-URS chemotherapy is safe and may be beneficial. The authors thus routinely give an intravesical single dose of chemotherapy (previously mitomycin-C [MMC], currently gemcitabine 1000 mg/50 mL) after URS management of UTUC.

Agent Selection

Similar to bladder cancer, adjuvant topical instillation following endoscopic treatment of UTUC includes chemotherapy in low-risk/intermediate-risk UTUC and bacillus Calmette-Guérin (BCG) for high-risk UTUC (including UTCIS, in which case BCG is the primary treatment and not an adjuvant). However, data supporting use of topical agents are limited to several series using heterogeneous application of different agents, instillation duration, and follow-up.[52,66] The most commonly used agents following endoscopic treatment of UTUC are BCG and MMC.

Patient Selection

Low-risk disease

Patients with elective indications for endoscopic management of UTUC, including low-risk (low-grade and low-volume) non–muscle-invasive UTUC tumors with a normal contralateral kidney and those with imperative indications (solitary functioning kidney, bilateral UTUC tumors, and baseline renal insufficiency) with high-grade tumors, are the best candidates for topical chemotherapy instillation following endoscopic management of their upper-tract tumors. Although the benefit of adjuvant topical instillations following endoscopic management in delaying UTUC recurrence or progression is not well defined, such practices can be extrapolated from observed benefits in bladder cancer. The authors have recently studied our experience with use of MMC as induction and maintenance

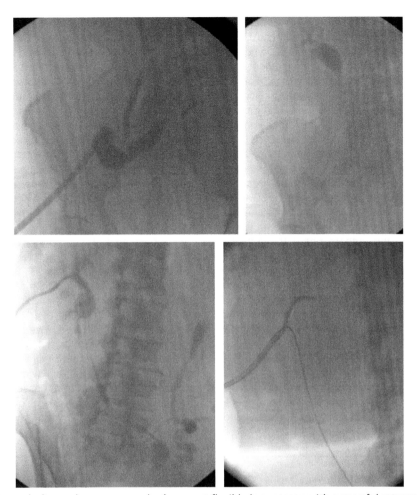

Fig. 7. Top 2 panels show a loopogram and subsequent flexible looposcopy with successful retrograde access to the right upper tract via an ileal conduit. Bottom 2 panels show a left-sided case in which this was not possible. Thus, after percutaneous nephrostomy placement, an antegrade diagnostic ureteroscopy is performed. The authors do not dilate the tract initially, but instead place a 10-F to 12-F short-access sheath through the nephrostomy site and use URS to perform the initial diagnostic evaluation and even biopsies. In rare cases in which these tumors are low grade and low volume, we can dilate the tract and perform more formal antegrade resection in a separate setting. However, in most postcystectomy cases, the tumors are high grade and high risk, so only a biopsy is taken at the initial diagnostic procedure. This technique minimizes patient morbidity and the risk of tract seeding. (*Courtesy of* S.F. Matin, MD, Houston, TX, 2017.)

for adjuvant therapy for endoscopically managed UTUC[67] using cystoscopically placed ureteral catheters (Royal Flush or Beacon Tip, Cook Medical, Bloomington, IN) in 67.9%, and nephrostomy tube in 32.1%, the route being chosen by patients. Induction with 6 doses was fully completed in 85.7% of patients and maintenance 1, 2, and 3 Courses in 60.7%, 35.7%, and 17.8% of patients. After a median follow-up of 19 months, 27 patients with 28 renal units had 3-year recurrence-free, progression-free, and nephroureterectomy-free survival rates of 60%, 80%, and 76%, respectively. The most common adverse events were ureteral or infundibular strictures, seen in 5 patients. With

a recent report showing efficacy of gemcitabine for adjuvant treatment of both low-grade and high-grade bladder cancers,[68] the authors have now switched to the use of gemcitabine as our standard topical therapy. Advantages of gemcitabine compared with MMC include efficacy against high-grade disease; a higher instilled volume (1000 mg/50 mL or 2000 mg/100 mL), which allows for possibly better surface coverage; and no need urinary alkalinization for optimal efficacy, as is needed with MMC. In addition, based on data from gemcitabine use in bladder cancer, the toxicity of gemcitabine seems considerably less than that of MMC.

High-risk disease

Patients with high-risk disease, including UTCIS or high-grade noninvasive tumors, who are considered for endoscopic management may be best served with BCG instillations. **Table 5** summarizes the available evidence relating to topical immunotherapy with BCG in patients with UTCIS. In the report by Metcalfe and colleagues,[67] 7 renal units received MMC as adjuvant after endoscopic management of high-grade disease, almost all treated under imperative indications. Two of these patients recurred for a 3-year recurrence-free survival of 60% and progression-free survival of 67%. In another unpublished work in preparation (Balasubramanian A et al, 2018), the authors noted that patients with UTCIS who fail BCG treatment are unlikely to respond to salvage topical therapy, whereas patients with papillary tumors that were endoscopically managed and who recurred after initial topical therapy still had an approximately 60% response rate to salvage therapy using a secondary agent.

Mode of Delivery

Various instillation techniques of topical agents into the upper urinary tract have been used, including a retrograde route via single-J stent or open-end ureteral catheter,[52,69] an intravesical route after creation of vesicoureteral reflux using either a double-J stent or following ureteral orifice resection,[70,71] and an antegrade route via a percutaneous nephrostomy tube.[72] Each of these techniques has its limitations in terms of reliable instillation and effective dwell time of the topical agents. However, a recent comparative study between these three upper-tract delivery techniques showed that retrograde instillation via open-ended ureteral catheter provided the highest exposure level to the greatest percentage of upper-tract urothelium in an ex vivo model.[73]

In our practice, the authors offer either weekly cystoscopically placed ureteral catheters or nephrostomy tube instillation (**Fig. 8**); we do not perform stent placement with intravesical instillation because this does not reliably provide upper-tract exposure. The first-ever drug-sponsored clinical study for UTUC is investigating the use of a thermosensitive hydrogel with reverse gelation properties and is currently enrolling patients as of this writing (https://www.clinicaltrials.gov/ct2/show/NCT02793,128, accessed 10/18/2017). In addition, preclinical work on drug-eluting ureteral stents is underway. These promising

---

Table 5
Oncologic outcomes of adjuvant bacillus Calmette-Guérin instillation following endoscopic management of upper-tract urothelial carcinoma for patients with a minimum of 20 months of follow-up

Study	N	Stage	Topical Agent	Follow-up (mo)[a]	Progression to Surgical Resection (%)	Oncologic Outcome (%)
Giannarini et al,[72] 2011	55	CIS: 42 RU Ta/T1: 22 RU	BCG	42	CIS: 5 pTa/pT1: 23	LR: CIS, 40; pTa/pT1, 59 Alive and NED: 36 DoD: 31
Miyake et al,[53] 2002	16	CIS	BCG	30	13	LR: 19 DOD: 0
Okubo et al,[69] 2001	11	CIS in 14 RU	BCG	60	29	RU with NED: 50 RU with LR: 14 RU negative response: 36 DOD: 9
Nonomura et al,[101] 2000	11	CIS	BCG	20[b]	9	LR: 11 DOD: 10
Hayashida et al,[66] 2004	10	CIS	BCG	51	10	LR: 50 DOD: 40
Irie et al,[70] 2002	9	CIS in 13 RU	BCG	36[b]	NR	LR: 33 DoD: NR

Abbreviations: CIS, carcinoma in situ; DoD, died of disease; LR, local recurrence; NED, no evidence of disease; RU, renal units.
[a] Median follow-up was reported except where marked.
[b] Mean follow-up was reported.

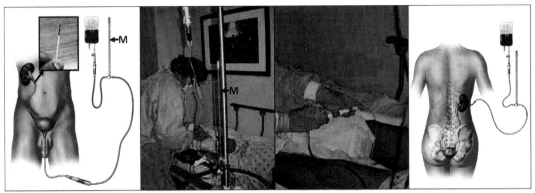

Fig. 8. Technique of retrograde and antegrade topical therapy instillation as performed in our center. For retrograde instillation (*left*), patients have weekly in-office cystoscopy under local anesthesia using intraurethral lidocaine jelly, with placement of a Royal Flush or Beacon Tip catheter, which have multiple side holes (*left*; inset); the ureteral catheter is tied to a Foley catheter to secure its position and positioning into the upper calyx can be performed using retrograde fluoroscopy, or correlating the bony landmarks on fluoroscopy to a prior retrograde pyelogram. Patients ambulate across the hallway to a treatment room, where nurses ensure the bladder is empty then plug the Foley, and attach the ureteral catheter to the prepared medication bag, with tubing running through a manometer (M), allowing monitoring of intrarenal pressure (*middle 2 panels*). At the end of treatment, the bladder is emptied, all catheters are removed, and the patient is discharged. Antegrade treatment is performed similarly through a nephrostomy tube (*right*), which is placed 1 to 2 weeks before treatment is initiated. This tube is left in for induction and maintenance, then changed at 3 months if additional maintenance treatments are planned. For both retrograde and antegrade methods, an initial urine culture is obtained. Additional cultures are sent only in the presence of new signs or symptoms, and patients take a prophylactic oral antibiotic the day before and on the day of each treatment. (*Courtesy of* S.F. Matin, MD, Houston, TX, 2017.)

approaches, which would work in both a chemo-ablative and an adjuvant fashion, have the potential for a paradigm shift in endoscopic management of UTUC.[74,75]

Oncologic Outcomes

The clinical evidence supporting the use of topical therapy is limited by retrospective studies of small cohorts of patients with heterogeneity in diagnosis (biopsy vs cytology used), variable mode of drug delivery (antegrade or retrograde or stent placement), inconsistent drug dose, as well as variability in follow-up schedules. For adjuvant therapy with MMC, Keeley and colleagues[52] instilled 40 mg of MMC via a retrograde route using a ureteral catheter clamped between 3 doses to achieve dwell time of 30 minutes for 21 renal units of 19 patients. Disease-free status was achieved in 11 of 19 renal units (58%), whereas 6 of 11 renal units (54%) had an ipsilateral local recurrence following a mean of 30 months of follow-up. Only 4 patients required RNU for persistent or recurrent disease. The oncologic outcomes for adjuvant BCG instillation following endoscopic treatment of UTUC are summarized in **Table 5**. The overall local recurrence rate following topical therapy is approximately 30%.

SURVEILLANCE AFTER ENDOSCOPIC TREATMENT OF UPPER-TRACT UROTHELIAL CARCINOMA

Surveillance after endoscopic intervention for UTUC is of the utmost importance given the high risk for local recurrence. Urinalysis, urine cytology, and FISH have traditionally been used in surveillance of these patients but retrospective data supporting their use are limited by low sensitivity and specificity, particularly for low-grade disease, with slightly improved results for FISH.[9,10] Various conventional imaging modalities have been used for initial diagnosis and follow-up following nephron-sparing approaches for UTUC, including intravenous pyelogram, retrograde pyelogram (RPG), CT scan, and MRI. There are limited data pertaining specifically to surveillance following endoscopic management of UTUC because most of the evidence on the sensitivity and specificity of imaging tests is derived from studies performed on the initial diagnosis of UTUC rather than surveillance following endoscopic resection. Novel imaging enhancement techniques, including narrow band imaging, Image1 S, and photodynamic techniques, might also be used to enhance early detection of recurrent disease[76] In contrast, ureteroscopic second-look surveillance is necessary to ensure no visible residual disease is present and thus prevent future recurrence and/or progression of untreated tumor areas. Second-look URS was advocated to be performed 6 to 8 weeks following initial URS ablation, whereas second-look antegrade nephroscopy was recommended within 4 to 14 days of a previous procedure.[77] Studies have shown cancer detection rates of 51% at second-look URS. Furthermore, the cancer detection rate significantly increased to 81% and decreased to 41% with positive and negative second-look URS, respectively.[78] Of course, the repetitive requirement for URS is a drawback that also increases the risk for strictures.

Our surveillance practice is intended to minimize interventions and their associated risks while maximizing detection of recurrence. We perform URS surveillance in the first 3 to 6 months after initial successful endoscopic management, and subsequently rely on CT or magnetic resonance urogram for surveillance, with URS to evaluate suspicious findings. Cytology is only obtained for follow-up of UTCIS or high-grade disease.

BLADDER SURVEILLANCE

Metachronous bladder cancer can occur following nephron-sparing treatment of UTUC in approximately 17% to 57%.[12,79–81] These rates of bladder recurrences are consistent with a 25% to 50% risk of bladder cancer recurrences after RNU.[36] Multiple factors have been investigated as potential causes for bladder recurrence, including multifocality, tumor pathologic stage, grade, size, and location, as well as surgical approach.[63] Cystoscopic surveillance remains the gold standard modality of bladder surveillance following treatment of UTUC. However, for patients without a prior history of bladder cancer and in whom a bladder tumor does not develop after a year, we rapidly deescalate the intensity of cystoscopy to every 6 to 12 months. The European Association of Urology guidelines seem to endorse this approach, except that they do not differentiate patients with or without a prior bladder cancer history, recommending urine cytology, CT urogram at 3 and 6 months and then annually, whereas cystoscopy, URS, and selective cytology are recommended at 3 and 6 months, then every 6 months for 2 years, and then annually.[2]

SUMMARY

Endoscopic management of UTUC remains challenging. For high-grade and invasive lesions, radical nephroureterectomy with lymphadenectomy is the treatment of choice. For patients with advanced disease, neoadjuvant chemotherapy should be considered based on renal function. For those with insufficient renal function, poor performance status, or low-grade disease, endoscopic management is a viable option. The techniques detailed in this article provide guidance on the complex management of this difficult disease.

SUPPLEMENTARY DATA

Supplementary data related to this article can be found online at https://doi.org/10.1016/j.ucl.2017.12.009.

REFERENCES

1. Siegel RL, Miller KD, Jemal A. Cancer statistics, 2017. CA Cancer J Clin 2017;67:7.
2. Roupret M, Babjuk M, Comperat E, et al. European Association of Urology guidelines on upper urinary tract urothelial carcinoma: 2017 update. Eur Urol 2018;73(1):111–22.
3. Sedlock DJ, MacLennan GT. Urine cytology in the evaluation of upper tract urothelial lesions. J Urol 2004;172:2406.
4. Messer J, Shariat SF, Brien JC, et al. Urinary cytology has a poor performance for predicting invasive or high-grade upper-tract urothelial carcinoma. BJU Int 2011;108:701.
5. Kleinmann N, Healy KA, Hubosky SG, et al. Ureteroscopic biopsy of upper tract urothelial carcinoma: comparison of basket and forceps. J Endourol 2013;27:1450.
6. Skolarikos A, Griffiths TR, Powell PH, et al. Cytologic analysis of ureteral washings is informative in patients with grade 2 upper tract TCC considering endoscopic treatment. Urology 2003;61:1146.
7. Williams SK, Denton KJ, Minervini A, et al. Correlation of upper-tract cytology, retrograde pyelography, ureteroscopic appearance, and ureteroscopic biopsy with histologic examination of upper-tract transitional cell carcinoma. J Endourol 2008;22:71.
8. Boorjian S, Ng C, Munver R, et al. Abnormal selective cytology results predict recurrence of upper-tract transitional-cell carcinoma treated with ureteroscopic laser ablation. J Endourol 2004;18:912.
9. Yu Q, Li Y, Li G, et al. Prospective evaluation of FISH for detecting upper tract urothelial carcinoma in voided urine specimens. Oncol Lett 2016;12:183.
10. Mian C, Mazzoleni G, Vikoler S, et al. Fluorescence in situ hybridisation in the diagnosis of upper urinary tract tumours. Eur Urol 2010;58:288.
11. El-Hakim A, Weiss GH, Lee BR, et al. Correlation of ureteroscopic appearance with histologic grade of

upper tract transitional cell carcinoma. Urology 2004;63:647.

12. Thompson RH, Krambeck AE, Lohse CM, et al. Endoscopic management of upper tract transitional cell carcinoma in patients with normal contralateral kidneys. Urology 2008;71:713.

13. Kulp DA, Bagley DH. Does flexible ureteropyeloscopy promote local recurrence of transitional cell carcinoma? J Endourol 1994;8:111.

14. Hendin BN, Streem SB, Levin HS, et al. Impact of diagnostic ureteroscopy on long-term survival in patients with upper tract transitional cell carcinoma. J Urol 1999;161:783.

15. Ishikawa S, Abe T, Shinohara N, et al. Impact of diagnostic ureteroscopy on intravesical recurrence and survival in patients with urothelial carcinoma of the upper urinary tract. J Urol 2010;184:883.

16. Sankin A, Tin AL, Mano R, et al. Impact of ureteroscopy before nephroureterectomy for upper tract urothelial carcinoma on oncologic outcomes. Urology 2016;94:148.

17. Waldert M, Karakiewicz PI, Raman JD, et al. A delay in radical nephroureterectomy can lead to upstaging. BJU Int 2010;105:812.

18. Nison L, Roupret M, Bozzini G, et al. The oncologic impact of a delay between diagnosis and radical nephroureterectomy due to diagnostic ureteroscopy in upper urinary tract urothelial carcinomas: results from a large collaborative database. World J Urol 2013;31:69.

19. Tawfiek E, Bibbo M, Bagley DH. Ureteroscopic biopsy: technique and specimen preparation. Urology 1997;50:117.

20. Guarnizo E, Pavlovich CP, Seiba M, et al. Ureteroscopic biopsy of upper tract urothelial carcinoma: improved diagnostic accuracy and histopathological considerations using a multi-biopsy approach. J Urol 2000;163:52.

21. Wason SE, Seigne JD, Schned AR, et al. Ureteroscopic biopsy of upper tract urothelial carcinoma using a novel ureteroscopic biopsy forceps. Can J Urol 2012;19:6560.

22. Verges DP, Lallas CD, Hubosky SG, et al. Endoscopic treatment of upper tract urothelial carcinoma. Curr Urol Rep 2017;18:31.

23. Cutress ML, Stewart GD, Zakikhani P, et al. Ureteroscopic and percutaneous management of upper tract urothelial carcinoma (UTUC): systematic review. BJU Int 2012;110:614.

24. Wang JK, Tollefson MK, Krambeck AE, et al. High rate of pathologic upgrading at nephroureterectomy for upper tract urothelial carcinoma. Urology 2012;79:615.

25. Keeley FX, Kulp DA, Bibbo M, et al. Diagnostic accuracy of ureteroscopic biopsy in upper tract transitional cell carcinoma. J Urol 1997; 157:33.

26. Brien JC, Shariat SF, Herman MP, et al. Preoperative hydronephrosis, ureteroscopic biopsy grade and urinary cytology can improve prediction of advanced upper tract urothelial carcinoma. J Urol 2010;184:69.

27. Brown GA, Matin SF, Busby JE, et al. Ability of clinical grade to predict final pathologic stage in upper urinary tract transitional cell carcinoma: implications for therapy. Urology 2007;70:252.

28. Smith AK, Stephenson AJ, Lane BR, et al. Inadequacy of biopsy for diagnosis of upper tract urothelial carcinoma: implications for conservative management. Urology 2011;78:82.

29. Tavora F, Fajardo DA, Lee TK, et al. Small endoscopic biopsies of the ureter and renal pelvis: pathologic pitfalls. Am J Surg Pathol 2009;33:1540.

30. Margulis V, Youssef RF, Karakiewicz PI, et al. Preoperative multivariable prognostic model for prediction of nonorgan confined urothelial carcinoma of the upper urinary tract. J Urol 2010;184:453.

31. Matin SF, Kamat AM, Grossman HB. High-frequency endoluminal ultrasonography as an aid to the staging of upper tract urothelial carcinoma: imaging findings and pathologic correlation. J Ultrasound Med 2010;29:1277.

32. Aboumarzouk OM, Ahmad S, Moseley H, et al. Accuracy of photodynamic diagnosis in the detection and follow-up of patients with upper urinary tract lesions: initial 3-year experience. Arab J Urol 2012; 10:138.

33. Traxer O, Geavlete B, de Medina SG, et al. Narrowband imaging digital flexible ureteroscopy in detection of upper urinary tract transitional-cell carcinoma: initial experience. J Endourol 2011;25:19.

34. Bus MT, Muller BG, de Bruin DM, et al. Volumetric in vivo visualization of upper urinary tract tumors using optical coherence tomography: a pilot study. J Urol 2013;190:2236.

35. Breda A, Territo A, Guttilla A, et al. Correlation between confocal laser endomicroscopy (Cellvizio®) and histological grading of upper tract urothelial carcinoma: a step forward for a better selection of patients suitable for conservative management. Eur Urol Focus 2017. [Epub ahead of print].

36. Raman JD, Park R. Endoscopic management of upper-tract urothelial carcinoma. Expert Rev Anticancer Ther 2017;17:545.

37. Sverrisson EF, Kim T, Espiritu PN, et al. The merits of cytology in the workup for upper tract urothelial carcinoma - a contemporary review of a perplexing issue. Int Braz J Urol 2014;40:493.

38. Adibi M, Youssef R, Shariat SF, et al. Oncological outcomes after radical nephroureterectomy for upper tract urothelial carcinoma: comparison over the three decades. Int J Urol 2012;19:1060.

39. Suh LK, Rothberg MB, Landman J, et al. Intrarenal pressures generated during deployment of various

antiretropulsion devices in an ex vivo porcine model. J Endourol 2010;24:1165.

40. Frees S, Bidnur S, Metcalfe M, et al. Effect of contrast media on urinary cytopathology specimens. Can Urol Assoc J 2016;10:228.

41. Fang D, Xiong G, Li X, et al. Incidence, characteristics, treatment strategies, and oncologic outcomes of synchronous bilateral upper tract urothelial carcinoma in the Chinese population. Urol Oncol 2015;33:66.e1.

42. Bagley DH, Grasso M 3rd. Ureteroscopic laser treatment of upper urinary tract neoplasms. World J Urol 2010;28:143.

43. Bader MJ, Sroka R, Gratzke C, et al. Laser therapy for upper urinary tract transitional cell carcinoma: indications and management. Eur Urol 2009;56:65.

44. Schilling A, Bowering R, Keiditsch E. Use of the neodymium-YAG laser in the treatment of ureteral tumors and urethral condylomata acuminata. Clinical experience. Eur Urol 1986;12(Suppl 1):30.

45. Wollin TA, Denstedt JD. The holmium laser in urology. J Clin Laser Med Surg 1998;16:13.

46. Traxer O, Thomas A. Prospective evaluation and classification of ureteral wall injuries resulting from insertion of a ureteral access sheath during retrograde intrarenal surgery. J Urol 2013;189:580.

47. Martinez-Pineiro JA, Garcia Matres MJ, Martinez-Pineiro L. Endourological treatment of upper tract urothelial carcinomas: analysis of a series of 59 tumors. J Urol 1996;156:377.

48. de la Rosette J, Denstedt J, Geavlete P, et al. The Clinical Research Office of the Endourological Society Ureteroscopy Global Study: indications, complications, and outcomes in 11,885 patients. J Endourol 2014;28:131.

49. Tyritzis SI, Wiklund NP. Ureteral strictures revisited…trying to see the light at the end of the tunnel: a comprehensive review. J Endourol 2015;29:124.

50. Smith AD, Preminger G, Badlani G, et al. Ureteroscopic diagnosis and treatment of upper urinary tract neoplasms. Smith's Textbook of Endourology 2012;1:436.

51. Thompson RH, Krambeck AE, Lohse CM, et al. Elective endoscopic management of transitional cell carcinoma first diagnosed in the upper urinary tract. BJU Int 2008;102:1107.

52. Keeley FX Jr, Bagley DH. Adjuvant mitomycin C following endoscopic treatment of upper tract transitional cell carcinoma. J Urol 1997;158:2074–7.

53. Miyake H, Eto H, Hara S, et al. Clinical outcome of bacillus Calmette-Guerin perfusion therapy for carcinoma in situ of the upper urinary tract. Int J Urol 2002;9:677.

54. Storm DW, Fulmer BR. Case report: percutaneous management of transitional-cell carcinoma of the upper urinary tract using the bipolar resectoscope. J Endourol 2007;21:1011.

55. Jabbour ME, Smith AD. Primary percutaneous approach to upper urinary tract transitional cell carcinoma. Urol Clin North Am 2000;27:739.

56. Liatsikos EN, Dinlenc CZ, Kapoor R, et al. Transitional-cell carcinoma of the renal pelvis: ureteroscopic and percutaneous approach. J Endourol 2001;15:377.

57. Argyropoulos AN, Tolley DA. Upper urinary tract transitional cell carcinoma: current treatment overview of minimally invasive approaches. BJU Int 2007;99:982.

58. Picozzi S, Ricci C, Gaeta M, et al. Upper urinary tract recurrence following radical cystectomy for bladder cancer: a meta-analysis on 13,185 patients. J Urol 2012;188:2046–54.

59. Wright JL, Hotaling J, Porter MP. Predictors of upper tract urothelial cell carcinoma after primary bladder cancer: a population based analysis. J Urol 2009;181:1035.

60. Azemar MD, Comperat E, Richard F, et al. Bladder recurrence after surgery for upper urinary tract urothelial cell carcinoma: frequency, risk factors, and surveillance. Urol Oncol 2011;29:130.

61. Tomaszewski JJ, Smaldone MC, Ost MC. The application of endoscopic techniques in the management of upper tract recurrence after cystectomy and urinary diversion. J Endourol 2009;23:1265.

62. Nelson CP, Wolf JS Jr, Montie JE, et al. Retrograde ureteroscopy in patients with orthotopic ileal neobladder urinary diversion. J Urol 2003;170:107.

63. Keeley FX Jr, Bibbo M, Bagley DH. Ureteroscopic treatment and surveillance of upper urinary tract transitional cell carcinoma. J Urol 1997;157:1560.

64. O'Brien T, Ray E, Singh R, et al. Prevention of bladder tumours after nephroureterectomy for primary upper urinary tract urothelial carcinoma: a prospective, multicentre, randomised clinical trial of a single postoperative intravesical dose of mitomycin C (the ODMIT-C Trial). Eur Urol 2011;60:703.

65. Ito A, Shintaku I, Satoh M, et al. Prospective randomized phase II trial of a single early intravesical instillation of pirarubicin (THP) in the prevention of bladder recurrence after nephroureterectomy for upper urinary tract urothelial carcinoma: the THP Monotherapy Study Group Trial. J Clin Oncol 2013;31:1422.

66. Hayashida Y, Nomata K, Noguchi M, et al. Long-term effects of bacille Calmette-Guerin perfusion therapy for treatment of transitional cell carcinoma in situ of upper urinary tract. Urology 2004;63:1084.

67. Metcalfe M, Wagenheim G, Xiao L, et al. Induction and maintenance adjuvant mitomycin C topical therapy for upper tract urothelial carcinoma: tolerability and intermediate term outcomes. J Endourol 2017;31:946.

68. Messing E, Tangen C, Lerner S, et al. A phase III blinded study of immediate post-TURBT instillation of gemcitabine versus saline in patients with newly diagnosed or occasionally recurring grade I/II non-muscle invasive bladder cancer: SWOG S0337. J Urol 2017;197:e914.

69. Okubo K, Ichioka K, Terada N, et al. Intrarenal bacillus Calmette-Guerin therapy for carcinoma in situ of the upper urinary tract: long-term follow-up and natural course in cases of failure. BJU Int 2001; 88:343.

70. Irie A, Iwamura M, Kadowaki K, et al. Intravesical instillation of bacille Calmette-Guerin for carcinoma in situ of the urothelium involving the upper urinary tract using vesicoureteral reflux created by a double-pigtail catheter. Urology 2002;59:53.

71. Yossepowitch O, Lifshitz DA, Dekel Y, et al. Assessment of vesicoureteral reflux in patients with self-retaining ureteral stents: implications for upper urinary tract instillation. J Urol 2005;173:890.

72. Giannarini G, Kessler TM, Birkhauser FD, et al. Antegrade perfusion with bacillus Calmette-Guerin in patients with non-muscle-invasive urothelial carcinoma of the upper urinary tract: who may benefit? Eur Urol 2011;60:955.

73. Pollard ME, Levinson AW, Shapiro EY, et al. Comparison of 3 upper tract anticarcinogenic agent delivery techniques in an ex vivo porcine model. Urology 2013;82:1451.e1.

74. Donin NM, Strauss-Ayali D, Agmon-Gerstein Y, et al. Serial retrograde instillations of sustained release formulation of mitomycin C to the upper urinary tract of the Yorkshire swine using a thermosensitive polymer: safety and feasibility. Urol Oncol 2017;35:272.

75. Barros AA, Browne S, Oliveira C, et al. Drug-eluting biodegradable ureteral stent: new approach for urothelial tumors of upper urinary tract cancer. Int J Pharm 2016;513:227.

76. Baard J, Freund JE, de la Rosette JJ, et al. New technologies for upper tract urothelial carcinoma management. Curr Opin Urol 2017;27:170.

77. Seisen T, Colin P, Roupret M. Risk-adapted strategy for the kidney-sparing management of upper tract tumours. Nat Rev Urol 2015;12:155.

78. Villa L, Cloutier J, Letendre J, et al. Early repeated ureteroscopy within 6-8 weeks after a primary endoscopic treatment in patients with upper tract urothelial cell carcinoma: preliminary findings. World J Urol 2016;34:1201.

79. Roupret M, Traxer O, Tligui M, et al. Upper urinary tract transitional cell carcinoma: recurrence rate after percutaneous endoscopic resection. Eur Urol 2007;51:709.

80. Hoffman A, Yossepowitch O, Erlich Y, et al. Oncologic results of nephron sparing endoscopic approach for upper tract low grade transitional cell carcinoma in comparison to nephroureterectomy - a case control study. BMC Urol 2014;14:97.

81. Grasso M, Fishman AI, Cohen J, et al. Ureteroscopic and extirpative treatment of upper urinary tract urothelial carcinoma: a 15-year comprehensive review of 160 consecutive patients. BJU Int 2012;110:1618.

82. Cutress ML, Stewart GD, Wells-Cole S, et al. Long-term endoscopic management of upper tract urothelial carcinoma: 20-year single-centre experience. BJU Int 2012;110:1608.

83. Pak RW, Moskowitz EJ, Bagley DH. What is the cost of maintaining a kidney in upper-tract transitional-cell carcinoma? An objective analysis of cost and survival. J Endourol 2009;23:341.

84. Lucas SM, Svatek RS, Olgin G, et al. Conservative management in selected patients with upper tract urothelial carcinoma compares favourably with early radical surgery. BJU Int 2008;102:172.

85. Krambeck AE, Thompson RH, Lohse CM, et al. Imperative indications for conservative management of upper tract transitional cell carcinoma. J Urol 2007;178:792.

86. Cornu JN, Roupret M, Carpentier X, et al. Oncologic control obtained after exclusive flexible ureteroscopic management of upper urinary tract urothelial cell carcinoma. World J Urol 2010; 28:151.

87. Johnson GB, Fraiman M, Grasso M. Broadening experience with the retrograde endoscopic management of upper urinary tract urothelial malignancies. BJU Int 2005;95(Suppl 2):110.

88. Gadzinski AJ, Roberts WW, Faerber GJ, et al. Long-term outcomes of nephroureterectomy versus endoscopic management for upper tract urothelial carcinoma. J Urol 2010;183:2148.

89. Daneshmand S, Quek ML, Huffman JL. Endoscopic management of upper urinary tract transitional cell carcinoma: long-term experience. Cancer 2003;98:55.

90. Matsuoka K, Lida S, Tomiyasu K, et al. Transurethral endoscopic treatment of upper urinary tract tumors using a holmium:YAG laser. Lasers Surg Med 2003;32:336.

91. Roupret M, Hupertan V, Traxer O, et al. Comparison of open nephroureterectomy and ureteroscopic and percutaneous management of upper urinary tract transitional cell carcinoma. Urology 2006;67:1181.

92. Reisiger K, Hruby G, Clayman RV, et al. Office-based surveillance ureteroscopy after endoscopic treatment of transitional cell carcinoma: technique and clinical outcome. Urology 2007;70:263.

93. Engelmyer EI, Belis JA. Long-term ureteroscopic management of low-grade transitional cell carcinoma of the upper urinary tract. Tech Urol 1996; 2:113.

94. Motamedinia P, Keheila M, Leavitt DA, et al. The expanded use of percutaneous resection for upper tract urothelial carcinoma: a 30-year comprehensive experience. J Endourol 2016;30:262.

95. Rastinehad AR, Ost MC, Vanderbrink BA, et al. A 20-year experience with percutaneous resection of upper tract transitional carcinoma: is there an oncologic benefit with adjuvant bacillus Calmette Guerin therapy? Urology 2009;73:27.

96. Palou J, Piovesan LF, Huguet J, et al. Percutaneous nephroscopic management of upper urinary tract transitional cell carcinoma: recurrence and long-term followup. J Urol 2004;172:66.

97. Patel A, Soonawalla P, Shepherd SF, et al. Long-term outcome after percutaneous treatment of transitional cell carcinoma of the renal pelvis. J Urol 1996;155:868.

98. Goel MC, Mahendra V, Roberts JG. Percutaneous management of renal pelvic urothelial tumors: long-term followup. J Urol 2003;169:925.

99. Clark PE, Streem SB, Geisinger MA. 13-year experience with percutaneous management of upper tract transitional cell carcinoma. J Urol 1999;161:772.

100. Plancke HR, Strijbos WE, Delaere KP. Percutaneous endoscopic treatment of urothelial tumours of the renal pelvis. Br J Urol 1995;75:736.

101. Nonomura N, Ono Y, Nozawa M, et al. Bacillus Calmette-Guerin perfusion therapy for the treatment of transitional cell carcinoma in situ of the upper urinary tract. Eur Urol 2000;38:701.

Perioperative Immunotherapy in Muscle-Invasive Bladder Cancer and Upper Tract Urothelial Carcinoma

Min Yuen Teo, MD, Jonathan E. Rosenberg, MD*

KEYWORDS

- PD1 • PD-L1 • Muscle-invasive bladder cancer • Urothelial carcinoma
- Renal pelvis urothelial carcinoma • Transitional cell carcinoma • Ureteral carcinoma

KEY POINTS

- Neoadjuvant cisplatin-based chemotherapy improves survival in patients with muscle-invasive bladder cancer but a significant proportion are not eligible owing to renal impairment or other medical comorbidities.
- The introduction of anti-programmed cell death protein 1/programmed death-ligand 1(PD1/PD-L1) checkpoint inhibitors has demonstrated clinical activity in a subset of patients with metastatic urothelial cancer, and a favorable toxicity profile.
- Extensive research activities are ongoing to investigate the role of perioperative immune checkpoint inhibition, including in the neoadjuvant and adjuvant settings.
- Urothelial cancers of the upper urinary tract and non-urothelial bladder cancers represent rare diseases that might benefit from similar strategies.

INTRODUCTION

Patients diagnosed with muscle-invasive bladder and upper tract urothelial (transitional cell) carcinoma have high rates of relapse despite primary therapy owing to early micrometastatic dissemination. Neoadjuvant cisplatin-based combination chemotherapy has become a standard of care for cT2-T4cN0cM0 patients based on 2 randomized trials that showed improved survival when chemotherapy was added to radical local therapy (surgery or radiotherapy) compared with radical local therapy alone.[1,2] In addition, meta-analysis of all the randomized trials have shown a benefit for this approach.[3] Adjuvant chemotherapy, in contrast, has not been clearly demonstrated to improve overall survival. Multiple trials have been attempted, and all modern trials closed early for lack of accrual. The largest trial comparing methotrexate, vinblastine, doxorubicin, and cisplatin (MVAC), dose-dense MVAC, or gemcitabine and cisplatin compared with treatment at relapse showed an improvement in progression-free survival, and a trend toward improved overall survival.[4] Meta-analysis of adjuvant cisplatin-based chemotherapy suggest a benefit for treatment, but the results must be interpreted with caution, because many flawed trials were included in the analyses.[5,6] The data supporting the use of perioperative chemotherapy for upper tract tumors is even more limited, with no prospective, randomized trials reported. Retrospective series suggest a benefit to perioperative therapy, but the level of evidence supporting it is poor.[7–9]

Disclosure Statement: M.Y. Teo has nothing to disclose. J.E. Rosenberg is a consultant for Merck, Roche/Genentech, EMD Serono, Inovio, BMS, Lilly, AstraZeneca, Bayer, and Gritstone.
Department of Medicine, Genitourinary Oncology Service, Memorial Sloan Kettering Cancer Center, 1275 York Avenue, New York, NY 10065, USA
* Corresponding author. 1275 York Avenue, New York, NY 10065.
E-mail address: rosenbj1@mskcc.org

urologic.theclinics.com

Although many patients with muscle-invasive urothelial carcinoma are fit for cisplatin-based therapy, about one-half are ineligible to receive it owing to comorbid health issues leading to a risk of excessive toxicity. These limiting factors include renal insufficiency, peripheral neuropathy, hearing loss, cardiomyopathy, or poor performance status.[10] Patients with non-metastatic muscle-invasive bladder cancer are generally not candidates for perioperative chemotherapy, because non-cisplatin regimens have never been shown to improve cure rates compared with radical local therapy alone. Patients with upper tract urothelial carcinoma frequently have impaired renal function owing to urinary tract obstruction, which frequently cannot be improved sufficiently for preoperative chemotherapy. These patient populations represent an unmet need for effective systemic therapy for micrometastatic spread.

IMMUNE CHECKPOINT BLOCKADE IN UROTHELIAL CARCINOMA

Although local immunotherapy with Bacille Calmette-Guérin has long played a key role in the treatment of non–muscle-invasive urothelial carcinoma, historically, there have been no effective systemic immunotherapy options available. The recognition that inhibition of the programmed cell death receptor pathway (PD1) on immune cells led to robust responses in metastatic urothelial carcinoma has led to a therapeutic revolution for patients with unresectable or metastatic disease not responsive or not eligible for cisplatin based chemotherapy.

Targeting the PD1 receptor as well as its ligand, programmed death ligand 1 (PD-L1), has been shown to lead to rapid and durable responses in some patients with advanced disease. A urothelial carcinoma expansion cohort in the phase I trial of atezolizumab demonstrated durable objective responses in a subset of patients, with higher responses rates (43%) observed in patients with greater numbers of immune cell staining positive for PD-L1 compared with 11% for those with lower numbers of immune cell staining.[11] Similarly, a phase I expansion cohort testing pembrolizumab showed objective responses in 26% of patients.[12] Both studies shows that patients could obtain complete responses, and that these responses were often quite durable compared with historically available second-line options such as taxanes, pemetrexed, and vinflunine.

These results spurred the development of several large single arm trials testing anti-PD1 and anti–PD-L1 antibodies in locally advanced or metastatic urothelial carcinoma (**Table 3**). Atezolizumab, an anti–PD-L1 antibody, was tested in 310 patients previously treated with platinum-based chemotherapy.[13] In this study, 15% of patients experienced objective responses, the majority of which have been durable for more than 1 year. Nivolumab, an anti-PD1 antibody, was tested in a phase I/II study of 78 patients with locally advanced or metastatic urothelial carcinoma previously treated with platinum-based chemotherapy.[14] Objective responses were noted in 24% of patients. This study led to a larger single arm phase II study enrolling 270 patients, which demonstrated a 20% objective response rate. Durvalumab, an anti–PD-L1 antibody, was tested in a phase I/II study of 191 patients with locally advanced or metastatic urothelial carcinoma after platinum-based chemotherapy.[15] Patients treated with durvalumab had a 17.8% objective response rate in this trial.[16] Avelumab, an anti–PD-L1 antibody, was tested in 242 patients previously treated with platinum-based chemotherapy.[17] Overall, 13% of patients experienced objective responses. Collectively, these trials each led to accelerated US Food and Drug Administration (FDA) approvals of atezolizumab, nivolumab, durvalumab, and avelumab for patients previously treated with platinum-based chemotherapy.

Pembrolizumab was tested in a phase III randomized trial compared with standard chemotherapy (paclitaxel, docetaxel, or vinflunine) in patients previously treated with platinum-based chemotherapy.[18] Patients treated with pembrolizumab had a higher response rate (21% vs 11%) and median survival (10.3 months vs 7.4 months; hazard ratio, 0.73; 95% confidence interval [CI], 0.59–0.91; $P = .002$). However, toxicity was lower with pembrolizumab compared with chemotherapy (15% vs 49%). This study led to the full FDA approval for pembrolizumab for patients with metastatic urothelial carcinoma previously treated with platinum-based chemotherapy. In contrast, atezolizumab was tested in a randomized phase III study against standard chemotherapy (docetaxel, paclitaxel, or vinflunine), with the primary endpoint of improved overall survival in the subset of patients with high PD-L1 expression on immune cells in their tumor.[19] This trial failed to meet the primary endpoint of improved survival in atezolizumab treated patients (hazard ratio, 0.87; 95% CI, 0.63–1.21; $P = .41$). In the entire population of patients treated regardless of PD-L1 status, the median survival was similar (8.6 months with atezolizumab vs 8.0 months with chemotherapy), but the hazard ratio was 0.85 (95% CI, 0.73–0.99; $P = .038$). Although this result has a P value of less than .05, it is not considered a positive result owing to the study design.

Single-agent therapy with anti-PD1 or anti–PD-L1 antibodies has been associated with a relatively modest rate of toxicity in the platinum-pretreated patient population, with grade 3 to 4 adverse events generally occurring in fewer than 25% of patients. This finding makes these treatments appropriate for patients with medical comorbidities or frailty. This safety profile led to the testing of pembrolizumab and atezolizumab in 2 phase II studies in patients with untreated metastatic urothelial carcinoma ineligible for cisplatin-based chemotherapy based on performance status or comorbid illness. Pembrolizumab was tested in 370 patients with untreated metastatic urothelial carcinoma ineligible for cisplatin-based therapy.[20] In an updated analysis,[21] the objective response rate was 29% (95% CI, 24–34), including 7% complete responses. The median duration of response was not reached at the time of reporting. Similarly, atezolizumab was tested in a phase II study of 119 patients unfit for cisplatin-based chemotherapy for untreated metastatic disease.[22] The objective response rate in this study was 24%, with a median overall survival of 15.9 months, which exceeds the historical survival in this patient population.[23] Based on these 2 studies, both atezolizumab and pembrolizumab received accelerated approval from the FDA for cisplatin-ineligible patients with metastatic urothelial carcinoma.

DEVELOPMENT OF IMMUNOTHERAPY IN PATIENTS WITH MUSCLE-INVASIVE UROTHELIAL CARCINOMA

The relatively modest toxicity profile from currently available immunotherapy agents targeting the PD1/PD-L1 axis warrants further testing in patients with muscle-invasive disease to improve cure rates. Several approaches are currently being explored to integrate these treatments into the standard paradigms.

Neoadjuvant Strategies

Neoadjuvant therapy entails the administration of systemic therapy before surgery. Multiple clinical trials are testing 2 general approaches: the addition of immunotherapy to chemotherapy before surgery, or instead of chemotherapy before surgery. There is evidence from lung cancer that chemotherapy and immunotherapy may have synergistic effects, and that improved clinical outcomes may be associated with this approach.[24] Preclinical evidence also suggests that there may be synergy between gemcitabine and immunotherapy owing to gemcitabine's effect on T-regulatory cells and myeloid-derived suppressor cells, and cisplatin's ability to increase CD8-mediated

killing of cancer cells (reviewed in[25]). Multiple phase II studies are combining gemcitabine and cisplatin with single-agent checkpoint blockade in cisplatin-eligible patients with muscle-invasive bladder cancer (**Table 1**). These single-arm studies are being compared with historical studies of cisplatin-based neoadjuvant chemotherapies using pathologic downstaging or complete response at cystectomy as the primary endpoint. Prior work has shown that both pathologic complete response and pathologic downstaging to less than muscle-invasive disease represent an intermediate endpoint associated with long-term clinical benefit after neoadjuvant therapy.[26]

Because many patients with muscle-invasive bladder cancer are not eligible for cisplatin-based therapy, the relatively benign toxicity profile of single-agent immunotherapy makes it an ideal modality to test as neoadjuvant therapy in this older and sicker patient population. These patients have no other proven treatment options for systemic therapy before cystectomy. In the phase II trials of metastatic disease discussed herein, rapid responses were seen in many patients, suggesting that a relatively short window of therapy may lead to clinically beneficial outcomes. Multiple single-agent anti-PD1 and anti–PD-L1 neoadjuvant trials are ongoing currently (see **Table 1**), however, to date, no data have been reported.

Ipilimumab, a checkpoint inhibitor targeting cytotoxic T-lymphocyte-associated protein 4 (CTLA4), was tested in a single agent neoadjuvant trial of 12 patients with cT1-2 N0 urothelial carcinoma treated at 2 dose levels.[27] Patients enrolled in this trial received 2 doses of preoperative ipilimumab. This trial demonstrated that ipilimumab can be administered safely as a single agent in the preoperative setting at the 3 mg/kg dose (the 10 mg/kg dose was associated with treatment-related delay in time to surgery). Interestingly, examination of the pathologic specimens demonstrated evidence of antitumor immune activation with increased infiltration of surgical specimens with activated T cells; however, conventional pathologic outcomes were not reported in this study.

Combined immune blockade of nonoverlapping mechanisms, such as PD1/PD-L1 and CTLA4, can lead to improved clinical outcomes as seen in metastatic melanoma and kidney cancers, albeit with higher rates of toxicity.[28,29] Encouraged by similar observations in metastatic urothelial cancers,[30] combination trials have been planned as neoadjuvant therapy in the nonmetastatic muscle-invasive setting (see **Table 1**). Because these combinations are expected to have higher levels of immune-mediated adverse events, many of these trials

Table 1
Selected neoadjuvant immunotherapy trials

Study ID	Agents	Phase	Expected Sample Size	Upper Tract Tumors Included?	Status	Primary Endpoint	Location
Immune checkpoint inhibitor(s)							
NCT03212651	Pembrolizumab	2	40	No	Accruing	Pathologic complete response rate	Paris, France
NCT02736266	Pembrolizumab	2	90	No	Accruing	Pathologic complete response rate	Milan, Italy
NCT03319745	Pembrolizumab	2	20	No	Not yet accruing	Toxicity	Houston, TX
NCT02662309	Atezolizumab	2	85	No	Accruing	Pathologic complete response and dynamic changes in CD8 and/or CD3 T-cells	London, UK
NCT02451423	Atezolizumab	2	42	No	Accruing	Pathologic complete response and change in $CD3^+$ T-cell count/μm^2	San Francisco, CA
NCT03234153	Durvalumab and tremelimumab	2	68	No	Not yet accruing	Pathologic response rate	Berne, Switzerland
NCT02812420	Durvalumab and tremelimumab	1	15	No	Accruing	Toxicity	Houston, TX
NCT02845323	Nivolumab ± urelumab	2	44	No	Accruing	$CD8^+$ T-cell density	Baltimore, MD
Immune checkpoint inhibitor plus cytotoxic chemotherapy							
NCT02365766	Pembrolizumab + gemcitabine ± cisplatin (2 arms)	1b/2	81	No	Accruing	Safety and pathologic downstaging	Cleveland, OH
NCT02690558	Pembrolizumab + gemcitabine + cisplatin	2	39	No	Accruing	Pathologic downstaging	Chapel Hill, NC
NCT03294304	Nivolumab + gemcitabine + cisplatin	2	41	No	Not yet accruing	Pathologic downstaging	Minneapolis, MN
NCT02989584	Atezolizumab gemcitabine cisplatin	2	30	No	Accruing	Pathologic downstaging	New York, NY

Data from U.S. National Library of Medicine. Available at: www.clinicaltrials.gov. Accessed Nov 26, 2017.

are pilot or safety studies in this patient population with potentially curable disease.

Adjuvant Immunotherapy

The addition of systemic therapy following surgery, or adjuvant therapy, is regularly used in many solid tumor types, but is not standard in the management of bladder cancers, largely owing to lack of clinical data, as discussed, and difficulties in administering cisplatin-based chemotherapy to patients who have compromised performance status and renal function after radical cystectomy. Nevertheless, it is not without its theoretic advantage: cystectomy is done immediately to avoid delays in definitive local therapy, and pathologic stage is available to optimize prognostication and patient selection for therapy.[4] The low rate of treatment-related toxicities associated with immune checkpoint inhibitors renders these agents an attractive therapeutic option in a postoperative setting.

To date, there are 3 ongoing clinical trials evaluating the role of adjuvant immune checkpoint inhibitors in urothelial cancers. The experimental arms consist of single-agent nivolumab, atezolizumab or pembrolizumab for up to a year, compared with placebo for the nivolumab study and observation in the other 2 trials (**Table 2**). These studies are unique in allowing patients with upper tract urothelial cancers to also be enrolled.

RARE DISEASES WITH UNMET NEEDS
Urothelial Cancers of the Upper Urinary Tract

Urothelial cancers of the upper urinary tract (UTUC) represent 5% to 10% of all urothelial cancers and are found in both patients with a history of bladder cancer and as an isolated site of de novo disease. Nephroureterectomy remains the main curative option for patients with localized disease. However, unlike its bladder equivalent, UTUC are more likely to harbor muscle-invasive disease (pT2 or higher) at surgery (42.1%–69.1%).[31–34] The risk of progression and prognosis strongly depends on disease stage, with survival rate at 5 years of 60.7% and 39.4% for pT2 and pT3-4 disease, respectively.[31] Prospective neoadjuvant cisplatin-based chemotherapy studies for UTUC are ongoing, but most patients with UTUC are not eligible for cisplatin owing to underlying renal impairment, frequently owing to obstruction from the primary tumor.

Although UTUCs are represented in studies of immunotherapy in the metastatic setting and have comparable response rates compared with urothelial cancers arising in the bladder (**Table 3**), existing neoadjuvant immunotherapy studies enroll only urothelial cancers that arise from the bladder. Although clinically treated as a similar disease entity, emerging evidence is suggestive of underlying molecular differences between UTUC and urothelial cancers of the bladder,[35] including high rates of association with microsatellite instability,[36] all of which point to an urgent need for UTUC-specific perioperative immunotherapy studies to improve the outcomes of these patients.

Non-urothelial Cancers of the Urinary Tract

Nonurothelial bladder cancers represent less than 7% of all bladder cancers and consist of a wide variety of histologic subtypes, including squamous cell carcinoma, both urachal and non-urachal adenocarcinomas and small cell carcinoma, many of which are chemoresistant and/or associated with poorer clinical outcomes,[37] with no optimal systemic therapeutic options to date. Furthermore, patients with nonurothelial histologies have been excluded routinely from existing and ongoing clinical trials, including the immunotherapy trials, representing a group of orphan diseases without evidence-driven treatment options.

More recently, a National Cancer Institute–initiated phase I study investigated cabozantinib

---

Table 2
Selected adjuvant immunotherapy trials

Study ID	Agents	Phase	Expected Sample Size	Upper Tract Tumors Included?	Status	Primary Endpoint	Location
NCT02632409	Nivolumab vs placebo	3	640	Yes	Accruing	Disease-free survival	Multicenter
NCT02450331	Atezolizumab vs observation	3	800	Yes	Accruing	Disease-free survival	Multicenter
NCT03244384	Pembrolizumab vs observation	3	739	Yes	Accruing	Disease-free survival and overall survival	Multicenter

Data from U.S. National Library of Medicine. Available at: www.clinicaltrials.gov. Accessed Nov 26, 2017.

Table 3
Anticancer activity of immune checkpoint blockade in metastatic urothelial carcinoma

Study	Balar et al,[22] 2017		Balar et al,[20] 2017		Rosenberg et al,[13] 2016		Sharma et al,[15] 2017 (Checkmate 275)		Sharma et al,[14] 2016 (Checkmate 032)		Bellmunt et al,[18] 2017		Apolo et al,[17] 2017		Powles et al,[16] 2017	
Line	1L		1L		2L		2L		2L		2L		2L		2L	
Agent	Atezolizumab		Pembrolizumab		Atezolizumab		Nivolumab		Nivolumab		Pembrolizumab		Avelumab		Durvalumab	
Total n	119		370		315		270		86		266		242		191	
ORR (%)	23		24		15		20		24		21		18		18	
	% of Cohort	ORR	% of Cohort	ORR	% of Cohort	ORR	% of Cohort	ORR	% of Cohort	ORR	% of Cohort	ORR	% of Cohort	ORR	% of Cohort	ORR
Renal pelvis	28	39	19	22	11	7	25	11	NA	NA	14	NA	23	11	NA	NA
Ureter					5	9										

Abbreviations: 1L, first-line treatment; 2L, second-line treatment; NA, not applicable; ORR, objective response rate.

(tyrosine kinase inhibitor targeting hepatocyte growth factor receptor [c-MET], vascular endothelial growth factor receptor [VEGFR], and tyrosine-protein kinase receptor UFO [AXL]), an anti-MET and anti–vascular endothelial growth factor inhibitor, plus nivolumab with or without ipilimumab across different rare genitourinary cancers. With 48 patients treated to date, an objective response rate of 37% was observed, including 2 of 2 squamous cell carcinomas and 1 of 4 urachal adenocarcinoma, hinting at possible clinical activity and worthy of further exploration in these tumors with rare histologies.[38]

SUMMARY/DISCUSSION

The introduction of anti-PD1/PD-L1 immune checkpoint inhibitors has significantly altered the treatment landscape of advanced urothelial cancers. A combination of durable clinical activity and tolerability has led to intense interest in exploring these agents in earlier disease states, including muscle-invasive disease, either as monotherapy or in combination with other agents.

To date, these studies are currently in varying levels of development or accrual. The results are eagerly awaited with the potential to improve patient outcomes, although they are likely to raise further questions. First, although most of these studies are developed based on the neoadjuvant chemotherapy paradigm as opposed to adjuvant approaches, it remains unknown whether this paradigm applies to immunotherapy. Second, many of these studies continue to use pathologic response as a primary endpoint, which has been associated with long-term clinical benefit[1,39]; however, it remains to be investigated if immunotherapy is likely to induce comparable rates of pathologic responses, or if pathologic responses are necessary for long-term disease control. Answers to some of these questions will become clearer as these studies begin to mature with clinical readouts.

In conclusion, perioperative immunotherapy has the potential to further revolutionize the field of bladder cancer and other urinary tract tumors. Given these agents' favorable toxicity profile and less intensive requirement for adequate end-organ functions, the benefit could potentially reach a larger patient population, many of whom might have impaired renal function owing to disease status and comorbidities.

REFERENCES

1. Grossman HB, Natale RB, Tangen CM, et al. Neoadjuvant chemotherapy plus cystectomy compared with cystectomy alone for locally advanced bladder cancer. N Engl J Med 2003;349(9):859–66.
2. International Collaboration of Trialists, Medical Research Council Advanced Bladder Cancer Working Party, European Organisation for Research and treatment of Cancer Genito-Urinary, et al. International phase III trial assessing neoadjuvant cisplatin, methotrexate, and vinblastine chemotherapy for muscle-invasive bladder cancer: long-term results of the BA06 30894 trial. J Clin Oncol 2011;29(16):2171–7.
3. Advanced Bladder Cancer (ABC) Meta-analysis Collaboration. Neoadjuvant chemotherapy in invasive bladder cancer: update of a systematic review and meta-analysis of individual patient data Advanced Bladder Cancer (ABC) Meta-analysis Collaboration. Eur Urol 2005;48(2):202–5 [discussion: 205-6].
4. Sternberg CN, Skoneczna I, Kerst JM, et al. Immediate versus deferred chemotherapy after radical cystectomy in patients with pT3-pT4 or N+ M0 urothelial carcinoma of the bladder (EORTC 30994): an intergroup, open-label, randomised phase 3 trial. Lancet Oncol 2015;16(1):76–86.
5. Advanced Bladder Cancer (ABC) Meta-Analysis Collaboration. Adjuvant chemotherapy for invasive bladder cancer (individual patient data). Cochrane Database Syst Rev 2006;(2):CD006018.
6. Leow JJ, Martin-Doyle W, Rajagopal PS, et al. Adjuvant chemotherapy for invasive bladder cancer: a 2013 updated systematic review and meta-analysis of randomized trials. Eur Urol 2014;66(1):42–54.
7. Hosogoe S, Hatakeyama S, Kusaka A, et al. Platinum-based neoadjuvant chemotherapy improves oncological outcomes in patients with locally advanced upper tract urothelial carcinoma. Eur Urol Focus 2017. https://doi.org/10.1016/j.euf.2017.03.013.
8. Porten S, Siefker-Radtke AO, Xiao L, et al. Neoadjuvant chemotherapy improves survival of patients with upper tract urothelial carcinoma. Cancer 2014;120(12):1794–9.
9. Leow JJ, Martin-Doyle W, Fay AP, et al. A systematic review and meta-analysis of adjuvant and neoadjuvant chemotherapy for upper tract urothelial carcinoma. Eur Urol 2014;66(3):529–41.
10. Galsky MD, Hahn NM, Rosenberg J, et al. Treatment of patients with metastatic urothelial cancer "unfit" for Cisplatin-based chemotherapy. J Clin Oncol 2011;29(17):2432–8.
11. Powles T, Eder JP, Fine GD, et al. MPDL3280A (anti-PD-L1) treatment leads to clinical activity in metastatic bladder cancer. Nature 2014;515(7528):558–62.
12. Plimack ER, Bellmunt J, Gupta S, et al. Safety and activity of pembrolizumab in patients with locally advanced or metastatic urothelial cancer (KEYNOTE-012): a non-randomised, open-label, phase 1b study. Lancet Oncol 2017;18(2):212–20.

13. Rosenberg JE, Hoffman-Censits J, Powles T, et al. Atezolizumab in patients with locally advanced and metastatic urothelial carcinoma who have progressed following treatment with platinum-based chemotherapy: a single-arm, multicentre, phase 2 trial. Lancet 2016;387(10031):1909–20.

14. Sharma P, Callahan MK, Bono P, et al. Nivolumab monotherapy in recurrent metastatic urothelial carcinoma (CheckMate 032): a multicentre, open-label, two-stage, multi-arm, phase 1/2 trial. Lancet Oncol 2016;17(11):1590–8.

15. Sharma P, Retz M, Siefker-Radtke A, et al. Nivolumab in metastatic urothelial carcinoma after platinum therapy (CheckMate 275): a multicentre, single-arm, phase 2 trial. Lancet Oncol 2017;18(3):312–22.

16. Powles T, O'Donnell PH, Massard C, et al. Efficacy and safety of durvalumab in locally advanced or metastatic urothelial carcinoma: updated results from a phase 1/2 open-label study. JAMA Oncol 2017;3(9):e172411.

17. Apolo AB, Ellerton JA, Infante JR, et al. Updated efficacy and safety of avelumab in metastatic urothelial carcinoma (mUC): Pooled analysis from 2 cohorts of the phase 1b Javelin solid tumor study. J Clin Oncol 2017;35(15_suppl):4528.

18. Bellmunt J, de Wit R, Vaughn DJ, et al. Pembrolizumab as second-line therapy for advanced urothelial carcinoma. N Engl J Med 2017;376(11):1015–26.

19. Powles T, Loriot Y, Duran I, et al. IMvigor211: a phase III randomized study examining atezolizumab vs. chemotherapy for platinum-treated advanced urothelial carcinoma. Florence, Italy: EACR-AACR-SIC; 2017.

20. Balar AV, Castellano D, O'Donnell PH, et al. First-line pembrolizumab in cisplatin-ineligible patients with locally advanced and unresectable or metastatic urothelial cancer (KEYNOTE-052): a multicentre, single-arm, phase 2 study. Lancet Oncol 2017;18(11):1483–92.

21. O'Donnell PH, Grivas P, Balar AV, et al. Biomarker findings and mature clinical results from KEYNOTE-052: first-line pembrolizumab (pembro) in cisplatin-ineligible advanced urothelial cancer (UC). J Clin Oncol 2017;35(15_suppl):4502.

22. Balar AV, Galsky MD, Rosenberg JE, et al. Atezolizumab as first-line treatment in cisplatin-ineligible patients with locally advanced and metastatic urothelial carcinoma: a single-arm, multicentre, phase 2 trial. Lancet 2017;389(10064):67–76.

23. De Santis M, Bellmunt J, Mead G, et al. Randomized phase II/III trial assessing gemcitabine/carboplatin and methotrexate/carboplatin/vinblastine in patients with advanced urothelial cancer who are unfit for cisplatin-based chemotherapy: EORTC study 30986. J Clin Oncol 2012;30(2):191–9.

24. Langer CJ, Gadgeel SM, Borghaei H, et al. Carboplatin and pemetrexed with or without pembrolizumab for advanced, non-squamous non-small-cell lung cancer: a randomised, phase 2 cohort of the open-label KEYNOTE-021 study. Lancet Oncol 2016;17(11):1497–508.

25. Funt SA, Rosenberg JE. Systemic, perioperative management of muscle-invasive bladder cancer and future horizons. Nature reviews. Clin Oncol 2017;14(4):221–34.

26. Sonpavde G, Goldman BH, Speights VO, et al. Quality of pathologic response and surgery correlate with survival for patients with completely resected bladder cancer after neoadjuvant chemotherapy. Cancer 2009;115(18):4104–9.

27. Carthon BC, Wolchok JD, Yuan J, et al. Preoperative CTLA-4 blockade: tolerability and immune monitoring in the setting of a presurgical clinical trial. Clin Cancer Res 2010;16(10):2861–71.

28. Wolchok JD, Chiarion-Sileni V, Gonzalez R, et al. Overall survival with combined nivolumab and ipilimumab in advanced melanoma. New Engl J Med 2017;377(14):1345–56.

29. Escudier B. Efficacy and safety of nivolumab + ipilimumab (N+I) v sunitinib (S) for treatment-naïve advanced or metastatic renal cell carcinoma (mRCC), including IMDC risk and PD-L1 expression subgroups. Madrid: ESMO Congress; 2017. LBA5.

30. Efficacy and Safety of Nivolumab Plus Ipilimumab in Previously Treated Metastatic Urothelial Carcinoma. First results from the phase I/II CheckMate 032 study. Journal for ImmunoTherapy of Cancer 2016;4(2-suppl):91. abstract O3.

31. Ploussard G, Xylinas E, Lotan Y, et al. Conditional survival after radical nephroureterectomy for upper tract carcinoma. Eur Urol 2015;67(4):803–12.

32. Roupret M, Hupertan V, Seisen T, et al. Prediction of cancer specific survival after radical nephroureterectomy for upper tract urothelial carcinoma: development of an optimized postoperative nomogram using decision curve analysis. J Urol 2013;189(5):1662–9.

33. Jeldres C, Sun M, Isbarn H, et al. A population-based assessment of perioperative mortality after nephroureterectomy for upper-tract urothelial carcinoma. Urology 2010;75(2):315–20.

34. Abouassaly R, Alibhai SM, Shah N, et al. Troubling outcomes from population-level analysis of surgery for upper tract urothelial carcinoma. Urology 2010;76(4):895–901.

35. Sfakianos JP, Cha EK, Iyer G, et al. Genomic characterization of upper tract urothelial carcinoma. Eur Urol 2015;68(6):970–7.

36. Carlo MI, Zhang L, Mandelker D, et al. Cancer predisposing germline mutations in patients (pts) with urothelial cancer (UC) of the renal pelvis (R-P),

ureter (U) and bladder (B). J Clin Oncol 2017; 35(15_suppl):4510.

37. Royce TJ, Lin CC, Gray PJ, et al. Clinical characteristics and outcomes of nonurothelial cell carcinoma of the bladder: results from the National Cancer Data Base. Urol Oncol 2017. https://doi.org/10. 1016/j.urolonc.2017.10.013.

38. Apolo AB, Mortazavi A, Stein MN, et al. A phase I study of cabozantinib plus nivolumab (CaboNivo) and cabonivo plus ipilimumab (CaboNivolpi) in

patients (pts) with refractory metastatic (m) urothelial carcinoma (UC) and other genitourinary (GU) tumors. J Clin Oncol 2017;35(15_suppl):4562.

39. Tully CM, Bochner BH, Dalbagni G, et al. Gemcitabine-cisplatin (GC) plus radical cystectomy-pelvic lymph node dissection (RC-PLND) for patients (pts) with muscle-invasive bladder cancer (MIBC): assessing impacts of neoadjuvant chemotherapy (NAC) and the PLND. Journal of Clinical Oncology, 2014;32(4_suppl):355.

Moving?

Make sure your subscription moves with you!

To notify us of your new address, find your **Clinics Account Number** (located on your mailing label above your name), and contact customer service at:

Email: journalscustomerservice-usa@elsevier.com

800-654-2452 (subscribers in the U.S. & Canada)
314-447-8871 (subscribers outside of the U.S. & Canada)

Fax number: 314-447-8029

**Elsevier Health Sciences Division
Subscription Customer Service
3251 Riverport Lane
Maryland Heights, MO 63043**

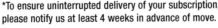

Printed and bound by CPI Group (UK) Ltd, Croydon, CR0 4YY

03/10/2024

01040302-0012